AF342046

VETERINARY ULTRASONOGRAPHY

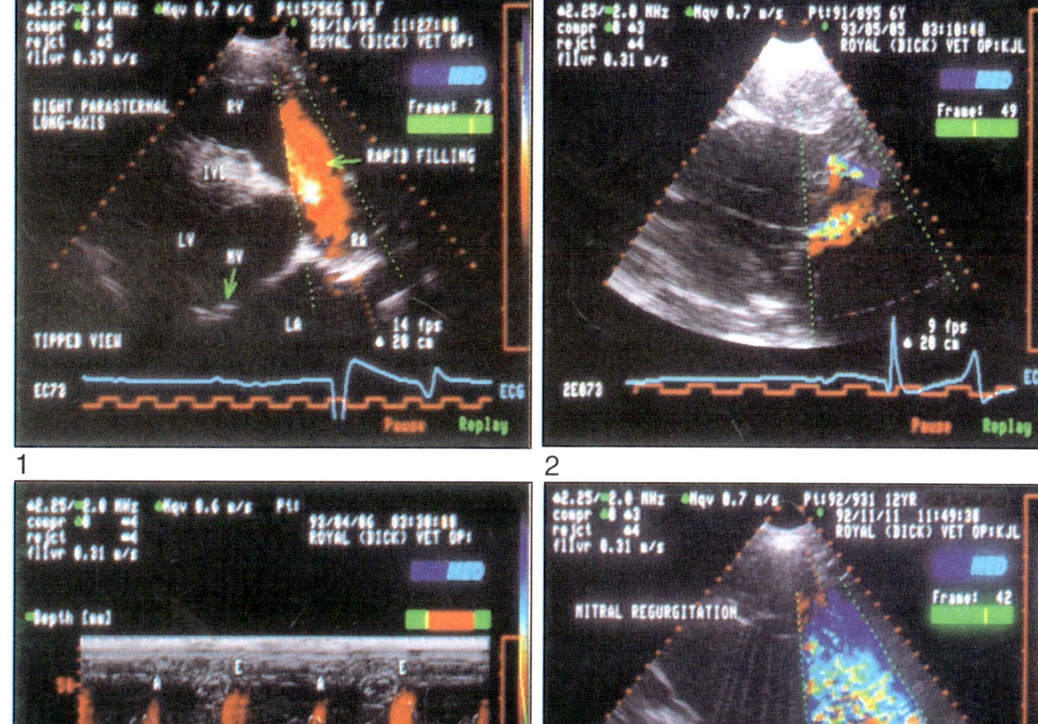

Plate 1: Colour flow Doppler study from a right parasternal long-axis view, showing a red flow signal in the right atrium, right ventricle and across the open tricuspid valve during early diastole. The lighter shades of red represent a central core of higher velocity flow. Two small pale blue areas seen in the centre of the high velocity flow do not represent blood flowing in the opposite direction, but are due to signal aliasing (see text). RA = right atrium; RV = right ventricle; LA = left atrium; LV = left ventricle; MV = mitral valve; IVS = interventricular septum.

Plate 2: Colour flow Doppler study from a left parasternal long-axis view, showing two jets of mitral regurgitation entering the left atrium at different angles. One jet, coded blue, is flowing away from the transducer towards the bottom of the screen, and the other jet, coded red, is flowing towards the transducer. The central cores of both jets are coded in green, indicating disturbed flow. Chordae tendineae are visible in the left ventricle on the left of this image.

Plate 3: Colour M-mode study recorded from the cursor shown in Plate 1, as a red dotted line passing through the right ventricle, tricuspid valve and right atrium. The images recorded along this line are displayed on the y-axis of the M-mode, and are plotted against time on the x-axis. The red flow signal (A) indicates the normal diastolic flow into the right ventricle following atrial contraction. To the right of this, a further red signal (VR) is displayed below the tricuspid valve. This signal represents the venous return during systole. The red flow signal (E) represents the flow from the right atrium across the tricuspid valve into the right ventricle during rapid filling of the ventricle.

Plate 4: Colour flow Doppler study from a horse with severe mitral regurgitation secondary to rupture of the chordae tendineae. This left parasternal long-axis view shows highly disturbed flow (coded green) throughout the left atrium. Compare the area of this signal to those shown in Plate 2. This flow Pattern was present throughout systole.

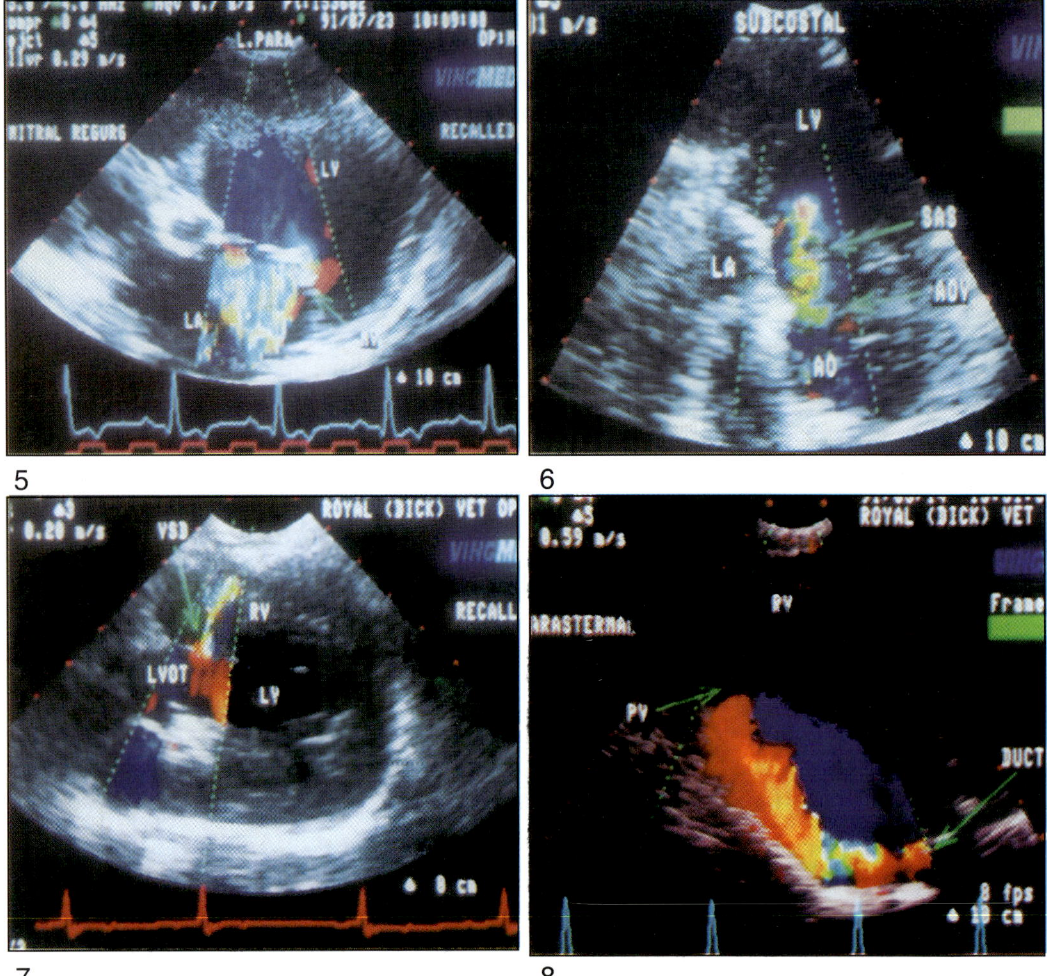

Plate 5: Two-dimensional echocardiogram with colour flow Doppler (right parasternal long-axis view) from a Cocker spaniel with mitral valve disease. The left ventricle is dilated. The colour Doppler shows the turbulent flow of mitral regurgitation during systole. The orientation here is not standard and should be reversed from left to right. LV = left ventricle; LA = left atrium; MV = mitral valve.

Plate 6: Two-dimensional echocardiogram with colour flow Doppler (subcostal view) from a: dog with subaortic stenosis. The colour Doppler shows turbulent flow through the stenosis during systole. LV = left ventricle; LA = left atrium; AO - aorta; SAS - subaortic stenosis; AOV = aortic valve.

Plate 7: Two-dimensional echocardiogram with colour flow Doppler (right parasternal long-axis view) from the dog in Fig. 6.19. The colour Doppler shows a jet of turbulent flow through the interventricular septal defect extending into the right ventricle. Note that the thick appearance of the left ventricular free wall is partly due to the papillary muscle. The orientation here is not standard and should be reversed from left to right. RV = right ventricle; LV = left ventricle; LVOT = left ventricular outflow tract; VSD = ventricular septal defect.

Plate 8: Two-dimensional echocardiogram with colour flow Doppler (right parasternal short-axis view) from a dog with a patent ductus arteriosus. The colour Doppler shows blood flowing from the ductus (origin arrowed but not visualized) upwards (coded red) to the pulmonic valve and circling clockwise and then down (coded blue) the pulmonary artery. Continuous blood flow is seen in real time. The orientation here is not standard and should be reversed from left to right. RV = right ventricle; PV = Pulmonic valve; DUCT = approximate location of the patent ductus arteriosus.

Veterinary Ultrasonography

Edited by

P. J. Goddard

The Macaulay Land Use Research Institute
Craigiebuckler
Aberdeen, UK

CAB INTERNATIONAL

CAB INTERNATIONAL
Wallingford
Oxon OX10 8DE
UK

Tel: +44(0)1491 832111
Telex: 847964 (COMAGG G)
E-mail: cabi@cabi.org
Fax: +44(0)1491 833508

A catalogue entry for this book is available from the British Library.

ISBN 0 85198 923 3

Disclaimer

Typeset by MFK Information Services Ltd.
Printed and bound in the UK at the University Press, Cambridge

Contents

Contributors

J.S. Boyd, *Department of Veterinary Anatomy, University of Glasgow, Veterinary School, Bearsden Road, Glasgow G61 1QH, UK.*

P. Boydell, *The Animal Medical Centre, 511 Wilbraham Road, Chorlton, Manchester M21 1UF, UK.*

G.C.W. England, *Department of Farm Animal and Equine Medicine and Surgery, Royal Veterinary College, University of London, Hawkshead Lane, North Mymms, Hatfield, Hertfordshire AL9 7TA, UK.*

P.J. Goddard, *The Macaulay Land Use Research Institute, Craigiebuckler, Aberdeen AB9 2QJ, UK.*

P.G. Griffin, *Lone Oak Veterinary Clinic Inc., 34775 Road 132, Visalia, California CA 93291, USA.*

C.R. Lamb, *Department of Small Animal Medicine and Surgery, Royal Veterinary College, University of London, Hawkshead Lane, North Mymms, Hatfield, Hertfordshire AL9 7TA, UK.*

K.J. Long, *Department of Veterinary Clinical Studies, Royal (Dick) School of Veterinary Studies, University of Edinburgh, Large Animal Hospital, Veterinary Field Station, Easter Bush, Roslin, Midlothian EH25 9RG, UK.*

S.J. Maddock, *Department of Clinical Veterinary Medicine, University of Cambridge, Madingley Road, Cambridge CB3 0ES, UK.*

C.M. Marr, *Valley Equine Hospital, Upper Lambourn Road, Lambourn, Berkshire RG16 7QG, UK.*

M.W.S. Martin, *Godiva Referrals, 207 Daventry Road, Cheylesmore, Coventry CV3 5HH, UK.*

J.P.M. Main, *O'Gorman, Slater and Main, Donnington Grove Veterinary Surgery, Oxford Road, Newbury, Berkshire RG13 2JB, UK.*

M.J. Meredith, *Department of Clinical Veterinary Medicine, University of Cambridge, Madingley Road, Cambridge CB3 0ES, UK.*

M. Porter, *4350 Harrodsburg Road, Lexington, Kentucky KY 40513, USA.*

A.J.F. Russel, *The Macaulay Land Use Research Institute, Hartwood Reseach Station, Hartwood, Shotts, Lanarkshire ML7 4JY, UK.*

Preface

Ultrasonography has rapidly become established as one of the principal imaging techniques used in veterinary practice. It allows the clinician to obtain instant information about a wide range of body systems and in some cases the dynamic function of organs can be assessed. New techniques and applications are regularly reported. In addition, ultrasonography has led to new insights into basic anatomy and physiological processes.

This book is intended as a general guide to the correct use and most advantageous application of ultrasonography by veterinary surgeons. The contributors all have considerable practical experience in the techniques they describe, and have attempted to provide sufficient guidance to allow investigations to be made for the first time. While every effort has been taken to ensure freedom from errors, the continued development of some of the techniques described inevitably means that advances in knowledge may render some procedures obsolete: we would encourage readers to indicate how future editions could be enhanced.

I would like to thank BCF Technology Ltd (8 Brewster Square, Brucefield Industrial Park, Livingston, West Lothian EH54 9BJ, Scotland) for a financial contribution towards the cost of including colour plates.

P.J. Goddard
Aberdeen
October, 1994

1 General Principles

P.J. Goddard
The Macaulay Land Use Research Institute,
Craigiebuckler, Aberdeen AB9 2QJ, UK

Modern ultrasound instruments are highly sophisticated pieces of equipment. Their complexity varies and, although it is possible for anyone to plug in, switch on and obtain an image, it is only by understanding the physics of ultrasound, its interactions with tissue and the functions of the controls of individual instruments that repeatable images of diagnostic quality can be obtained: the quality of the image is very dependent upon the skill of the sonographer. Linked to this is the need to be aware of artifacts which have the potential to confuse the viewer and impair diagnosis.

Although ultrasound is considered a safe system, patient exposure should not be extended unnecessarily and consequently correct scanning techniques should be employed to allow rapid visualization of target structures.

This chapter will primarily consider B-mode systems. Although the principles of operation are essentially similar, other systems are also employed both in clinical veterinary practice and research environments. These will be discussed where appropriate, in this chapter and in those which subsequently cover their application. It is likely that technological advances in the human field will rapidly filter through to find veterinary application, for example the use of contrast agents.

A glossary of terms can be found at the end of this chapter.

What is Ultrasound?

Ultrasound is a high-frequency sound wave. Audible sounds are of the order 20–20,000 hertz (Hz) (cycles per second) while ultrasound waves are of a higher frequency. For diagnostic applications, frequencies of 1–10 MHz are employed. Like audible sound, ultrasound cannot be propagated in a vacuum and in gas transmission is poor. Reflection of ultrasound occurs between substances of different acoustic impedance (defined as the product of the velocity of sound in a substance and the density of the latter). Even the short distance between the transducer (which emits and receives ultrasound signals) and the patient must be bridged by a suitable coupling agent. Ultrasound can be propagated in an elastic medium primarily as longitudinal compression waves. By means of the echo principle, an image can be produced on the display of the scanner which relates to the acoustic impedance of tissues encountered by the ultrasound beam and the depth/distance of tissue interfaces.

How is Ultrasound Generated and Detected?

By means of the piezoelectric effect, crystal(s) in the transducer (scan head) are deformed when a high-voltage electrical current is applied and ultrasound is generated (Fig. 1.1). The high voltage is applied to the back face of the crystal while

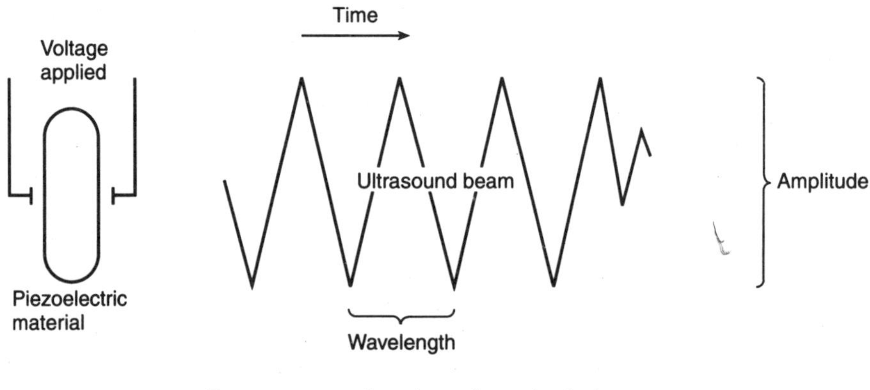

Fig. 1.1. Ultrasound beam characteristics.

the front face is earthed. The magnitude of the deformation (vibration) is proportional to the applied voltage and results in the power of the ultrasound beam. The conversion efficiency of the transducer relates electrical power to acoustic power. The intensity of the beam (in watts per unit area) relates to the area over which this power is available and is thus a function of the cross sectional area of the beam, being maximal at the defined focal length. The frequency of vibration of the ultrasound waves is related primarily to crystal characteristics although it may be influenced electronically. The natural resonant frequency of the crystal is related to its thickness. Frequency of emission and wavelength are inversely proportional. At 2 MHz the wavelength of the beam is around 0.8 mm. This relationship has consequences for penetration of tissue and definition of detail: as frequency increases, the ability to differentiate objects along the path of the beam (axial resolution) increases, but the beam is more rapidly attenuated (reduced in power).

Ultrasound is transmitted to the patient from the transducer and propagates through the tissues. The velocity of propagation is independent of frequency but depends on the tissue characteristics. It is reflected by structures normal to the beam axis, and nearer boundary echoes return first. The returning ultrasound meets with and deforms the crystals in the transducer. This mechanical energy is converted back to an electrical signal proportional to the strength of the echo and delayed by a time roughly proportional to the distance travelled. The reflected signal is interpreted by the instrument as variations in brightness displayed on the cathode ray tube of a B-mode system (or as variation in amplitude on the x-axis of an A-mode oscilloscope screen). In some Doppler systems a simple audio output is produced. Since ultrasound travels in a straight line, a composite two-dimensional image can be achieved with a linear array of a large number of precisely aligned crystals or a single crystal in a mechanical transducer. Movement of the beam may be achieved electronically with multiple transducers or mechanically with a single transducer. Both methods are used to produce linear and sector scans.

Ultrasound is not emitted from the transducer continuously in B-mode diagnostic situations (although it is in some Doppler and therapy applications). If it were it would be impossible to interpret the returning signals. A pulse–echo system is employed. A pulse of ultrasound (comprising around 5–6 wave cycles typically lasting less than one microsecond) is emitted and its reflection received prior to emission of the next pulse. (For pulsed Doppler ultrasonography 5–20 cycles are used lasting around 2 μs, while for therapy instruments the pulse duration of around 0.2 ms approximates to the off-time duration). The frequency of pulse emission is governed by the speed of ultrasound in tissue (approximately 1540 m s^{-1}; equivalent to 6.5 μs cm^{-1}) and the total time needed for the ultrasound pulse to cover its outward and return journeys (the round-trip time). For real-time (live) ultrasonography, as high a pulse frequency as possible is adopted up to a theoretical maximum of around 2000 Hz. It is important to use a high quality pulse of uniform frequency. Because of sub-optimal performance of the crystals at the beginning and end of each pulse, they do not have long to achieve their resonant frequency, and sometimes this is not achieved (Fig. 1.2). For Doppler ultrasonography uniform frequency is particularly important because the

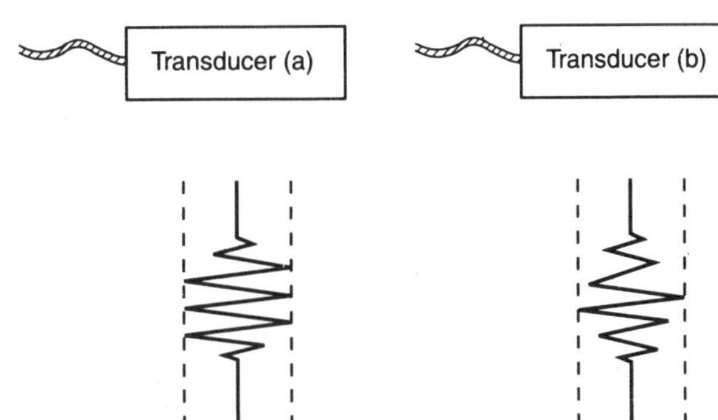

Fig. 1.2. Representation of ultrasound pulses of different quality. Both transducers operate for the same time. A greater proportion of the pulse from transducer (a) is at the resonant frequency, and is thus of higher quality.

frequency of the returning signal is measured. Low quality transducers often make better receivers. The maximum intensity in relation to the period of ultrasound pulse generation is termed the temporal peak. Such measures are important when considering the effects of the beam on biological tissue.

The ability of the system to differentiate two structures along the length of the beam is described as the axial resolution (Fig. 1.3). It is improved by a shorter pulse duration. Since the number of cycles in each pulse is usually fixed by the design of the instrument, the only way the sonographer can improve axial resolution is to increase the frequency. Lateral resolution, the ability of the system to differentiate two structures lying side-by-side, is related to the size of the transducer elements and the frequency. It is optimal at the focal length, where the beam is thinnest, and, like axial resolution, improves as frequency increases. In practice, reducing the gain (and thus the strength of close echoes) may improve lateral resolution.

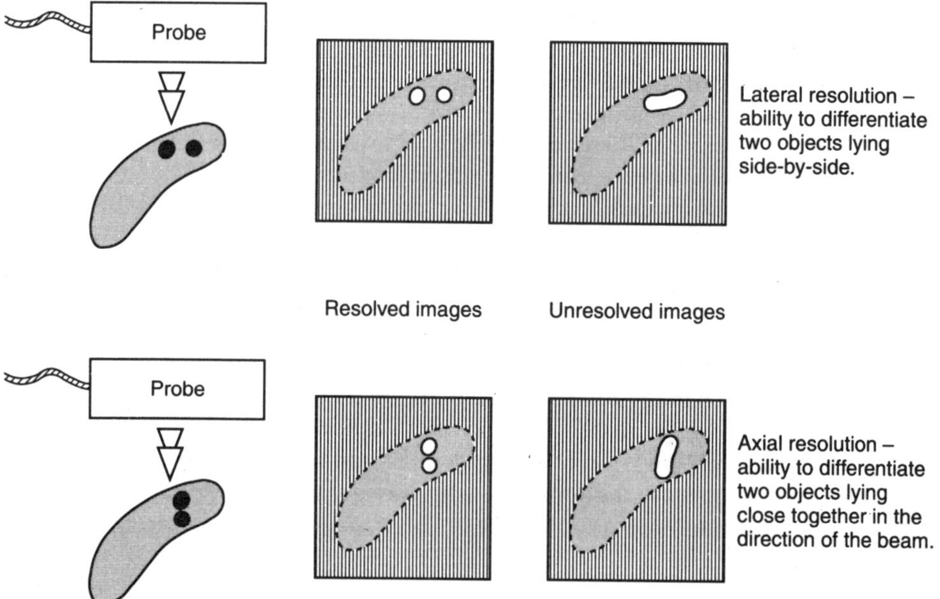

Fig. 1.3. Resolution of the ultrasound image.

How do Tissues Interact with Ultrasound?

The display on the ultrasound system presents an interpretation of returning ultrasound signals. The strength of the reflected ultrasound beam depends upon a number of factors, but of primary importance are the differences in tissue acoustic impedance it encounters on its journey, the angle at which it meets tissue boundaries and the distance travelled. If the beam were to pass through a homogeneous structure then there would be no reflection. However, even relatively homogeneous tissues, such as the liver, present a matrix of small structural and density variations and consequently an image of apparently uniform brightness is produced. At tissue interfaces the density gradient may be marked (a large acoustic impedance difference) and from such areas a strong echo is generated (e.g. soft tissue/air interfaces). Although tissues of similar acoustic density are not themselves easily differentiated, serosal surfaces often provide strong lines of demarcation. These acoustically reflective surfaces normal to the ultrasound beam are termed specular reflectors. Here the character of the reflected signal is dependent upon the ratio of reflector size and wavelength of the beam. Specular reflectors are large compared to the beam width. Scatter occurs when the beam meets very small objects (relative to the wavelength of the beam) or irregular interfaces. As the wavelength decreases, this effect increases. Consequently attenuation increases as frequency increases and leads to the inability of higher frequency ultrasound to penetrate deeply into tissue even though its resolving power is greater. This type of scatter may provide a measure of tissue quality. The size of these small scatterers is an important determinant of tissue echogenicity. For example, the abnormal structure within organs caused by tumour growth may lead to atypical echogenicity and hence be visible sonographically.

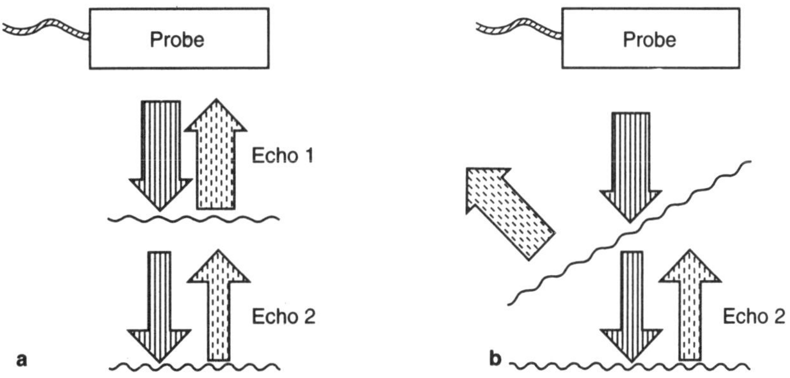

Fig. 1.4. Major interactions of the ultrasound beam. **(a)** When the beam meets a highly reflective surface perpendicular to it, much is reflected and not available for further tissue penetration. Both echoes return to the probe. **(b)** If the angle of incidence is not perpendicular then the reflected signal is not available for recapture. The beam, passing deeper into the tissue, may be refracted if the tissues are of different acoustical density. Only echo 2 is received by the probe.

The angle at which the beam strikes an acoustically reflective surface is important, since if the beam is perpendicular to this surface then much of the reflection is recaptured by the transducer (Fig. 1.4). As the angle is altered less of the beam is reflected to the transducer. The reflected beam is not available for further tissue penetration. An ultrasound shadow may be cast if a high percentage of beam energy is lost at an interface.

The velocity of ultrasound in tissue varies with tissue density between around 1500 and 1600 m s^{-1}. If the ultrasound beam is subject to a velocity change across a tissue boundary at angles other than perpendicular, refraction of the beam may occur. This leads to the potential for mislocation of structures on the display (Fig. 1.5).

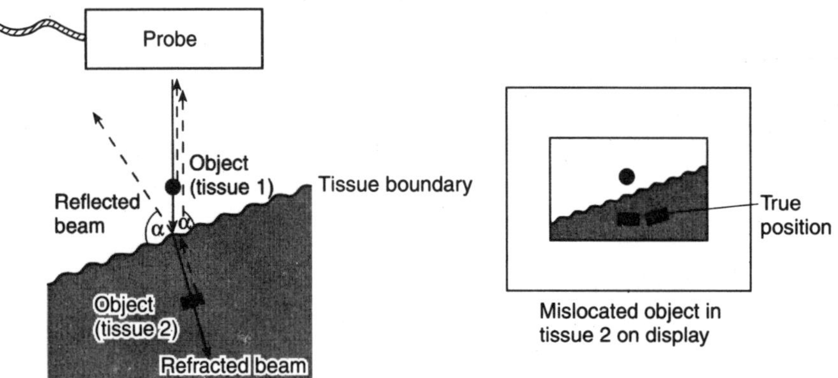

Fig. 1.5. Refraction of the ultrasound beam may lead to mislocation of structures on the display, since the instrument 'assumes' the beam travels in a straight path. The ultrasound beam is refracted when it enters a tissue of different acoustical density. The angle of refraction depends on the relative velocity of sound in the two tissues.

Useful energy is lost from the beam in a variety of ways and the beam is attenuated as it passes deeper into tissue. As described above, reflection is the chief reason why the beam does not penetrate further into tissue (although, of course, it is needed for generation of the image). Also as noted above, scatter is responsible for some loss of beam energy by dispersing the ultrasound beam. This dispersion also has the effect of spreading the beam and so reduces lateral resolution. Ultrasound is absorbed by some tissues through which it passes, due to hysteresis: the compression and relaxation forces of the ultrasound wave are not transmitted with complete efficiency because of frictional effects, and the beam becomes phase-shifted. Heat may be generated within the tissue. Up to a point, absorption due to hysteresis increases with frequency. Passage through a gas-filled structure (e.g. lung or bowel) also attenuates the beam due to scatter and absorption and will have a masking effect on more deeply situated structures. Thus cardiac examination must be made at sites where the heart is not masked by the lungs or the ribs.

As it travels beyond its focal length divergence occurs and the beam loses intensity (geometric attenuation).

How are Images Generated on the Display?

Images are usually generated from the system's scan converter or frame store, which processes the reflected ultrasound into a form required for screen presentation. Storage is not essential to create an image, although it is now the norm.

Information is displayed regarding distance and amplitude, in relation to either the individual element in a linear array scan head or the alignment of the crystal in a mechanical scan head (essentially location across the width of the scan). Each echo position is represented as a dot on the screen. Thus a two-dimensional image is generated. The brightness (and hence B-mode: brightness-mode) of each dot is related to the amplitude of the reflection and is referred to as a grey scale display. Individual instruments can vary in the number of divisions of the grey scale (from black to white) they are able to generate.

An analogue scan converter or frame store allows the display to be generated by means of a stored charge on a dielectric matrix. There are problems with long-term stability. A digital scan converter or frame store allows greater flexibility in electronic handling of the image subsequently (post-processing) which may be required in some applications. A scan converter changes the format of the scan from the way it is produced at source to the way it is displayed. In electronic terms it may be described as being six or eight bits deep, allowing 64 or 256 shades of grey respectively in each pixel on the screen. Digital scan converters predominate due to the common requirement to display in standard television (TV) format, thus taking advantage of TV recording accessories.

Because of attenuation, deeper tissues could be expected to produce less reflection and consequently less bright images on the screen, regardless of their density. In order not to confuse visual interpretation, instruments adopt a time-gain compensation adjustment which automatically amplifies signals which have a longer round-trip time.

Although the image appears to be live (real-time), it is in fact a constantly updated fixed image, the speed of which is defined by the frame rate. There are usually two frame rates, the scanning frame rate and the display frame rate. Visual flicker is most influenced by the latter, and where this is satisfactory (usually more than 20 frames per second) the scanning frame rate can be ignored except in extreme cases. The importance of the scanning frame rate is more related to the speed at which a search scan can be made, the resolution in a relatively stable image or the ability to resolve movement as distinct from structure. Thus lower frame rates may be selected to provide enhanced detail, while higher frame rates facilitate the study of moving structures. Since the product of the frame rate and the number of elements in the display (lines) represents the minimum pulse frequency needed, and since this frequency must be finite given the obligatory round-trip time, the frame rate generally never exceeds 60 frames per second, and a much lower rate is usually adopted.

Types of Instrument

In the main, sonography for veterinary work is accomplished using B-mode, real-time scanning as described in the preceding pages, producing the illusion of a live, two-dimensional image representing a slice through the tissue, the thickness of which is related to the size of the transducer element. The movement of structures greatly assists tissue identification and to some extent function as well as structure may be studied. All instruments have a conventional cathode ray tube display which may be augmented by a high-resolution video monitor, valuable for replaying video recordings. M-mode scanning allows the motion of tissues, principally the heart, to be studied by creating a one-dimensional image that is displayed on the vertical axis with time on the horizontal axis. This image is rapidly updated. Continuous output may be saved by using a chart recorder or videotape.

Doppler ultrasound, a further specialized technique often employed for studies of haemodynamics and pregnancy diagnosis, especially in pigs, registers the increase or decrease in frequency caused by structures moving, respectively, towards or away from the transducer. These differences may be displayed in a variety of ways including audio and duplex systems, the latter of which overlay Doppler information on a conventional two-dimensional, real-time display. Some information can be displayed with the benefit of colour flow enhancement. Doppler ultrasound is increasingly being used in human medicine, for example to locate flow disturbances due to stenotic vessels. The Doppler shift of frequency (F_d) can be simply calculated as the difference between the transmitted (F_t) and received (F_r) signal:

$$F_d = F_r - F_t$$

or by:

$$F_d = F_t\,(2u/v)$$

where v is the velocity of ultrasound in the medium and u is the velocity of movement of the target (e.g. red blood cells). In practice the transformation of Doppler shift into velocity is carried out automatically. If the precise flow rate is required, it is necessary to know the angle at which the beam impinges on the vessel, since maximum Doppler shift occurs when the flow is directly towards or away from the transducer (Fig. 1.6). The formula:

$$F_d = F_t\,(2u/v)\cos\Theta$$

where Θ is the angle of incidence, provides the required adjustment. The output from the transducer may be continuous, using a separate receiving transducer, and such systems have become widely used to monitor fetal heartbeat and enhanced maternal blood flow, for example when performing pregnancy diagnosis in sows. Portable battery-powered systems are available which have an audio output. Pulsed Doppler systems have the advantage of being able to study specific tissues (since depth information is also generated) by a process called range gating.

B-mode instruments generally incorporate an on-screen measurement facility. This may also allow areas to be calculated. Electronic callipers are superior to making measurements manually from a hard copy. It is important to recognize some limitations. Accuracy may be affected if the velocity of the ultrasound beam in the tissue concerned is different from that in the calibration medium. This particularly affects measurements along the beam axis. Refraction of the beam may affect measurements across the beam axis. Accuracy will also depend on the number of pixels in the display. It is also important to ensure that on-screen cursor placement is accurate, especially if areas are to be calculated.

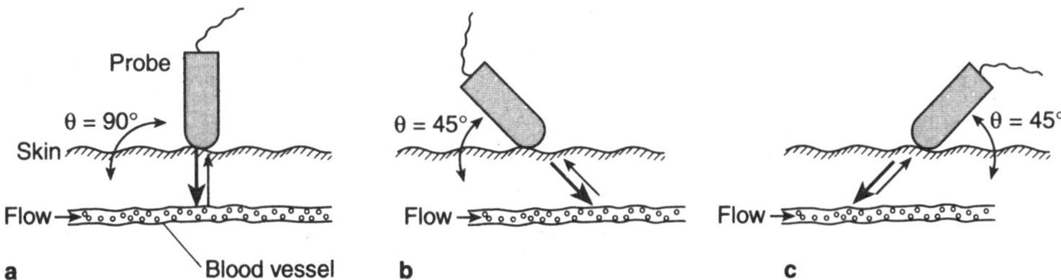

Fig. 1.6. Using Doppler shift to estimate velocity. **(a)** If the incident beam is perpendicular to the moving target, there is no Doppler shift of the returning beam. **(b)** If the incident beam is at an angle of 45° in the direction of the flow, the returning beam will be of reduced frequency (negative Doppler shift). **(c)** If the incident beam is at an angle of 45° against the flow, the returning beam will be of increased frequency (positive Doppler shift).

Transducers

The heart of the transducer is the piezoelectric material which generates the ultrasound pulses across its narrow axis and sends a thin beam of ultrasound into a receptive tissue. A number of piezoelectric materials exist naturally or have been manufactured. Lead zirconate-titanate (PZT) is considered one of the best, although it is not naturally piezoelectric but made so during manufacture. The resonant frequency of the transducer is generally fixed and is related to the thinness (usually less than 1 mm) of the piezoelectric material. For diagnostic work frequencies of 1–10 MHz are adopted. Linear transducers consist of a number (64–256) of such piezoelectric crystals precisely aligned along the long axis of the probe. When excited, these produce a plane wavefront of ultrasound emission. A layer of damping material behind the crystal array (e.g. epoxy resin with tungsten powder and rubber) reduces pulse duration and thus improves axial resolution. A matching layer at the transducer face improves the quality of the signal and the transmission of the ultrasound to the subject by reducing reflection back to the transducer. In a linear array multi-element transducer, not all the crystals may be excited simultaneously. They are either triggered sequentially along the length or segmentally in overlapping blocks (Fig. 1.7). Segmental activation optimizes beam quality.

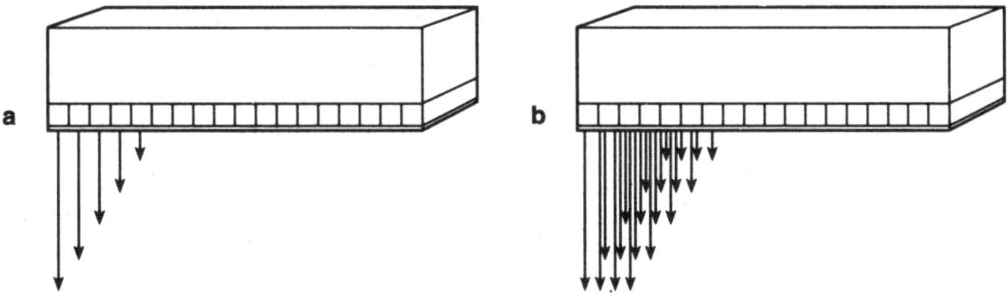

Fig. 1.7. Transducer array activation. **(a)** Sequential activation of a linear transducer array. **(b)** Segmental activation produces a flatter wavefront.

Although ultrasound is a sound wave, it can be focused. Resolution is maximal at the defined focal length. In multi-element transducers focusing can be achieved by adjusting the physical shape of the transducer face, which may have a superficial concave acoustic lens. However, the focal length is then permanently fixed. Although focusing across the narrow axis of the transducer is thus fixed mechanically, focusing along the length of the linear probe may also be accomplished electronically, by suitably altering the time frame of activation of individual elements (Fig. 1.8). Since this is a dynamic process, it may, in some equipment, be varied by the sonographer in relation to the study being undertaken, although the optimal longitudinal and transverse focal lengths may then not coincide.

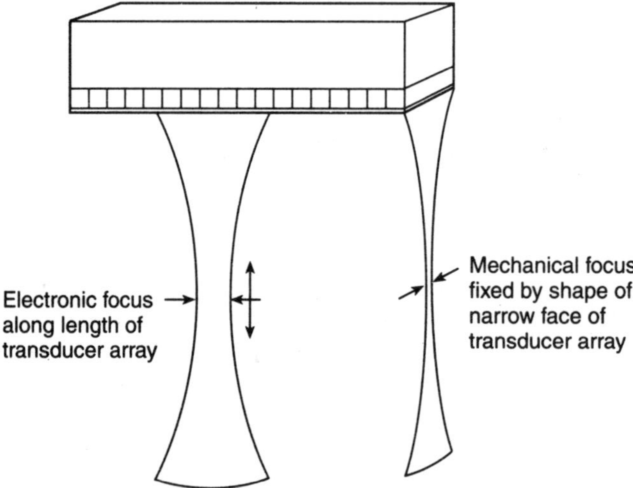

Fig. 1.8. Focusing of linear array transducers. Electronic focal length can be varied but will then not coincide with mechanical focal length. Electronic focus in the receiving mode can be continuously varied to give dynamic focusing.

Despite electronically sophisticated designs, the very near field always suffers from variation in ultrasound intensity, while the far field suffers from beam divergence. At the interface of these two fields beam quality is optimal and the best diagnostic images are obtained. The intensity of the beam is greatest at the defined focal length.

Linear array transducers require a relatively large area of patient contact. Sector transducers only require a small area (they are said to have a small footprint) and thus facilitate visualization of some structures inaccessible to the linear array transducer (e.g. viewing between ribs). Mechanical sector probes consist of a small number of rotating transducer crystals, a single fixed crystal with an oscillating mirror, or a single oscillating crystal (Fig. 1.9). These cover the field of view and produce a sector image, on the screen. The ultrasound beam source is at a short distance from the probe surface and is usually mounted in a sealed unit

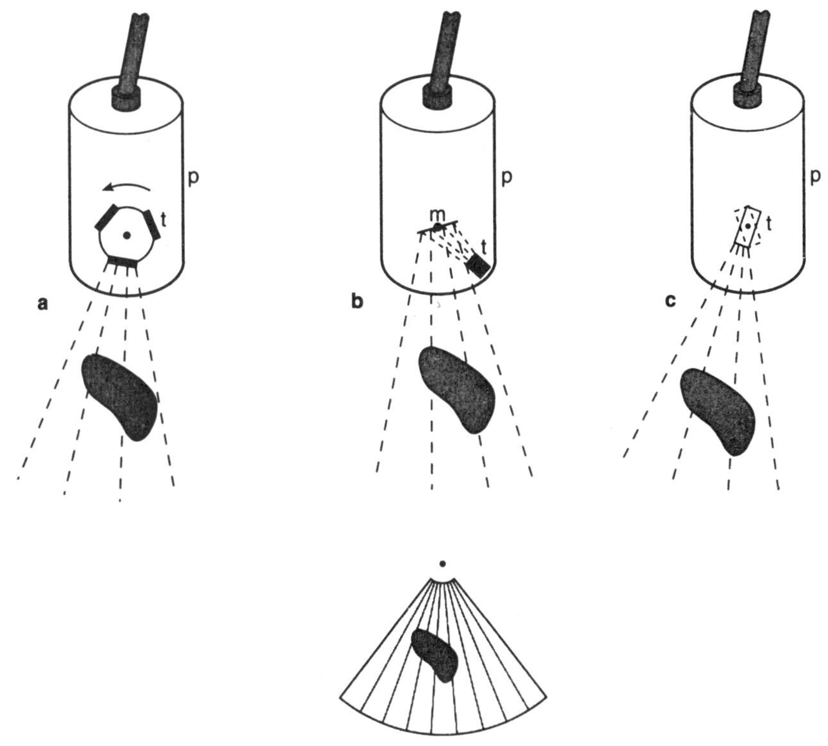

Fig. 1.9. Mechanical sector probes. **(a)** Three-element rotating transducer bathed in acoustic coupling oil. **(b)** Single fixed transducer with oscillating mirror. **(c)** Single oscillating transducer. t = transducer, m = mirror, p = probe.

surrounded by oil. The beam is projected through an acoustic window. Oscillating devices suffer from a variability in the speed of scanning at the extremities of the image.

It is possible to create the illusion of a sector output from a linear array using an electronically phased excitation of the elements. Similarly, linear array beams can be permanently steered. With mechanical sector scanners, the line density is no longer controlled by the number of piezoelectric crystals in the array but by the number of pulses emitted with each sweep across the field of view. The amount of missing information increases with tissue depth due to beam divergence.

Doppler transducers in pulsed systems usually contain a single crystal, while for continuous-wave Doppler systems separate transmitting and receiving crystals are needed.

Specialized probes exist which have been designed to look inside cavities or allow positioning of biopsy instruments. In the latter case, practice using some form of phantom is valuable before targeting on a patient.

Probe components are sealed to prevent entry of moisture and ensure electrical safety. Although probes should be cleaned between patients, it may be necessary to sterilize the probe and cable, in which case the manufacturer's guidance should be obtained. Other solutions to problems of disease transmission involve covering the probe with gel and inserting it in a disposable plastic sleeve.

Coupling Agents

If high-quality images are to be obtained it is crucial to ensure maximum ultrasound transmission to and from the patient. Ultrasound travels poorly through air, and so a coupling agent is needed to bridge the small gap between the transducer face and the patient. This agent is usually a coupling gel applied to the contact area of the patient. Gels should be of suitable impedance to reduce contact artifacts and should not contain materials likely to damage the patient, or the scan head on long-term exposure. Since hair traps air it is important to clip hairy parts of the patient closely and, if necessary, to shave them closely prior to applying the gel. The skin should then be degreased. (Veterinary surgeons are often requested to part, rather than to clip, the hair of show animals. Under such circumstances the owner should be made aware of the constraint this imposes on the examination.) The gel should be rubbed into the patient to ensure optimum penetration. Gel should always be washed from the patient after the investigation to reduce the chance of allergic reaction, although the risk is minimal with gels known to be free of skin irritants and sensitizers. Gels may also contain antimicrobial agents. Vegetable oils have been used as coupling agents and allow reasonable sound transmission, but are messy to use and may damage some materials, particularly rubber or flexible plastics.

Although gel is still needed for trans-rectal examinations, it is important to remove as much faecal material as possible from the rectum first, particularly if this is relatively dry. The procedure may need to be repeated during the examination.

To improve the resolution of superficial structures, a short-focus probe should be employed. It may additionally be necessary to increase the distance between the transducer and the patient and ensure conformity of the contact area between a rigid probe and a relatively firm tissue by means of a stand-off gel. Stand-offs are essentially blocks of acoustically transparent material and may come pre-formed in a carrier which attaches to the probe for ease of manipulation. Some probes may be designed for obligatory use of stand-offs.

Safety

Safety of the sonographer (and patient)

Electrical safety of the equipment is initially the responsibility of the manufacturer. However, the manufacturer has little control over subsequent use. It is important that the instrument and associated cables are routinely examined and treated with due care during storage and use. Cables in particular should be checked regularly for worn areas or splits, and probe cables especially should not be tightly coiled during storage. Inappropriate coupling agents may cause probe cables to become brittle and even crack. If damage has occurred or a fault is suspected, the manufacturer should be contacted before the system is used again. In addition, most manufacturers will provide routine servicing and other support facilities.

In some veterinary applications the electrical supply to the scanning site is substandard and thus its suitability should be investigated before connection. Most instruments have the facility for supplementary earth connections and if they can be set up to operate from a lower voltage supply this will improve safety in the event of a fault developing. A number of safety devices can be inserted in line between the supply and the scanner and advice on the value of these should be obtained. Since water and electricity are especially dangerous in combination, every effort must be made to prevent moisture entering the instrument.

Instruments should be protected from physical injury. This may be facilitated by the provision of long cables to the transducer, although the sonographer will still need to see the screen! Adequate handling facilities contribute to safe operation.

Safety of the patient (and sonographer)

Ultrasonography is a painless procedure. No harmful effects of diagnostic ultrasound (the power of which is around 1% of that used therapeutically) have been reported, despite large epidemiological studies. Since ultrasound does interact with tissues in a variety of ways, prolonged exposure may have deleterious thermal or mechanical effects on tissue, and consequently in human medicine there are guidelines to limit patient exposure. From the description of ultrasound in the preceding pages, however, it should be clear that there is great difficulty in dosimetry (accurately defining the dose received by the patient).

Ultrasound may cause tissues to heat. Indeed, this is one of the effects exploited in therapeutic applications. The rate of heating in a given tissue is dependent upon a number of factors, but principally the intensity and duration of the insonation and the conduction of heat away from the area, for example by blood flow. Thus tissues with a poor blood supply will tend to heat more quickly. At some point, tissues will reach an equilibrium temperature. The surface of bone may reach a high temperature due to its high attenuation of the ultrasound beam. These remarks apply particularly to some Doppler instruments. Fluids may be set in motion by insonation and move in the direction of the beam, and this streaming effect is also used therapeutically.

Cavitation can occur when gas bubbles expand and contract by rapid diffusion of gas from surrounding structures. This cavitation may be stable and cause minimal effect, but if unstable or transient the bubbles may collapse, causing tissue disruption. Cavitation is unlikely to constitute a serious problem with pulsed ultrasound.

Thus, while the net result of the physical effects of ultrasound on tissues is often employed therapeutically, its potentially harmful effects are less well understood. Much interest centres on the potential for genetic damage, but again there is no hard evidence of harmful effects. However, the guidelines of the British Medical Ultrasound Society and the American Institute of Ultrasound in Medicine uphold the principle that only examinations likely to benefit the patient should be undertaken. On a practical note, since much time is spent examining on-screen frozen images, it is important to establish whether the probe is still insonating the patient at this time. If so, it should be removed until the examination is interactive again.

Obtaining the Best Images

An adequate knowledge of the anatomy of the area under investigation is vital to image production and interpretation. Prior practice with cadavers is a valuable teaching aid. Movement of tissues, either spontaneously or by pressure from surrounding structures, is a great help in identification and is one of the main reasons for loss of information on hard copy prints. By making use of acoustic windows (e.g. a fluid-filled bladder) some structures may be more clearly visualized, although the beam should ideally still be as perpendicular as possible to the target structures. Identification of landmarks also facilitates orientation. Sufficient time must be allowed for patient preparation if high quality images are to be obtained. Investigations should always be performed in a standard manner.

By understanding the functions of the control panel optimum images can be achieved. Once set up there should be little need to adjust settings for standard investigations, particularly for the display parameters, brightness and contrast. These should always be set first, before gain and power adjustments are made. Many instruments have on-screen grey scale displays which allow optimum screen adjustment. By limiting the number of adjustments made comparative information is much easier to obtain. An increase in received ultrasound can be achieved by either increasing the power output (and consequently increasing patient exposure) or increasing the gain (and consequently amplifying the effect of signal noise). Viewing is improved by positioning the screen away from direct light.

Regular care of the instrument, particularly the probe, is important. Daily checks should be made to ensure safe operation and promote longevity. Individual elements in linear array probes may be damaged by rough use, with the result that lines of information are lost. Initially this goes unnoticed but the cumulative effect proceeds until image quality markedly deteriorates. The damping material behind the transducer array may also be damaged. It is important to wash gel from the probe after each session (as it may become brittle) and to avoid contact with corrosive substances. Gel should not be spilt on the instrument, particularly near ventilation slots, and operators should wash gel from their hands before adjusting controls.

Although only recently commercially available, contrast agents may be used to enhance the quality of information obtained from certain studies. These small particulate echogenic agents are primarily used for cardiovascular studies. They are injected into the circulation and an ultrasound study is undertaken on their first pass through the target organ (usually the heart). They tend to be filtered out by the first capillary bed they pass through, and so need to be suitable for subsequent elimination (generally by being soluble). A similar, though less standardized, effect can be obtained following the injection of a bolus of saline which was vigorously shaken prior to administration. For a review of these agents, see Schlief (1991).

Manufacturers use complex phantoms, often perspex blocks with embedded objects or wires, to perform quality control reference tests. These allow quantification of resolving power and assessment of the accuracy of on-screen measurement facilities. Measurements of power output are also made. The term 'registration' is used to describe the accuracy of on-screen location of an object. In the human field these checks are routinely performed but in most veterinary applications this does not yet occur. The most difficult faults to appreciate are those of an insidious nature, particularly when standard quality control checks are not available. Sonographers with specific needs for precision in these areas should consult the manufacturer.

Artifacts

Artifacts may mislead the sonographer, since they are representations on the screen of structures that do not exist in the place shown. They may arise from effects within the instrument or from the use of electrical equipment nearby, or be due to tissue effects. They may also depend on the technique of the sonographer. As has previously been discussed, it is important that the instrument is set up correctly. If the gain is too great, for example, spurious reflection may be seen from homogeneous structures. If the time-gain compensation does not truly represent the tissue attenuation, deeper tissues will be misread. Poor patient contact results in poor transmission of ultrasound, while excessive pressure may distort anatomical relationships.

Artifacts due to tissue effects are less easily dealt with. Refraction, as has already been described, may lead to the misplacement of a structure on the screen. It often occurs when fat intervenes between the transducer and the target object, due to its low transmission velocity. In addition, in unusual circumstances a small object may be displayed at more than one location on the screen. Repositioning the transducer generally resolves this problem.

Reverberation artifacts are commonly seen when highly reflective surfaces bounce reflected signals back into the patient, causing second- and higher-order copies of the true structures to appear at increasing depths, but with decreasing intensity, on the scanner display. Such effects may be seen when the ultrasound beam impinges upon the bladder wall or gas in the lumen of the gut. Within-organ reverberation may also occur. Reverberation echoes may be seen close to the top of the display if initial transmission from the probe to the patient is poor. Rotating probes have problems of close-range reverberation due to reflection from the near face of the acoustic window. Multiple reflection artifacts may not always be recognized as such, but generally decrease the contrast of the image. Problems may be corrected in practice by altering the viewing angle or resiting the probe altogether.

Real variations in attenuation will not be adequately compensated for by the fixed time-gain compensation of the instrument. Thus relative densities of some tissues will be misread.

Shadowing can occur when the ultrasound beam meets a highly reflective or absorbing (attenuating) structure. Objects distal to this can only be seen by altering the angle of the incident beam. Gas in the lumen of the gut, calcified structures or very dense objects are primarily responsible. Shadows due to refraction by the edges of rounded objects may also arise.

Enhancement of the beam may occur if it passes through areas of below average attenuation on its way to and from the object of interest, thus enhancing the object's apparent echogenicity.

Because of the effect of beam focal width, small structures in front of and beyond the defined focal zone will appear slightly larger than they truly are.

If a fast-moving object is scanned at too low a frame rate aliasing artifacts may be seen, leading to malpresentation of the object. Although this is not generally a problem with real-time ultrasonography, it may affect Doppler or duplex systems where there may be an incorrect registration of flow rate or direction.

Storing Images

Images may be stored in a number of ways. Since permanent copies may be the subject of legal inquiry, they should be captured only after appropriate on-screen annotation (rather than hand written information added subsequently). The principles of ownership of such hard copies will probably be deemed to equate to that of radiographs. In most cases the image quality of the print is poorer than that on the screen. The loss of information due to tissue movement is also a significant detraction.

A common way to store images is by use of an appropriate Polaroid camera attached to the display panel of the scanner. This is a straightforward method and the result is rapidly available. If a large number of hard copies are to be made, the method is relatively expensive. It is important to ensure that the screen controls are correctly set with the help of the grey scale prior to photography. It is also important to understand the correct functioning of the camera itself and be aware of factors which may influence subsequent film development, e.g. cold processing conditions. Increasing the f stop will darken the image, as will decreasing the exposure time. Generally black and white prints are taken, but colour Polaroid film is available for use with some more sophisticated instruments. Polaroid images fade with time, particularly if exposed to strong light.

Thermal imaging can be used by attaching a printer to the video output. This option is not available for instruments with digital frame stores. The printer has controls for adjusting brightness and contrast which, like the scanner display, should generally be left at a standard setting.

Multiformat cameras may be used but they are expensive and not in general veterinary use.

The video output can also be taken to a video recorder. This allows live images to be recorded, but reviewing to find specific information may be slow, and yet another bulky piece of equipment must be transported to the site, in the case of field work. It may be possible to make hard copies subsequently when optimum images can be chosen.

Glossary

Absorption — Loss of energy (principally due to molecular friction forces and the production of heat). As frequency increases, absorption increases.

Acoustic coupling — Since ultrasound is poorly transmitted through air it is necessary to exclude air and link the transducer to the surface of the subject with a suitable coupling gel.

Acoustic enhancement — Tissues distal to an anechoic structure may display enhanced echogenicity.

Acoustic interface — Junction of two tissues with different acoustic impedances. This leads to the reflection of a proportion of the incident beam and possible diffraction of much of the remainder of the beam. The greater the difference in acoustic impedance, the stronger the reflection.

A-mode — Amplitude modulation. A one-element (one-dimensional) display with time (distance) on the horizontal axis. The relative strength of the echo is registered as amplitude on the vertical axis.

Amplitude — Height of the ultrasound waveform.

Anechoic (sonolucent) — A tissue failing to reflect the ultrasound beam produces no echoes (e.g. a fluid-filled viscus).

Array — Distribution of crystals along the length of a linear scan head.

Artifact — An on-screen representation of a structure which does not exist or is incorrectly located.

Attenuation — Decrease in power of the ultrasound beam, caused principally by absorption, scatter and reflection.

Axial resolution — Measure of the ability of the system to differentiate two structures lying closely together along the path of the ultrasound beam.

B-mode — Brightness modulation. A compound A-mode scan with amplitude translated into a brightness scale. Location on the display is related to position and depth.

Callipers — A system for measurement of distance and area is provided on most instruments.

Diffuse reflection — An echo from a target(s) less than one wavelength in size.

Doppler ultrasound — When an ultrasound beam meets a moving object the reflected ultrasound is either of increased or decreased frequency, depending on whether the motion is towards or away from the transducer. Either continuous or pulsed Doppler can be used and some systems can display compound information.

Echogenic — A structure causing a marked reflection of the ultrasound beam. A change in echogenicity in a homogenous structure may indicate a pathological change.

Focal area — Region of the scanned field where resolution is greatest. Focusing can be achieved by electronic or physical means.

Frame rate — The frequency with which images are updated on the screen. Altering the frame rate may improve image quality in some applications.

Frequency — Number of ultrasound waves emitted per second. 1 cycle per second = 1 hertz (Hz).

Gain — The amplification level of a returned signal. On some instruments different depths of the field are handled separately. Incorrect setting of gain controls will lose detail from fine structures.

Grey scale — Range of intensities displayed on the cathode ray tube.

Hyperechoic — Showing increased echogenicity.

Hypoechoic — Showing decreased echogenicity.

Lateral resolution — Measure of the ability of the system to differentiate two structures lying side-by-side at the same distance from the transducer.

Linear array — Distribution of piezoelectric crystals along the length of a scan head. The image produced is generally rectangular.

M-mode — Motion mode. Essentially a rapidly updated one-dimensional B-mode display with time on the second axis to allow study of moving structures. Used principally in cardiology.

Piezoelectric crystals — Crystals of materials such as lead zirconate-titanate, capable of converting applied electrical energy to mechanical deformation and vice versa.

Power — Energy of the ultrasound beam. It is generally expressed in watts (or as intensity in watts cm^{-2}). The minimum power consistent with good image quality should be employed.

Probe — The transducer array and its housing.

Real-time — Images generated from reflected ultrasound following sequential activation of the transducer array are displayed on the screen at sufficient speed to give the appearance of a live image.

Reverberation echo — An artefact created by the retransmission of a strongly reflected ultrasound signal. The display may show several images of a single structure, which appear at increasing distances from the transducer.

Scan converter — A component of the processing system which converts the electrical output of the transducer to the cathode ray tube image, essentially by aggregating sequential arrays across the screen. A scan converter allows for subsequent analysis beyond the screen display (post-processing) and the use of standard TV accessories.

Scatter — When the ultrasound beam encounters a small object in its path the beam energy is spread in all directions.

Sector scan — A pieslice/sector-shaped image is produced on the screen. The initial signal is produced by a single vibrating piezoelectric crystal or a small number of rotating crystals (although an electronic phased linear array can produce a sector image). The scan head only needs a limited contact area (small footprint).

Shadowing — Caused by severe attenuation of the ultrasound beam such that it fails to penetrate sufficiently deeply.

Specular reflection — A strong echo created by a highly reflective tissue interface representing an area significantly larger than one wavelength.

Time-gain compensation (TGC) — Since the ultrasound beam is increasingly attenuated as it travels deeper into tissue, by applying TGC tissues of similar reflectivity are presented with similar brightness, regardless of distance from the transducer.

Transducer — The piezoelectric crystal or element which converts electrical to mechanical energy.

Ultrasound — Sound of a frequency above that perceived by the human ear. Diagnostic ultrasound lies in the 1–10 MHz region.

Velocity — Speed of travel of the ultrasound wave. In tissue this is usually density dependent and ranges from 1500 to 1600 m s^{-1}. An average of 1540 m s^{-1} is usually adopted.

Acknowledgement

The advice and comments of Brian Fraser, BCF Technology Ltd, are gratefully acknowledged.

Reference

Schlief, R. (1991) Ultrasound contrast agents. *Current Opinion in Radiology*, 3, 198–207.

Further Reading

Bushong, S.C. and Archer, B.R. (1991) *Diagnostic Ultrasound: Physics, Biology and Instrumentation.* Mosby Year Books, St Louis.

Docker, M.F. and Duck, F.A. (eds) (1991) *The Safe Use of Diagnostic Ultrasound.* British Institute of Radiology, London.

Fish, P. (1990) *Physics and Instrumentation of Diagnostic Medical Ultrasound.* John Wiley & Sons, Chichester.

Sanders, R.C. (ed.) (1991) *Clinical Sonography: A Practical Guide*, 2nd edn, Little, Brown & Company, Boston.

Abdominal Ultrasonography in Small Animals

C.R. Lamb

Department of Small Animal Medicine and Surgery, Royal Veterinary College, University of London, Hawkshead Lane, North Mymms, Hatfield, Hertfordshire AL9 7TA, UK

Introduction

Ultrasonography has made a major impact on the diagnosis of abdominal diseases in small animals. First used for pregnancy diagnosis, abdominal ultrasonography is now established as a rapid, non-invasive technique for obtaining information about an increasing number of abdominal disorders. Many applications of ultrasonography pertain to situations in which radiographic techniques are limited; hence ultrasonography complements radiography. Those with experience in abdominal ultrasonography are frequently asked by colleagues whether to request radiography or ultrasonography for a certain case, because it is perceived that one may be more sensitive than the other for the expected abnormality. Often one modality can be rationally selected; however, for a large number of common clinical presentations, both ultrasonography and radiography prove to be necessary. For example, an old dog has an abdominal tumour: the mass may be detectable using ultrasonography, but any metastasis to the lungs and/or sternal lymph node will be apparent only on radiographs.

When both radiography and ultrasonography are planned for an animal with signs of abdominal disease, the radiographs are best obtained first and examined before the ultrasound scan. This is principally because radiographs alone enable assessment of important thoracic and/or skeletal lesions that may occur secondary to certain abdominal diseases. Radiographs often provide more easily interpretable data about the stomach and intestine. Also, it is often easier to recognize displacement of abdominal organs when the entire abdomen is visible on a single image; the ultrasound scan may be facilitated by prior knowledge of organ displacement, for example, when selecting appropriate acoustic windows for the study.

Ultrasonography of the abdomen is particularly useful for the following:

- Measurements of organs, e.g. renal length or intestinal wall thickness, without the need for radiographic magnification correction or contrast media.

- Obtaining anatomical information not easily obtainable by other means, e.g. identifying the biliary tract or pancreas.
- Investigating peritoneal fluid, which obscures radiographic detail and may mask the underlying cause.
- Determining the origin and structure of masses, which may be invisible radiographically.
- Guiding biopsy to obtain definitive diagnosis of lesions identified by physical examination, radiography or ultrasonography.

Principles of Ultrasound Scan Interpretation

Interpretation of abdominal radiographs is based on the recognition of certain visual signals ('Roentgen signs'), namely, abnormalities of organ number, size, shape, position, opacity and margination. Similarly, when performing and interpreting abdominal ultrasound scans, attention must be paid to specific visual signals that represent the ultrasonographic signs of disease. These signs include abnormalities of organ number, size, position, shape and echotexture.

Organ number

Determination of organ number in the abdomen depends partly on the ability to recognize organs that are diseased and therefore abnormal in appearance. Hence, the determination of organ number partly depends upon other ultrasonographic signs, including position, shape and echotexture. Errors in organ number determination may occur when an organ is not recognized because it has been displaced or damaged by disease. Despite these potential limitations, ultrasonography can usually confirm the presence of, for example, both kidneys even when they are hypoplastic or shrunken. Other small organs such as the adrenal glands may both be identified in many instances. Intra-abdominal lymph nodes are not amenable to number determination because some are not identifiable unless enlarged, and others, for example the mesenteric nodes, do not form separate, distinct structures.

Position

Organ position is normally described on ultrasound scan images relative to adjacent organs or blood vessels. Depending upon the position of a mobile organ such as the spleen, a detailed multiplanar examination may be required to determine its relationship with adjacent organs. A three-dimensional anatomical description based on ultrasonography is inherently more useful than the radiographic equivalent. Radiographic descriptions of organ position and borders are limited because they are usually inferred from only one or two projections and because unrelated, extra-abdominal structures such as the lumbar vertebrae are normally used as reference points, e.g. in statements of the form 'the left kidney lies ventral to the third lumbar vertebra'. Furthermore, ultrasonography enables the important distinction to be made between structures that are adjacent to, as opposed to continuous with each other. There is a fundamental difference between a mass adjacent to the spleen versus a mass continuous with the spleen: the latter is a splenic mass.

Size

Ultrasonography enables direct, multiplanar measurements to be made of abdominal organs. However, problems arise when making and interpreting abdominal organ measurements, including: difficulty in knowing what measurement to take of an irregular organ such as the liver and how to achieve consistency (Barr, 1992a); the lack of correlation between simple linear measurements and organ volume (Godshalk *et al.*, 1988); the necessity to correct for body weight in the dog (Barr *et al.*, 1990; Barr, 1992b); the lack of correlation between organ size and functional status, for example in the case of the common bile duct (Raptopoulos *et al.*, 1985) or adrenal glands (Kelly *et al.*, 1971).

Shape

Compared to radiography, ultrasonography has the advantage of enhancing recognition of abnormal organ shape because it can show more of the contour of certain organs, e.g. the liver, especially in the presence of peritoneal fluid. On the other hand, an abnormal shape might not be recognized if repeatable standard views of an organ are not routinely obtained. When using a cross-sectional imaging technique such as ultrasonography, it is easy to overinterpret a strange appearance due to oblique positioning.

Echotexture

Perhaps the most striking difference between survey radiographs and ultrasonography in the abdomen derives from the fact that radiographs show only part of the outline of overlapping or adjacent organs such as the liver, spleen or kidney, whereas ultrasonography provides a cross-sectional view of these organs and therefore enables examination of details of their internal anatomy without superimposition. This difference accounts for the higher sensitivity of ultrasonography for lesions affecting parenchymal organs. For example, in humans the sensitivity of ultrasonography for focal hepatic lesions >2 cm is 80% (Zeman *et al.*, 1985) and 73% for hepatocellular carcinomas <5 cm (Choi *et al.*, 1989). Survey radiography cannot approach this.

In a typical abdominal ultrasound image there are relatively few large acoustic interfaces to produce the high-amplitude, specular echoes seen when scanning the heart, for example. The major part of a typical abdominal ultrasound image is composed of non-specular echoes. Non-specular echoes are the low amplitude echoes (backscatter) that give organs their characteristic echotexture (Thijssen and Oosterveld, 1990). There are two points arising from this observation: first, appropriate ultrasound machine settings for abdominal ultrasonography are those which promote detection of variations in non-specular echoes (see below). Second, it may be useful to have at least a basic understanding of the physical features of tissue which influence backscatter, so that some correlation may be attempted between abnormalities on an ultrasound scan image and likely structural abnormalities in the tissue concerned. Histological features known to influence backscatter levels include fat (Taylor *et al.*, 1986; Afschrift *et al.*, 1987), water content (Cloostermans *et al.*, 1986), vascularity (Rubaltelli *et al.*, 1980; Tanaka *et al.*, 1983; Marchal *et al.*, 1985), collagenous tissue (Landini *et al.*, 1987), and calcification (Lin *et al.*, 1989).

Scatterer size is an important physical factor influencing backscatter. For example, fat produces relatively strong backscatter because of the large size of adipocytes compared to other cells (Bondestam *et al.*, 1992). Individual mammalian adipocytes can reach more than 0.1 mm in diameter. Hence, fat accumulation in the liver can produce a hyperechoic appearance whereas a focal reduction in fat content (e.g. due to displacement by a tumour nodule) can produce a hypoechoic lesion. Other tissue types do not contain cells as large as adipocytes; however, when cells clump together they may produce a similar effect (Feleppa *et al.*, 1986). Echotextural changes in tissue may therefore result from changes in the arrangement of cells rather than changes in the cell population *per se*.

Despite many detailed studies, attempts to correlate the grey-scale ultrasonographic appearance of various lesions with their histology have failed to provide reliable diagnostic guidelines (Taylor and Wells, 1989). Lesions of very different histological type may appear similar enough to prevent even a basic differentiation of malignant from insignificant lesions. For example, hyperechoic hepatic nodules may be due to primary tumour, metastasis, nodular hyperplasia, steroid hepatopathy, extramedullary haematopoiesis, focal fat deposition, or calcification. The lack of correlation between cell type and ultrasonographic appearance supports increased use of guided biopsy (Hager *et al.*, 1985; Leveille *et al.*, 1993) coordinated with the imaging study.

Technique

There are few specific equipment requirements for abdominal ultrasonography. A small transducer contact area (footprint) is desirable because it enables use of small acoustic windows such as intercostal spaces, and because it makes it easier to indent the abdominal wall with the transducer, necessary for bringing small structures into the focal zone of higher frequency transducers. For cats and small dogs, and for superficial structures, a 7.5 MHz transducer is recommended. A 5 MHz transducer is suitable for most medium-sized and some large dogs. For scanning the liver of a large dog a 3.5 MHz transducer may be necessary to achieve adequate penetration. Use of transducers with variable receiving frequency (e.g. 4–6 MHz and 6–9 MHz) and/or a variable focal zone can help maximize ultrasound examination quality in patients of greatly differing size.

Before scanning the abdomen, the ultrasound machine should be adjusted to enhance detection of variations in non-specular echoes. The complement of adjustable controls varies between machines; however, examples of appropriate settings for abdominal ultrasonography include a low reject level, a high dynamic range, a low frame rate (unless breath motion is rapid), low contrast post-processing option, and careful adjustment of time-gain compensation. For further discussion of these factors, the reader is referred to other sources (Kremkau, 1989).

Animals for abdominal ultrasonography should ideally be fasted to empty the gastrointestinal tract. A full stomach or intestine may prevent adequate examination of the liver, and distend the abdomen, sometimes preventing use of optimal approaches to such deep-seated organs. Nervous animals or those in pain should have sedation and/or analgesia to relax them and to inhibit panting or abdominal splinting, both of which can hamper the ultrasonographic examination.

Careful removal of hair is essential prior to abdominal ultrasonography. The ventral aspect should be clipped from the xiphoid to the pelvic brim, and as far dorsally as necessary to examine the retroperitoneal organs. In a cat the abdominal wall may be flexible enough to allow a complete examination through a relatively small clipped area; however, the larger the patient, the more will have to be clipped in order to achieve optimal transducer positions.

Some veterinary ultrasonographers prefer to scan the abdomen with the animal in dorsal recumbency, supported in a V-shaped trough. Others lay the dog or cat in lateral recumbency on a flat table, a position that many animals seem to prefer. In the presence of excessive intestinal gas or a large volume of peritoneal fluid which causes gas-filled intestine to float, scanning from the non-dependent aspect of an animal in dorsal recumbency may be difficult due to interference by the gas. Scanning from the dependent aspect, for example through a cut-out in the tabletop or with the animal standing, may avoid this problem. Also, certain mobile lesions such as intestinal masses are most visible using this approach because they fall to the dependent aspect of the abdomen.

Should the entire abdomen be scanned in every case? Or, to restate the question with reference to a specific example, should the adrenal glands be examined ultrasonographically in animals without clinical signs of adrenal gland disease? Although opinions on this subject differ (Mills *et al.*, 1989), there is not a strong indication to do so. Many adrenal neoplasms in dogs are non-functional so may be identified unexpectedly during ultrasonography (Schelling, 1991); however, pursuing incidental findings risks diverting attention from the current clinical problem and incurring additional expense for the animal owner that may prove to be unnecessary for a variety of reasons. Also, as abdominal ultrasonography has developed, its scope has enlarged to include examination of small parts such as the adrenal glands, which often are difficult to image, as well as duplex or colour-flow Doppler techniques for examination of blood flow in vessels such as the portal vein. With these developments, the average time required for a complete study has greatly increased. Principally for this reason, one recommendation is not to routinely attempt a total abdominal examination with every ultrasound scan, but rather to focus attention on sites of potential lesions based on the animal's clinical signs and any clinicopathological data that may be available. This requires the ultrasonographer to have a detailed understanding of the case before starting the scan. Additional studies may be chosen later as more data become available.

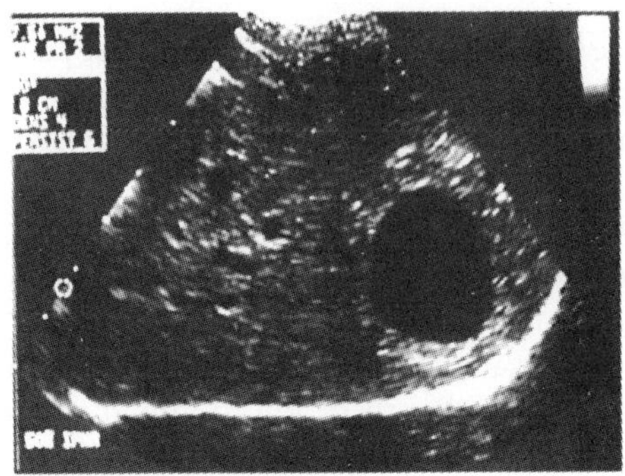

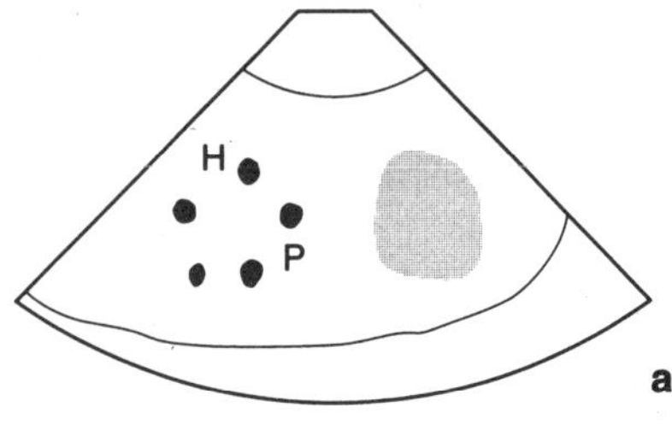

H
P
a

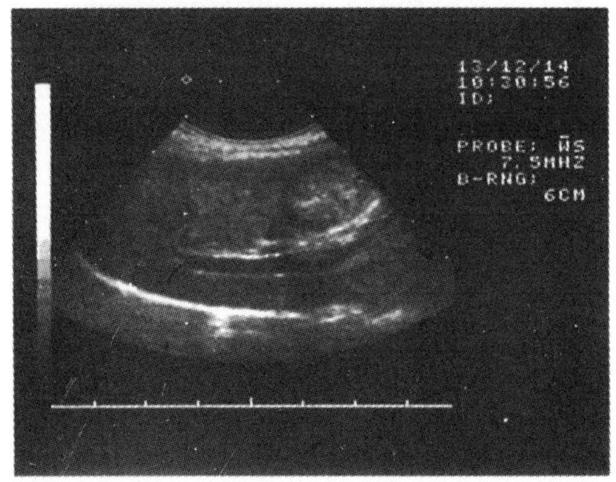

13/12/14
10:30:56
ID:
PROBE: MS
7.5MHZ
B-RNG:
6CM

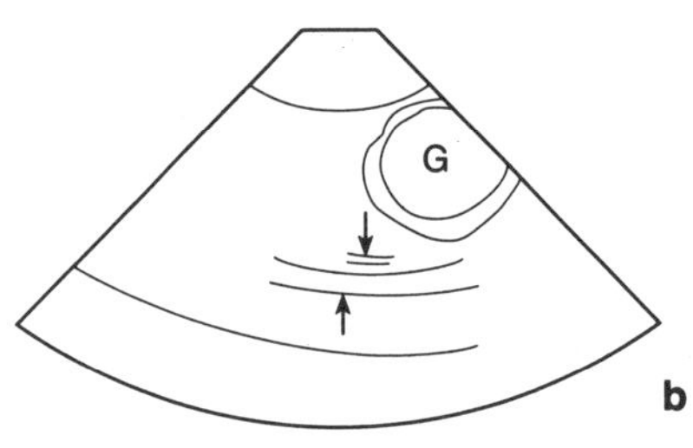

G
b

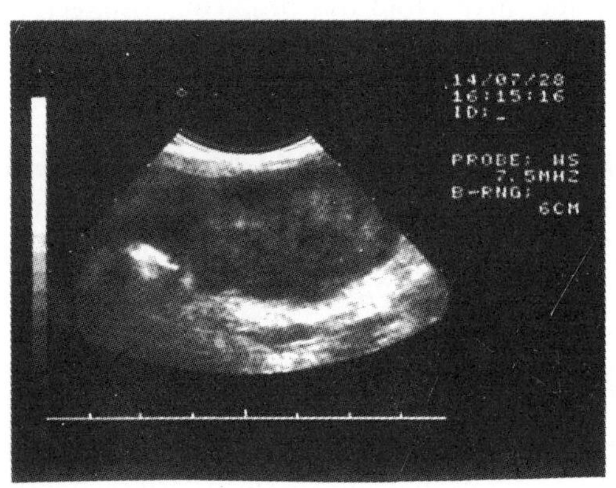

14/07/28
16:15:16
ID:
PROBE: MS
7.5MHZ
B-RNG:
6CM

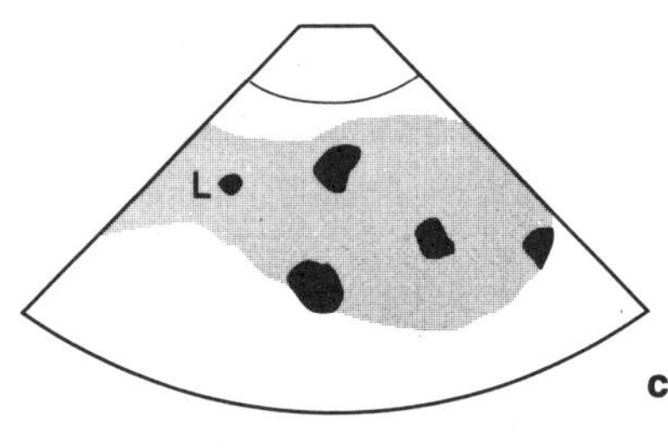

L
c

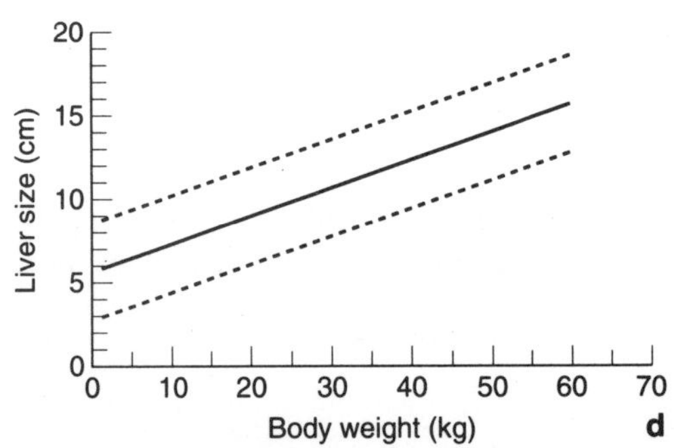

20
15
10
5
0
Liver size (cm)
0 10 20 30 40 50 60 70
Body weight (kg)
d

Normal Ultrasonographic Anatomy of the Abdomen

Liver

The majority of the liver is examined by positioning the transducer on the ventral midline immediately caudal to the xiphoid and scanning craniodorsad. Complete sweeps through the liver should be routinely made in both sagittal and transverse planes. The following normal structures may be identified.

The gall bladder lies to the right of the midline, close to the diaphragm (Fig. 2.1a). It is an oval or tear-shaped anechoic structure with a barely visible wall in young animals. In older dogs, or when the gall bladder is contracted, the wall may be visible because it is thicker. There are various methods available for measuring gall bladder volume ultrasonographically (Finn-Bodner *et al.*, 1993).

The cystic duct and the common bile duct may be identified. The common bile duct may be visible ventral to the portal vein when using a ventral or right intercostal approach (Nyland and Hager, 1985). It normally measures less than 3 mm in diameter (Zeman *et al.*, 1981; Raptopoulos *et al.*, 1985) and could be confused with a hepatic artery which has a similar position and appearance (Fig. 2.1b).

The portal vein lies close to the midline and branches as it passes cranially. The portal vein and its branches normally have echogenic walls due to adjacent fat and fibrous tissue (Fig. 2.1b).

The caudal vena cava is dorsal to the portal vein. In large or deep-chested breeds, it is most clearly visible on views obtained from a right intercostal approach.

The left and right branches of the hepatic veins are normally visible entering the caudal vena cava just caudal to the diaphragm. Hepatic veins have no discernible wall and their tributaries cross peripheral portal vein branches.

The diaphragm is closely applied to the cranial aspect of the liver. It is visible as a distinct structure only when there is peritoneal and pleural fluid to isolate it. The echogenic interface on the cranial aspect of the liver normally corresponds to the surface of the (air-filled) lung.

Symmetrical changes in hepatic volume may be estimated by measuring the maximal distance from the caudal tip of the liver on the ventral midline to the

Fig. 2.1. The liver. **(a)** Transverse image of the liver in a young dog. The hepatic parenchyma has a uniform echotexture. Large hepatic veins (H) and portal veins (P) are visible; the portal veins have more echogenic walls and in real-time may be traced back to the main portal vein at the porta hepatis. The gall bladder has anechoic contents and no discernible wall. **(b)** Sagittal image of the porta hepatis showing the portal vein (lower arrow) passing dorsal to the gastric antrum (G) into the liver. The narrow duct (upper arrow) immediately ventral to the portal vein is the common bile duct, although without Doppler ultrasonography it cannot be reliably distinguished from the hepatic artery. **(c)** Sagittal image showing a mass protruding from the caudal border of the liver (L) of a cat. The mass has a blotchy hypoechoic echotexture and is well-demarcated from fat in the surrounding omentum/mesentery. The histological diagnosis was hepatocellular carcinoma. **(d)** Graph showing the maximal distance from the caudal tip of the liver on the ventral midline to the diaphragm on a sagittal or transverse image ('liver size'), plotted against body weight in normal dogs. There is an approximately linear relationship between this dimension and body weight. The dashed lines indicate 95% confidence limits. Reproduced from Barr, 1992b, with the permission of the publishers.

14/11/22
15:49:18
ID:
SPLEEN
LIVER
ANNOT
*1 COMM
2 HOSP

a

14/08/04
16:34:11
ID:
PROBE: S
5.0MHZ
B-RNG:
9CM

b

13/12/13
13:44:46
ID:
PROBE: S
5.0MHZ
B-RNG:
6CM

c

14/03/03
09:53:54
ID:
PROBE: WS
7.5MHZ
B-RNG:
6CM

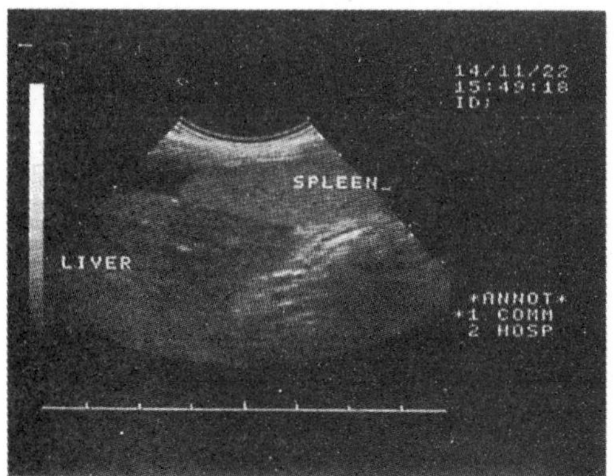

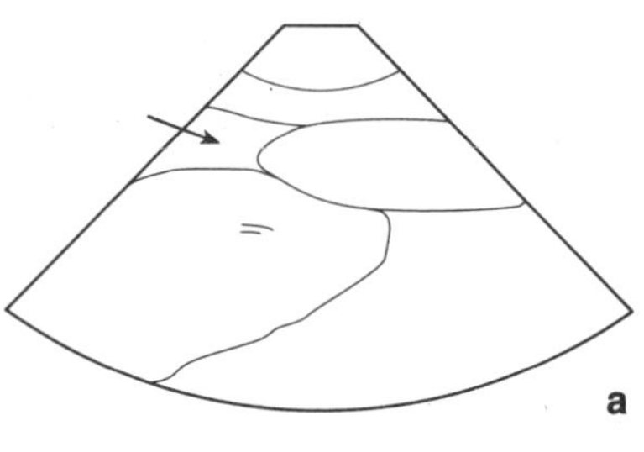

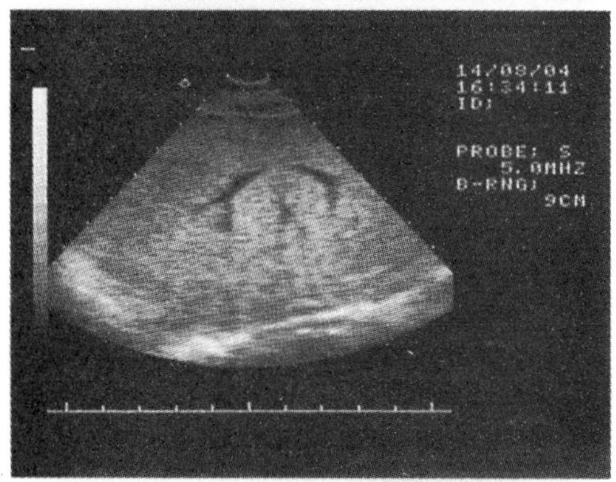

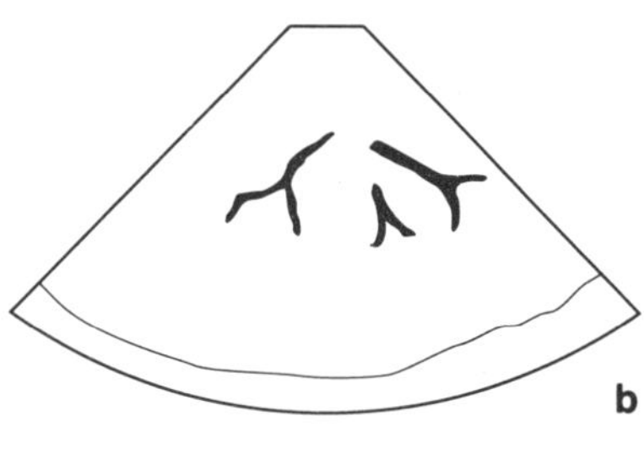

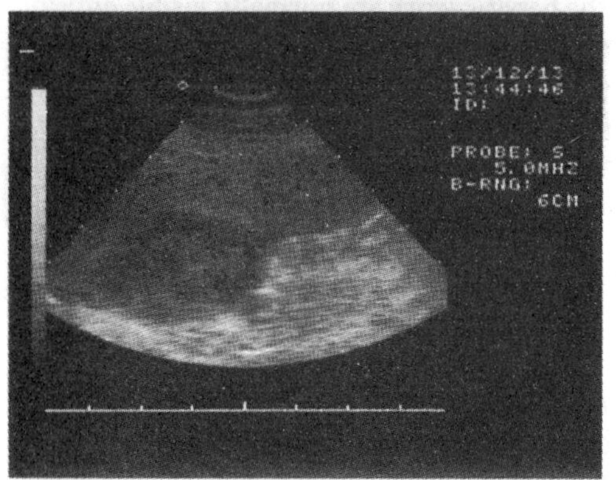

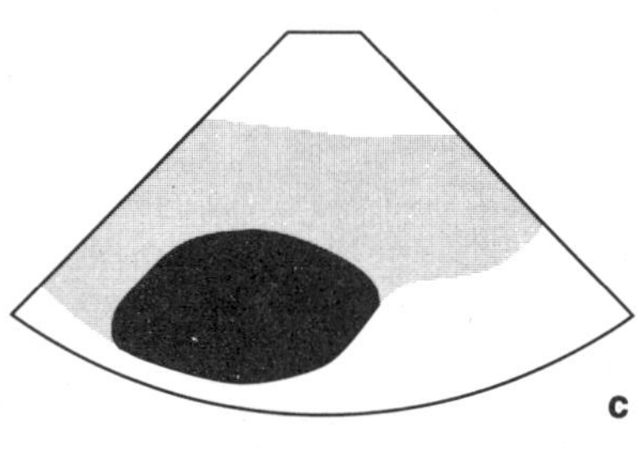

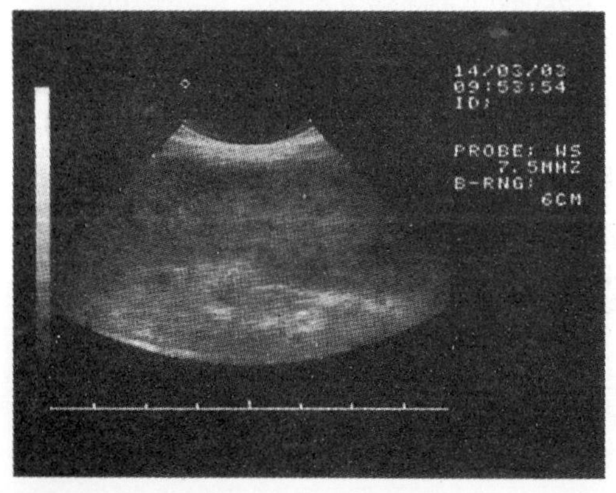

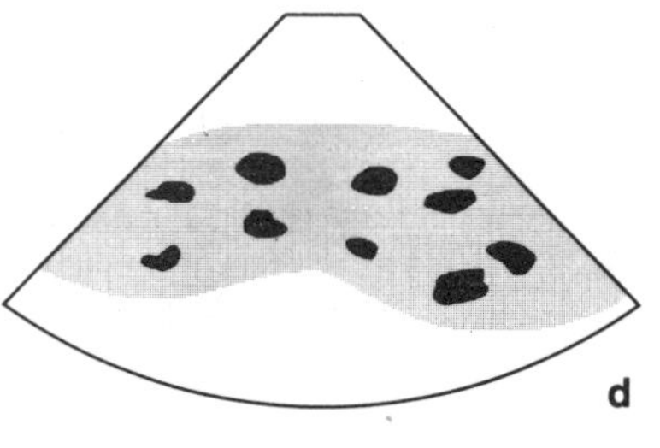

d

diaphragm on a sagittal or transverse image (Barr, 1992a). There is an approximately linear relationship between this dimension and body weight (Fig. 2.1d) (Barr, 1992b).

Spleen

The spleen is examined by scanning along the caudal aspect of the left 13th rib. Its dorsal part may be located under the ribs, particularly if the stomach is empty, necessitating an intercostal approach in some cases. The ventral part is mobile and may lie in contact with the liver or as far caudal as the neck of the bladder. The flattened shape of the normal spleen and its superficial position allow use of higher frequency transducers, e.g. 7.5 MHz, which enables higher resolution images to be obtained. Splenic veins are visible on its medial aspect but are not normally visible deep within the parenchyma. The splenic parenchyma is normally hyperechoic compared to the liver (Fig. 2.2a). There are no established quantitative measurements for assessment of splenic size; determination of splenomegaly is therefore subjective and probably inaccurate.

Kidneys

The left kidney is found by scanning caudal to the dorsal part of the spleen. In cats and small dogs, both kidneys are normally visible from a ventral approach, while in fat or deep-chested dogs a lateral approach is often necessary, scanning through intercostal spaces to find the right kidney. The normal kidney has a uniformly echogenic cortex clearly demarcated from the hypoechoic medulla. Interlobar vessels and renal diverticula subdivide the medulla. In dogs undergoing diuresis the medulla may increase in size (Konde, 1985) and there may be mild dilatation of the pelvis (Pugh *et al.*, 1994). This effect is less apparent in the cat (Walter *et al.*, 1987a, c). The renal sinus normally contains an echogenic fat pad.

The ultrasonographic appearance of the kidneys varies according to the plane of imaging, transducer frequency and fat content. From a right intercostal approach, the echogenicity of the right kidney may be compared with the caudate lobe of the liver (Fig. 2.3a). Studies in humans (Platt *et al.*, 1988) and dogs (Hartzband *et al.*, 1991) have shown that the renal cortex may normally be hypo-, iso- or hyperechoic compared to the liver parenchyma. A larger proportion of kidneys appear hyperechoic when imaged at 7.5 MHz than at 5 MHz. This difference in backscatter generated by the kidney and liver at different ultrasound frequencies is due to differences in the relative sizes of scatterers in these tissues.

The fat content of the kidney has been correlated with its echogenicity in

Fig. 2.2. The spleen. **(a)** Sagittal image of a dog showing adjacent parts of the liver and spleen. The spleen is normally hyperechoic compared to the liver. A small amount of anechoic peritoneal fluid is present (arrow). **(b)** Sagittal image of a dog showing an enlarged spleen and dilated intrasplenic veins. This combination is compatible with congestion. Note that the parenchyma has an apparently normal echotexture; hypoechoic splenic parenchyma due to congestion is seen only in extreme cases. **(c)** Hypoechoic nodule bulging from the surface of the spleen in a sagittal image from a dog. The histological diagnosis was lymphoid hyperplasia. **(d)** Dorsal image of a cat with multicentric lymphoma showing a thickened, hypoechoic spleen with blotchy echotexture.

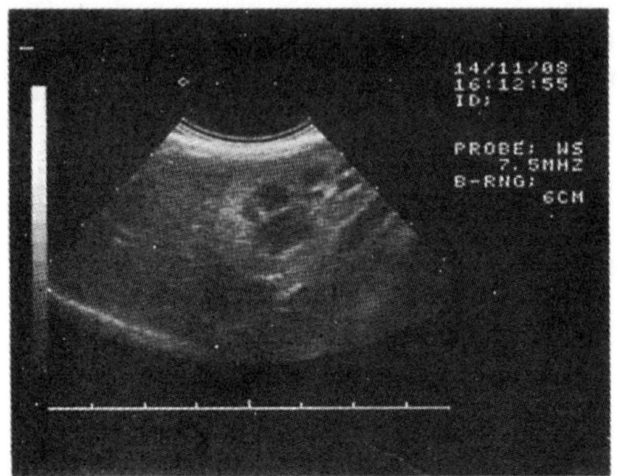
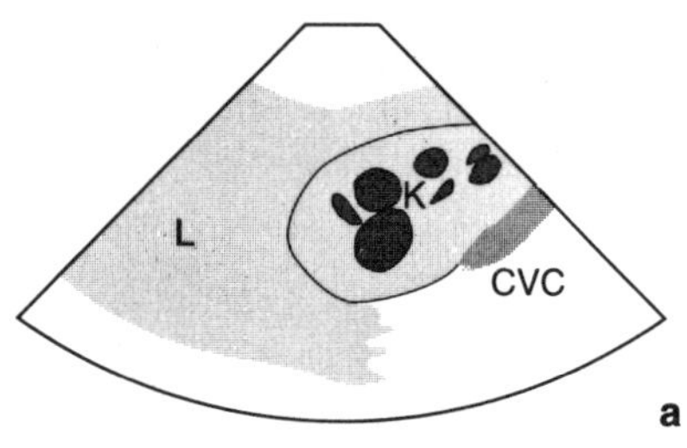
L
K
CVC
a

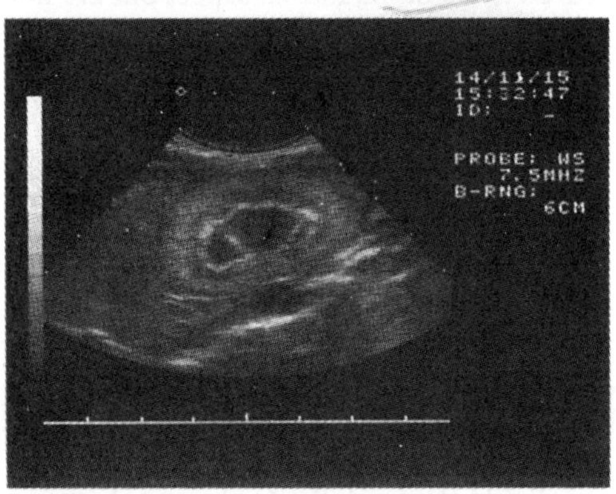
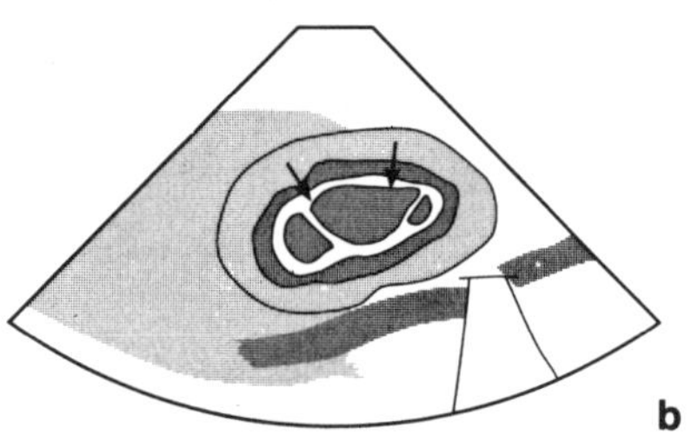
b

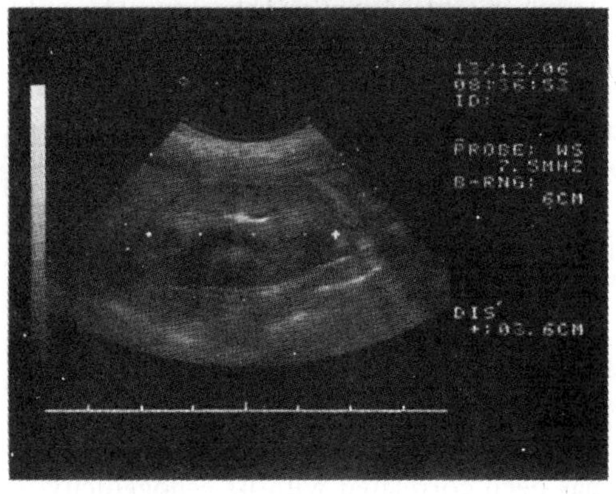
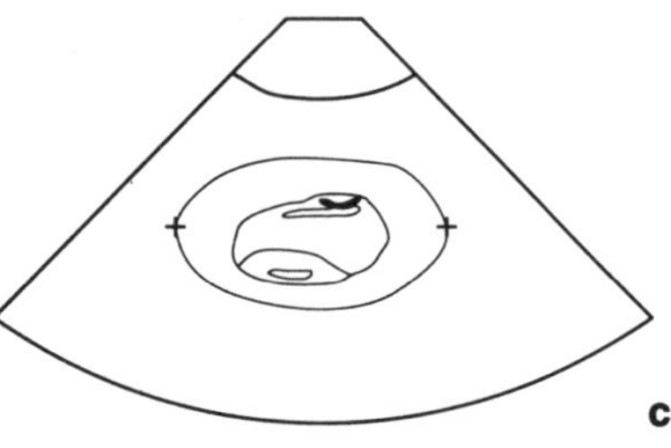
c

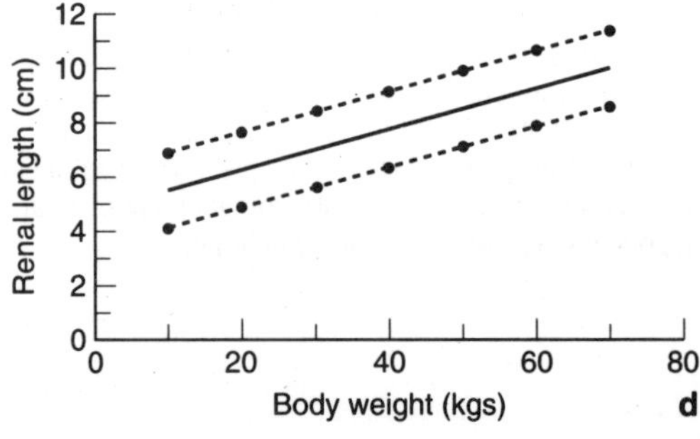
12
10
8
6
4
2
0
Renal length (cm)
0   20   40   60   80
Body weight (kgs)
d

cats. Male and pregnant female cats have increased cortical echogenicity because of normal fat deposition (Yeager and Anderson, 1989). Some normal cats also have a well-defined echogenic line in the medulla parallel to the corticomedullary junction, known as the medullary rim sign (Fig. 2.3b). This represents deposits of crystalline material in the renal tubules (Yeager and Anderson, 1989).

Renal size may be assessed using measurements of length or volume (Nyland *et al.*, 1989; Barr, 1990). Ultrasonographic volume determinations require careful measurement of at least three dimensions and tend to underestimate true renal volume, hence simple linear measurements are usually considered sufficient. Longitudinal renal length may be determined from a sagittal image, i.e. an image showing the parallel bars of the renal diverticuli (Walter *et al.*, 1987c). The normal feline kidney measures 38–44 mm in maximal sagittal dimension (Schummer *et al.*, 1979). In the dog there is a linear relationship between renal length and body weight (Fig. 2.3d) (Barr *et al.*, 1990).

Adrenal glands

The adrenal glands occupy the cranial retroperitoneum. Their small size necessitates use of a high-resolution transducer (usually 7.5 MHz), but their deep position may be beyond its focal zone. Therefore, the adrenal glands are difficult to examine in large dogs.

In dogs, the left adrenal gland lies lateral or ventrolateral to the aorta and medial to the cranial pole of the left kidney. The right adrenal gland lies dorsal or dorsolateral to the caudal vena cava and medial to the cranial pole of the right kidney (Voorhout, 1990). Both glands are flattened dorsoventrally with the left sometimes having a 'dumb-bell' shape and the right being thicker at its cranial aspect (Figs 2.4a and 2.4b) (Schelling, 1991). The medulla of the normal gland is slightly hyperechoic compared to the cortex. The maximal longitudinal dimension of a normal canine adrenal gland is typically 15–25mm; however, this varies with body size. The normal ultrasonographic appearance of feline adrenal glands has not been established.

Pancreas

The pancreas is a thin, flat organ lying adjacent to the greater curvature of the stomach, medial to the proximal duodenum, ventral to the portal vein and cranial

Fig. 2.3. The kidneys. **(a)** Dorsal image of a cat without clinicopathological evidence of hepatic or renal disease. The right kidney (K) is visible adjacent to the caudate lobe of the liver (L). The renal cortex and medulla are clearly demarcated. In this instance the cortex is hyperechoic compared to the liver. CVC = caudal vena cava. **(b)** Dorsal image of a cat showing a well-demarcated echogenic line (arrows) parallel to the corticomedullary junction ('medullary rim sign'). This is a potentially normal finding in cats, but may also be associated with nephrosis or hypercalcaemia (see text). **(c)** Sagittal image of a cat with chronic renal failure showing a small kidney with loss of definition of the internal structure and overall increased echogenicity. The ultrasonographic appearance is typical of non-specific, end-stage renal disease. **(d)** Graph showing sagittal renal length, as determined by ultrasonography, plotted against body weight. In the normal dog there is a linear relationship between kidney length and body weight. The dashed lines indicate 95% confidence limits. Reproduced from Barr *et al.*, 1990, with permission of the publishers.

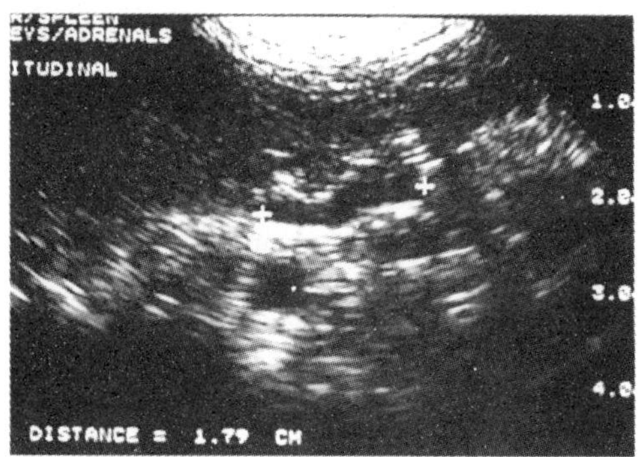
R/SPLEEN
EYS/ADRENALS
ITUDINAL
DISTANCE = 1.79 CM

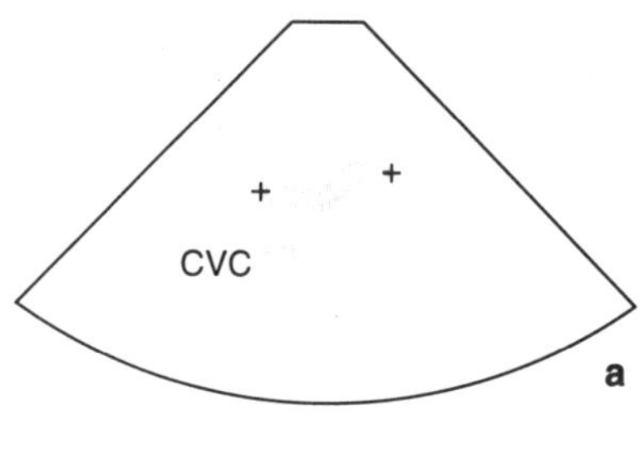
CVC
a

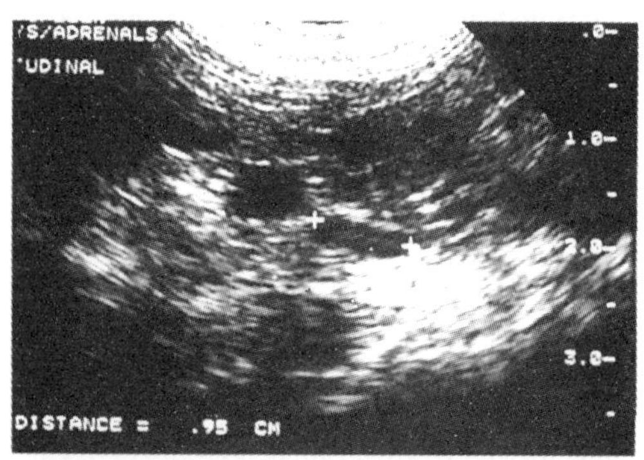
/S/ADRENALS
UDINAL
DISTANCE = .95 CM

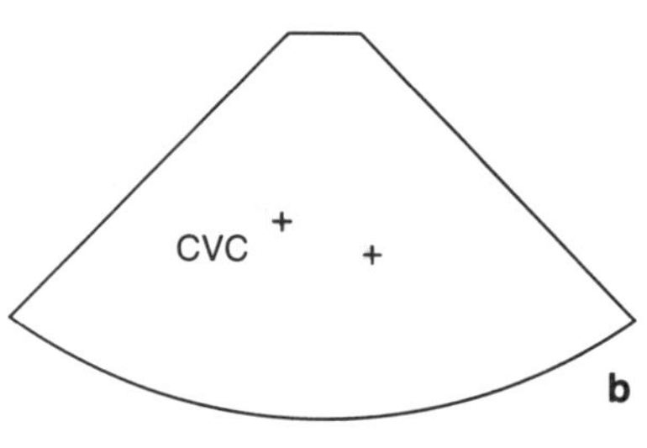
CVC
b

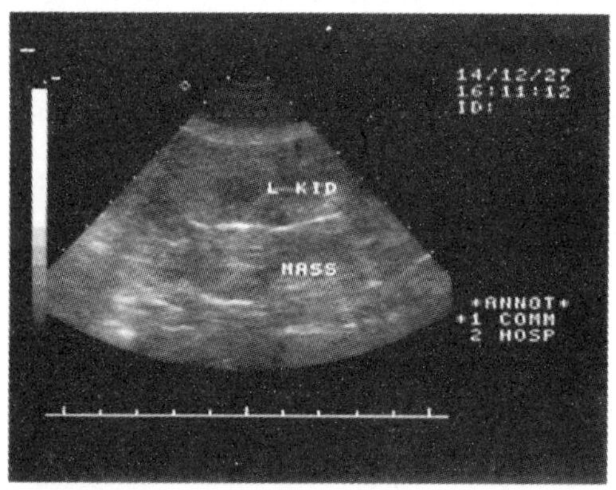
14/12/27
16:11:12
ID:
L KID
MASS
ANNOT
1 COMM
2 HOSP

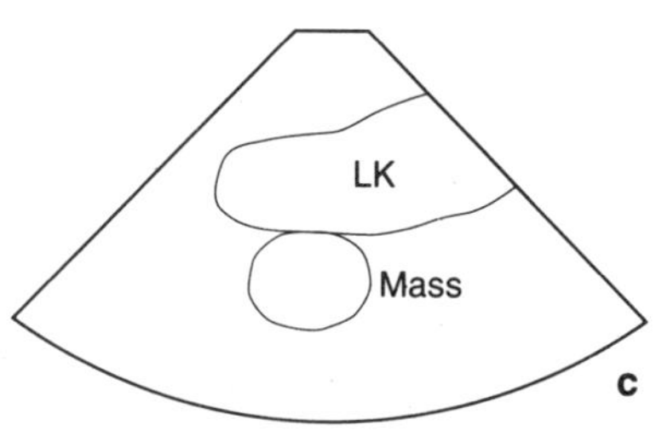
LK
Mass
c

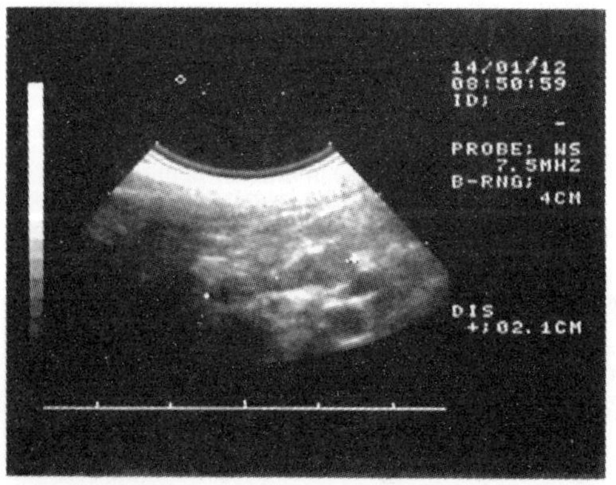
14/01/12
08:50:59
ID:
PROBE: WS
7.5MHZ
B-RNG:
4CM
DIS
+:02.1CM

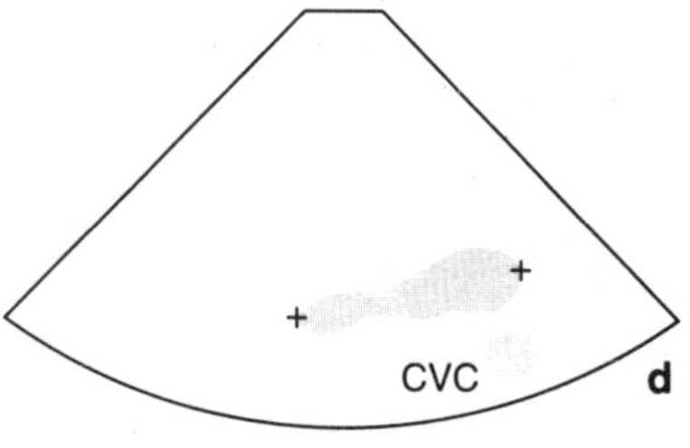
CVC
d

to the transverse colon (Fig. 2.5a). It is identified with some difficulty in normal dogs and cats, requiring a high-resolution transducer and careful attention to probe position. The left lobe may be visible between the stomach and transverse colon from a ventral or left lateral approach. The right lobe is identified using the duodenum, portal vein and right kidney as landmarks. The duodenum may be traced caudally from the stomach on a ventral approach or identified medial to the right kidney on a right lateral approach. It is usually necessary to indent the abdominal wall with the transducer in order to displace other parts of the small intestine and to bring the area of interest into the focal zone of the transducer. Once the duodenum is located, the right lobe of the pancreas may be visible dorsomedial to it. The pancreas is normally slightly hyperechoic compared to the liver (Saunders, 1991). The pancreaticoduodenal vein passes through the right lobe and is visible in some instances.

Stomach and intestine

Gas in the gastrointestinal tract may interfere with transmission of the ultrasound beam and produce artifacts; however, in many cases this is not a problem. When examining the stomach, water (preferably degassed) should be administered by tube into an otherwise empty stomach to distend it and to displace gas. The stomach, proximal duodenum and large intestine may be identified because of their consistent anatomical locations; other levels of the small intestine cannot be specifically identified. Therefore, when an intestinal lesion is suspected, it is necessary to scan the whole abdomen methodically to ensure that no part is overlooked.

The gastric and intestinal walls have a layered structure which is visible using a high resolution transducer. The five layers normally visible correspond to the mucosal surface, mucosa, submucosa, muscularis and serosa (Fig. 2.6a) (Penninck *et al.*, 1989). The thickness of the gastric wall is variable depending on the degree of distension and so it is difficult to interpret measurements of thickness unless the stomach has been filled with water (Worlicek *et al.*, 1989). The normal duodenal wall is 5 mm thick; the jejunal wall is 3 mm thick (Penninck *et al.*, 1989). Peristalsis may be observed in real-time.

Mesentery and peritoneum

The mesentery is a flexible thin sheet of fat, vessels and lymph nodes within a fold of visceral peritoneum. Not normally identifiable as a distinct structure, the mesentery may be visible when peritoneal fluid is present (Fig. 2.7a).

Fig. 2.4. The adrenal glands. **(a)** Oblique image of a dog showing the normal left adrenal gland. CVC = caudal vena cava. **(b)** Oblique image of a dog showing the normal right adrenal gland. **(c)** Dorsal image of a dog with left adrenal adenoma causing a spherical mass adjacent to the cranial pole of the left kidney (LK). **(d)** Oblique image of a dog with pituitary-dependent hyperadrenocorticism showing a thickened, hypoechoic left adrenal gland. The gland subjectively appears larger than normal but its normal shape is preserved, compatible with hypertrophy.

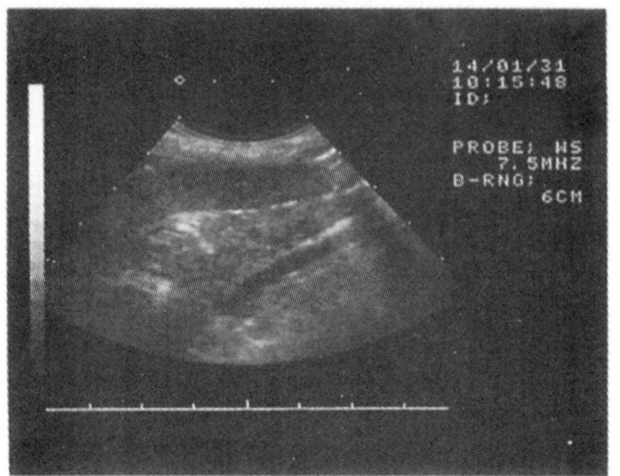
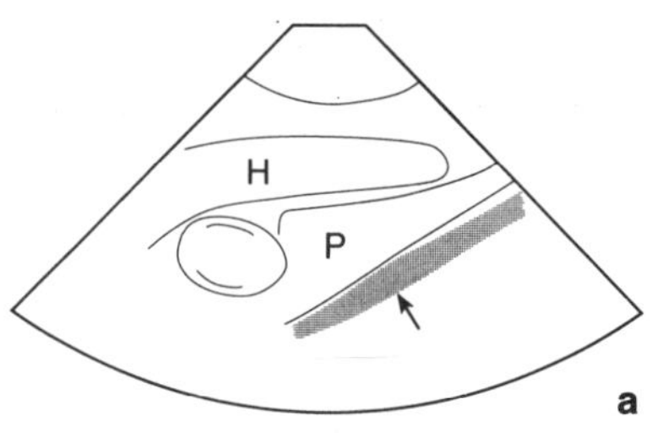

a

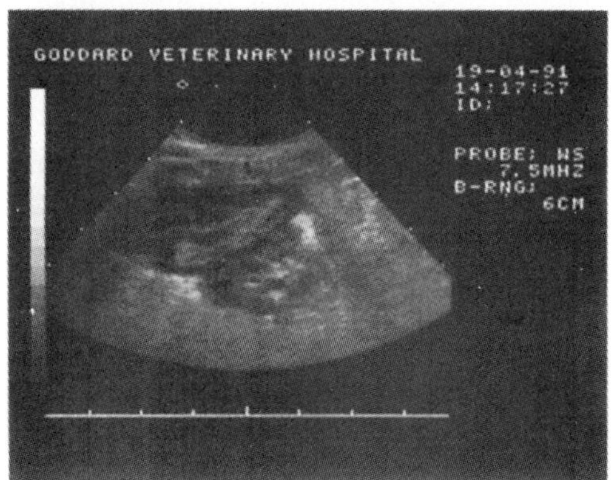

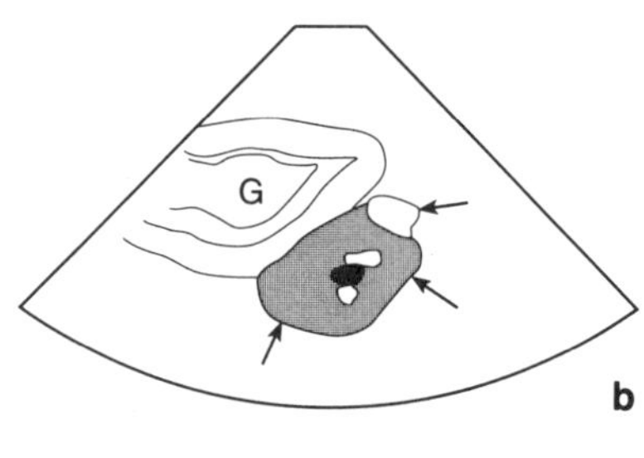

b

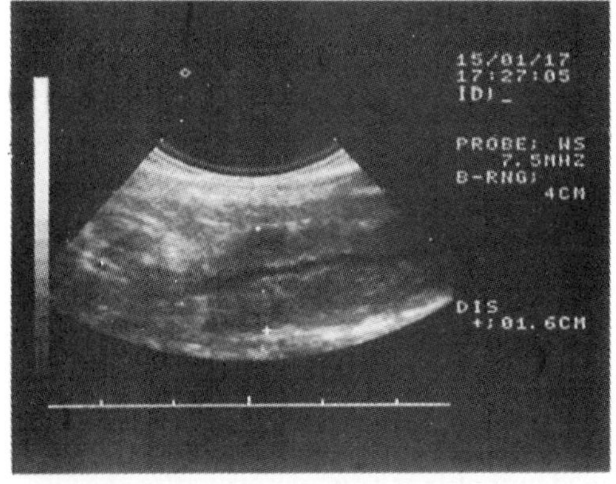
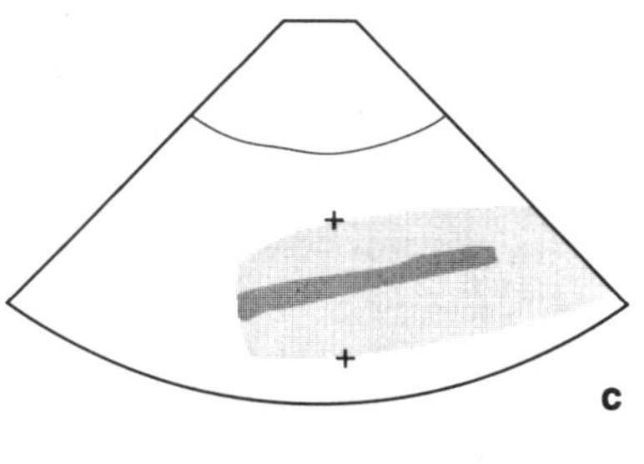

c

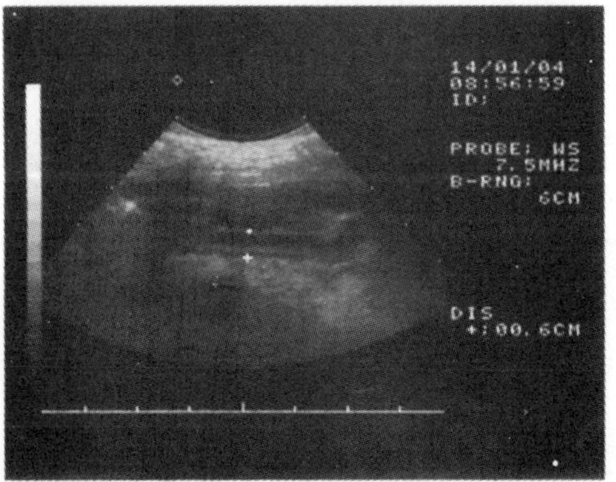
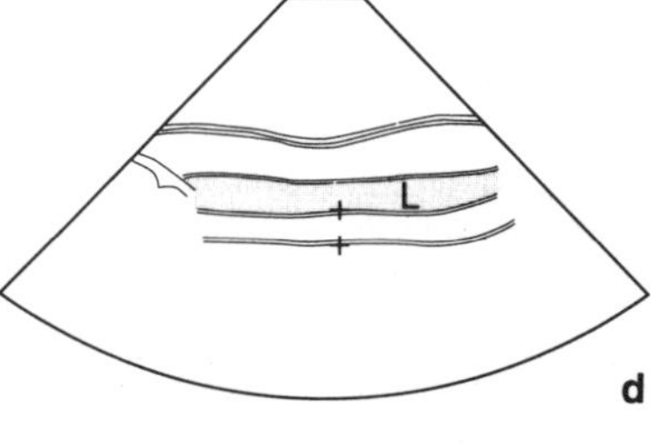

d

Urinary bladder

The urinary bladder normally appears as a rounded anechoic space bounded by a thin wall. The wall is normally 1–2 mm thick and may have a faint layered appearance. When almost empty, the bladder wall is thicker and slightly irregular on its mucosal surface. The ureterovesicular junctions are normally visible as small convex structures on the dorsal surface of the bladder (Douglass, 1993). Peristalsis of the distal ureters and flow of urine into the bladder ('ureteral jets') may be visible (Lamb and Gregory, 1994).

Ultrasonography of Abdominal Diseases

Liver

Hepatic lesions may be identified by ultrasonography when they alter the size and shape of the liver, its surface contour, parenchymal echogenicity, or vasculature, or the biliary tract.

Size and shape

Assessment of hepatic volume is based on either quantitative or subjective criteria. Neither method is perfect: a quantitative method (Barr, 1992a, b) uses a single linear measurement from which the volume is extrapolated, and therefore cannot account for asymmetrical changes in hepatic shape or volume; subjective evaluation depends on operator experience and probably is inaccurate.

Surface contour

The cranial border of the liver lies against the diaphragm while the ventral and much of the caudal border are visible as an interface with adjacent fat. When peritoneal fluid is present a greater proportion of the surface of the liver, i.e. the lobar borders, is visible, and minor surface irregularities may be more easily detected. The lateral lobe tips are normally sharp; hepatomegaly produces a rounded contour (Biller *et al.*, 1992b). Nodules of various types (e.g. hyperplastic, or neoplastic) may cause bulges on the surface of the liver (Fig. 2.1c).

Fig. 2.5. The pancreas. **(a)** Sagittal image of a dog showing part of the normal right lobe of the pancreas (P) between an enlarged hepatic lobe (H) and the portal vein (arrow). The pancreas is slightly hyperechoic compared to the liver. **(b)** Sagittal image of a dog showing a hypoechoic structure (arrows) containing small hyperechoic foci adjacent to the gastric antrum (G). The acutely or chronically inflamed pancreas typically becomes hypoechoic; hyperechoic foci may represent gas (i.e. necrosis) in severe, acute pancreatitis or fibrosis and/or fat saponification in chronic cases. **(c)** Dorsal image of the right lobe of the pancreas in a dog showing diffusely hypoechoic parenchyma and longitudinal duct-like structure, which may represent a dilated pancreatic duct or the pancreaticoduodenal vein. These possibilities may be distinguished using Doppler ultrasonography to identify venous blood flow; lack of a Doppler signal supports the diagnosis of dilated pancreatic duct. **(d)** Sagittal image of the proximal duodenum in a dog with acute pancreatitis. The duodenum is dilated (L = lumen) and the walls are diffusely thickened (6 mm between cursors; normal thickness 5 mm).

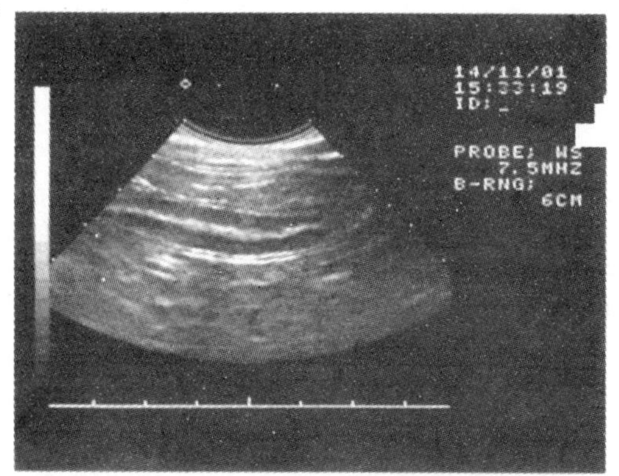

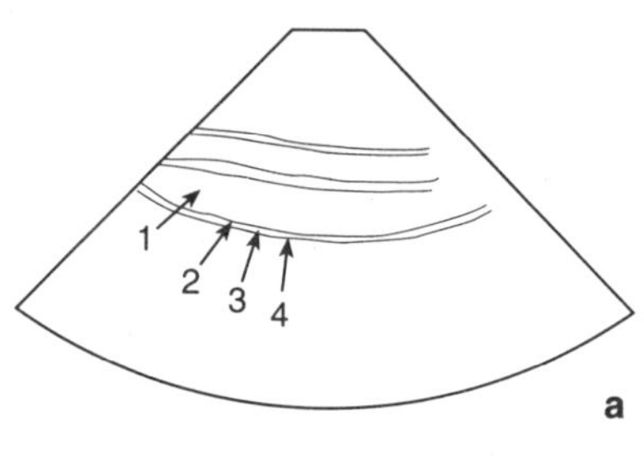
1
2 3 4
a

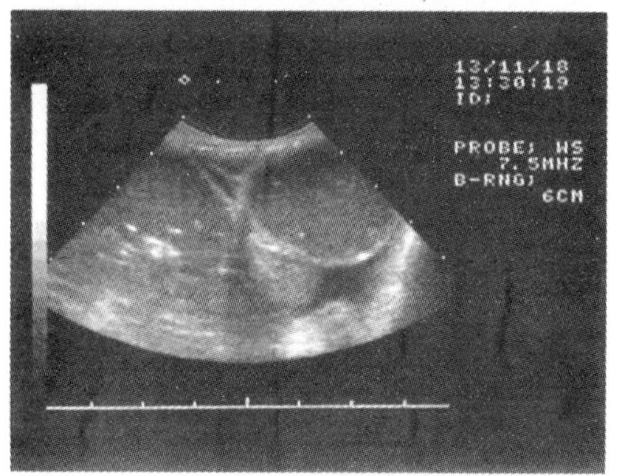

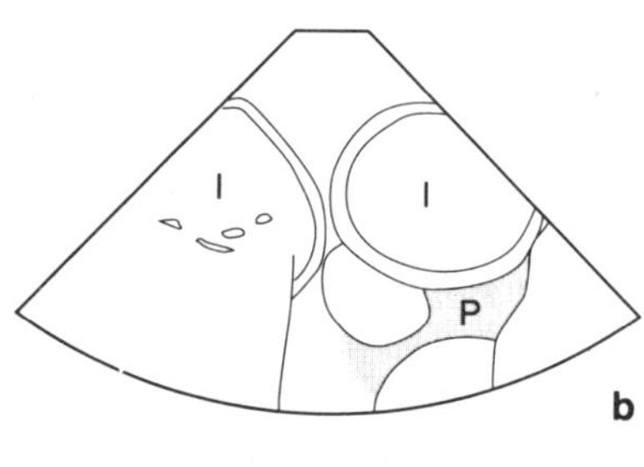
I
I
P
b

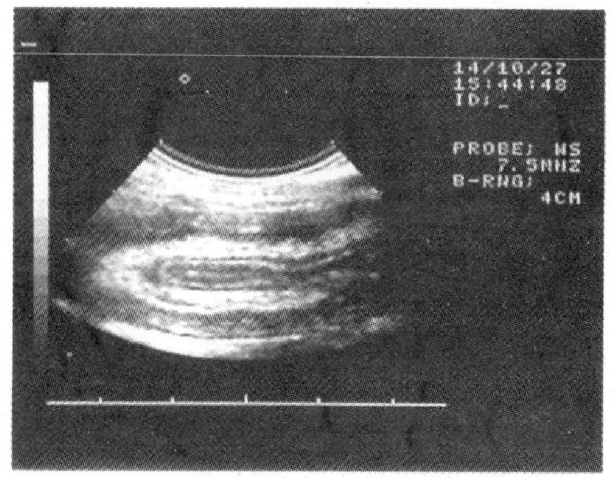

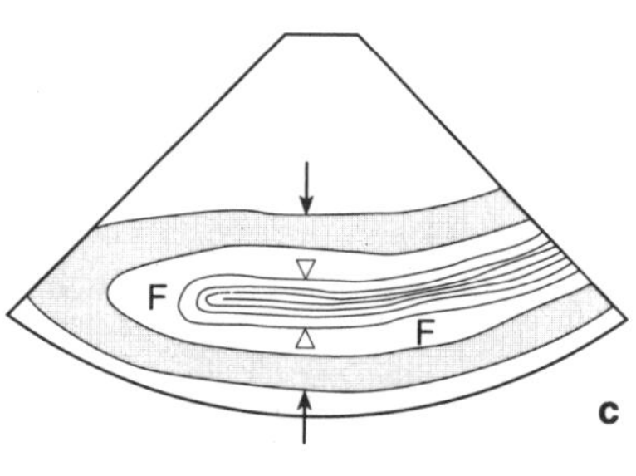
F
F
c

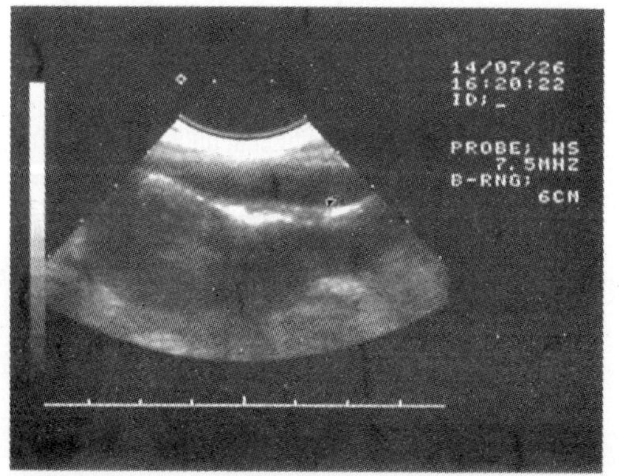

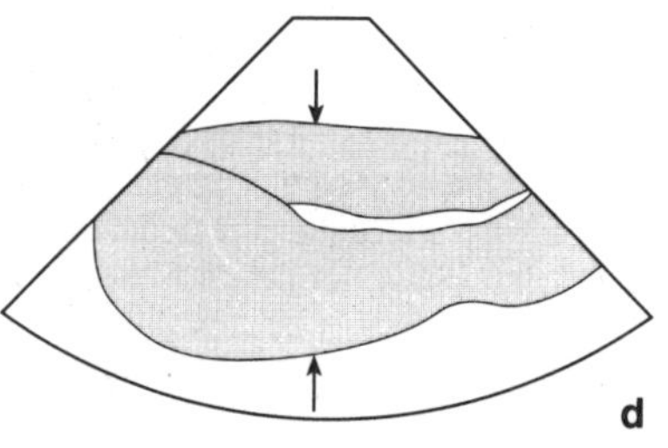
d

Parenchymal abnormalities

Hepatic parenchymal abnormalities may be classified as focal or diffuse, hypo- or hyperechoic (Table 2.1) (Nyland and Hager, 1985; Whiteley *et al.*, 1989; Lamb, 1991; Biller *et al.*, 1992b). In addition, cavitary lesions may represent primary or secondary neoplasia, hepatic nodular hyperplasia, abscess or haematoma. Lesions that have a combination of component parts, for example part cavitary and part solid-appearing, are termed complex. There is considerable overlap in the appearance of mass lesions due to a variety of causes. However, a lesion with relatively specific diagnostic significance is the target lesion, a nodular lesion which has a hyperechoic rim and hypoechoic centre (or hypoechoic rim and hyperechoic centre). Target lesions in the liver are correlated with malignancy (Wernecke *et al.*, 1992a, b)

Table 2.1. Classification of hepatic lesions identified by ultrasonography.

	Hypoechoic	Hyperechoic
Focal/multifocal lesions	Primary neoplasm Metastasis Lymphoma Hepatic nodular hyperplasia Hepatitis Cyst Telangiectasia Abscess Haematoma	Primary neoplasm Metastasis Hepatic nodular hyperplasia Steroid hepatopathy Fat deposit Extramedullary haematopoiesis
Diffuse lesions	Lymphoma Histoplasmosis	Lymphoma Lipidosis Cirrhosis

Fig. 2.6. The small intestine. **(a)** Longitudinal image of the normal jejunum showing the layered appearance of the wall. The central echogenic line is the lumen containing a small amount of gas and mucus; the other layers are: 1 = mucosa (hypoechoic); 2 = submucosa (hyperechoic); 3 = muscularis (hypoechoic); 4 = serosa (hyperechoic). **(b)** A sonogram from a puppy with an intussusception showing transverse sections through dilated small intestine (I) and a small amount of anechoic peritoneal fluid (P). Monitoring the same part of the intestine for a few minutes enables motility to be assessed. In this instance, no peristalsis was observed. **(c)** Longitudinal image of an intussusception showing the intussusceptum (arrowheads) and mesenteric fat (F) within the intussuscipiens (arrows). Transverse images of these lesions have a target-like appearance due to multiple concentric layers of intestinal wall and fat. **(d)** Longitudinal image of a neoplasm causing severe localized, eccentric thickening of the intestinal wall and loss of the normal layered appearance. The lumen is represented by the thin echogenic line. In transverse images these lesions have a doughnut- or horseshoe-like appearance. The histological diagnosis was lymphoma.

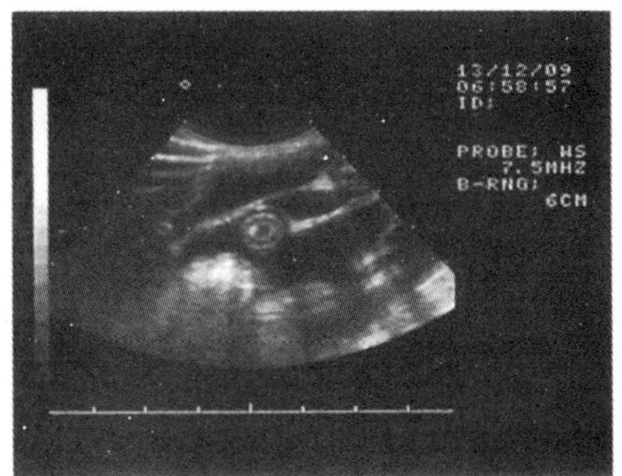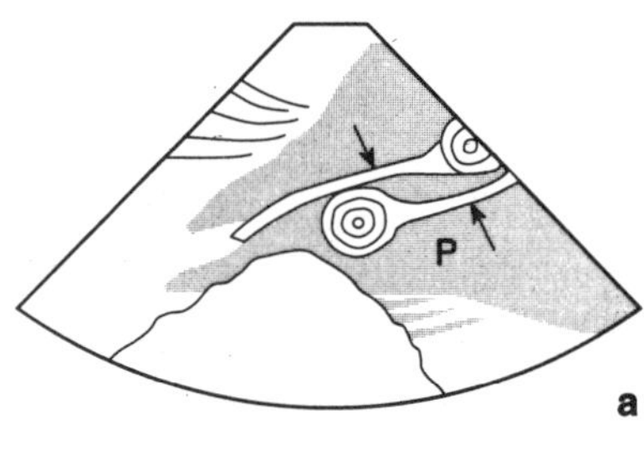

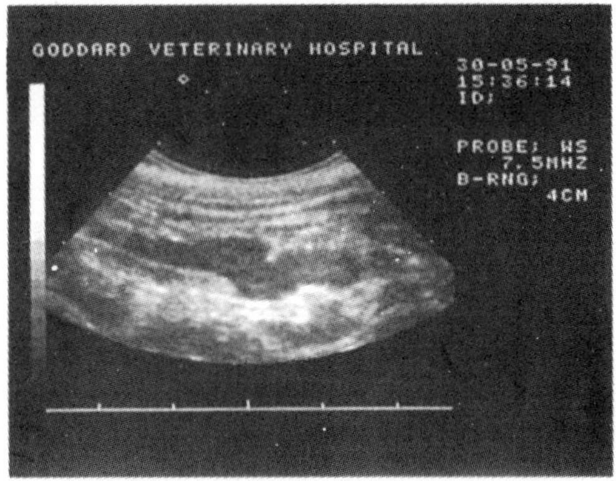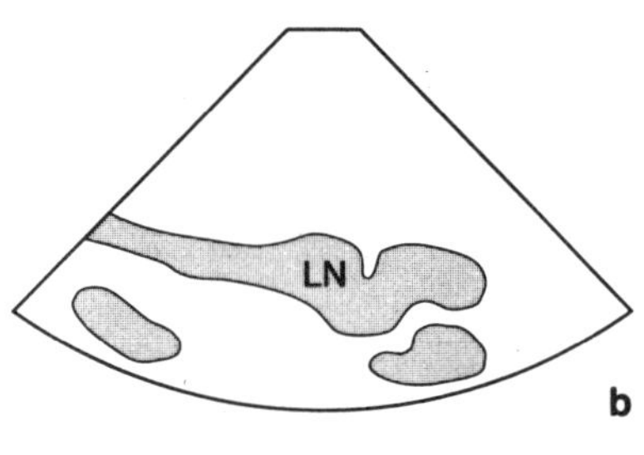

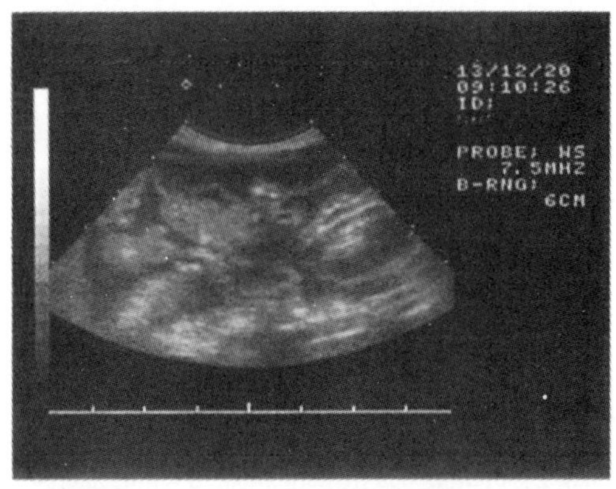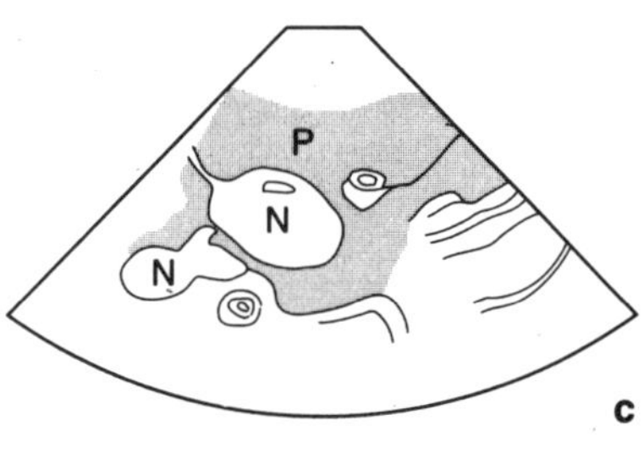

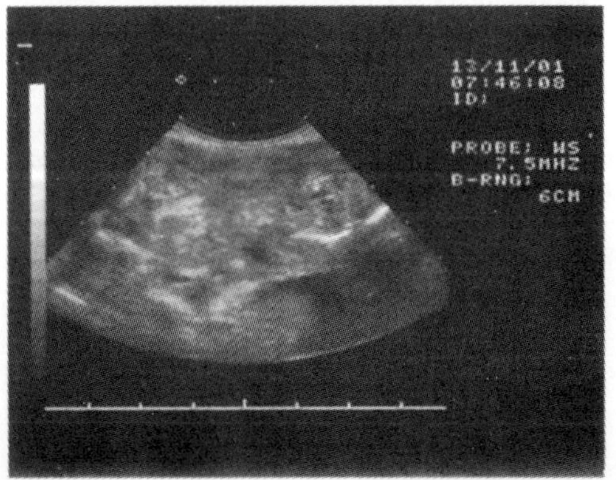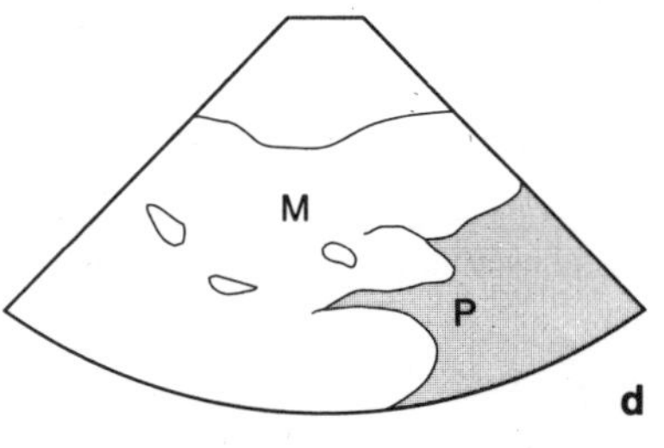

Two important limitations of ultrasonography have been demonstrated with respect to parenchymal abnormalities of the liver. The first is non-specificity: there is limited potential for making a specific diagnosis based on the echotextural features of a lesion. For example, unimportant age-related lesions such as hepatic nodular hyperplasia can mimic neoplasia (Stowater *et al.*, 1990), and a study of 48 dogs with hepatic neoplasms could not provide reliable guidelines for predicting cell type based on the ultrasonographic image (Whiteley *et al.*, 1989). Obtaining a biopsy remains the only reliable diagnostic method.

The other limitation is insensitivity for diffuse lesions. Infiltrative diseases such as lymphoma may be undetected because mild diffuse changes in hepatic echotexture do not occur or are not recognized (Lamb *et al.*, 1991). A normal-appearing liver on ultrasonography does not rule out the possibility of significant disease. Again, biopsy is required when infiltrative disease is suspected.

Vasculature

Abnormalities of the hepatic vessels include dilatation of hepatic veins, for example, due to right-sided cardiac insufficiency or pleural effusion; small or absent intrahepatic portal vein branches in some dogs with congenital portacaval shunts; anomalous intra- or extrahepatic vessel due to portacaval shunt (Wrigley *et al.*, 1987; Lamb., 1994) or arteriovenous fistula (Bailey *et al.*, 1988); and dilated main portal vein and/or decreased blood flow velocity due to portal hypertension, e.g. secondary to cirrhosis (Goyal *et al.*, 1990; Nyland and Fisher, 1990).

Biliary tract

The gall bladder may be relatively large in fasted or anorexic animals. Occasionally, congenital abnormalities of the gall bladder are identified, including septa or double gall bladder. Echogenic 'sludge', which settles in the dependent aspect of the gall bladder (Fig. 2.8a), is a very common finding of no apparent clinical significance (Murray *et al.*, 1992).

The gall bladder wall may be thick, echogenic and nodular-appearing in many old dogs due to mucinous hyperplasia, an insignificant age-related change. The gall bladder also has a thicker wall when it is contracted (Fig. 2.8b). Pathological thickening of the gall bladder wall, sometimes producing a double or layered appearance, may be due to cholecystitis or various non-biliary tract diseases (Wegener *et al.*, 1987; Teefey *et al.*, 1991).

Fig. 2.7. The mesentery and peritoneum. **(a)** A sonogram of a cat with peritoneal fluid (P) showing the normal appearance of the mesentery (arrows). **(b)** Enlarged mesenteric lymph node (LN) in a cat with lymphoma. This appearance, of a uniformly hypoechoic, elongated structure surrounded by hyperechoic fat, is typical of enlarged mesenteric lymph nodes. **(c)** A sonogram of the mid-abdomen of a cat with feline infectious peritonitis, showing peritoneal fluid (P) and two small irregular, nodule-like lesions (N) attached to the peritoneum. These correspond to fibrin aggregates and represent a non-specific sign of high-protein peritoneal effusion. **(d)** A sonogram of the mid-abdomen of a dog with carcinomatosis, showing replacement of normal mesentery and intestine by amorphous tissue with variable echogenicity (M). This poorly circumscribed lesion may be distinguished from normal mesentery by the abnormal echotexture and lack of attached intestine. Peritoneal fluid (P) is present.

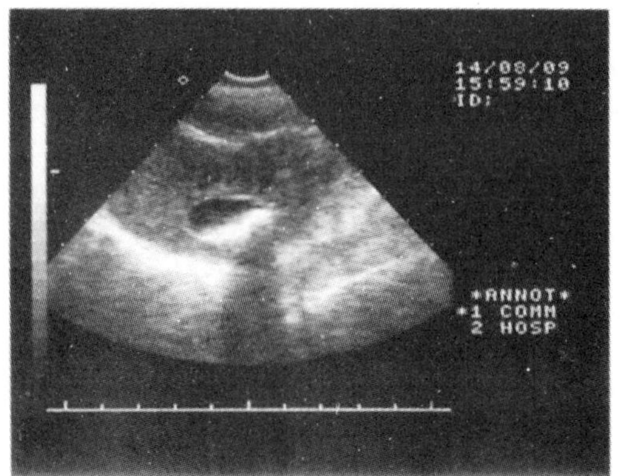
14/08/09
15:59:10
ID:
ANNOT
*1 COMM
2 HOSP

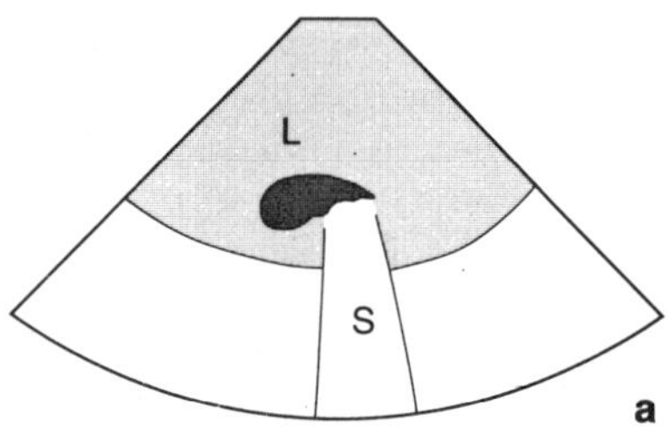
L
S
a

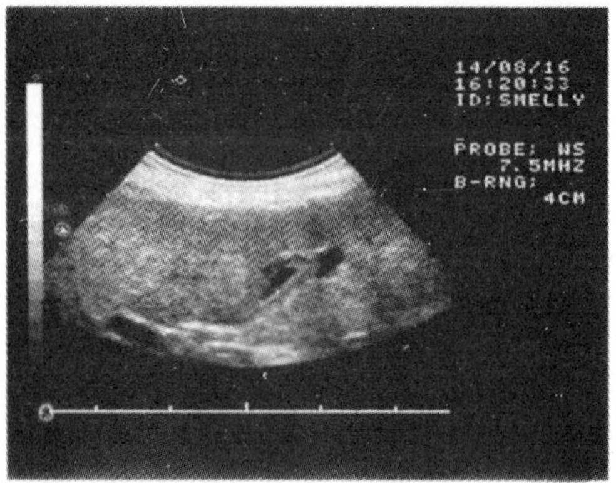
14/08/16
16:20:33
ID:SMELLY
PROBE: WS
7.5MHZ
B-RNG:
4CM

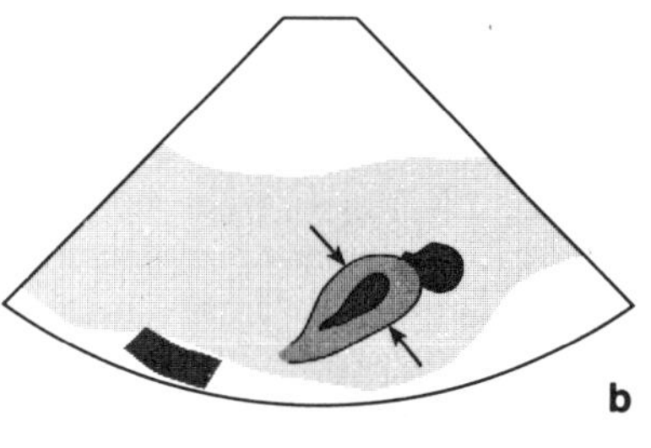
b

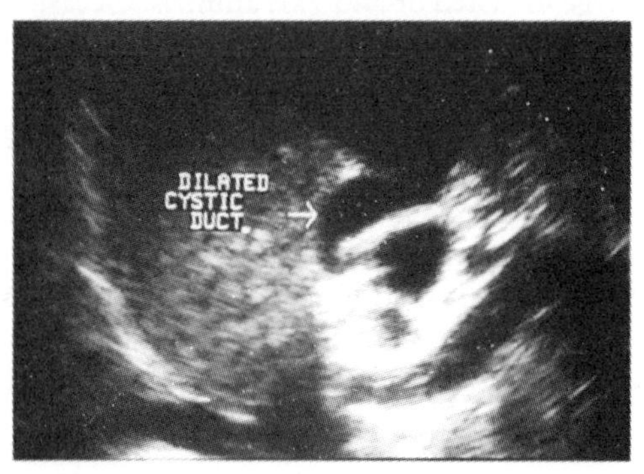
DILATED
CYSTIC
DUCT.

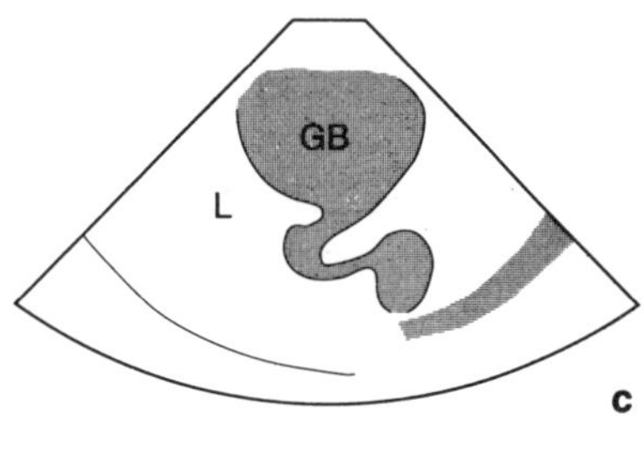
GB
L
c

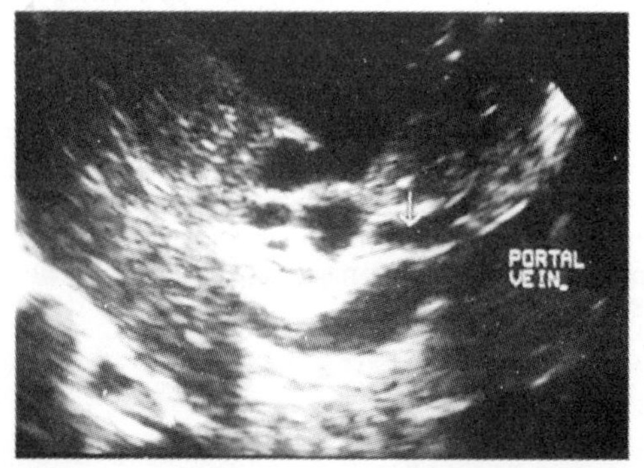
PORTAL
VEIN.

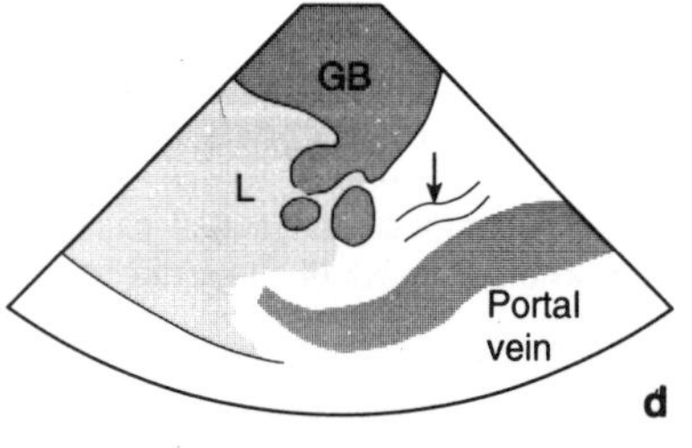
GB
L
Portal
vein
d

Ultrasonography may be used to attempt diagnosis of obstructive jaundice (Figs 2.8c and 2.8d). After experimental bile duct ligation in dogs, dilatation of the common bile duct and intrahepatic bile ducts may become visible within a few hours (Zeman *et al.*, 1981; Raptopoulos *et al.*, 1985), although in some cases intrahepatic duct enlargement is apparent only after seven days (Nyland and Hager, 1985). Pancreatitis is the commonest cause of extrahepatic biliary obstruction in dogs and cats. In clinical cases the diagnosis of biliary obstruction is often difficult, because it may be difficult to identify the common bile duct, and because dilatation of the duct does not necessarily indicate current obstruction. The common bile duct gradually becomes less elastic due to ageing, inflammation or chronic dilatation, and once the duct has been dilated, it may remain dilated for a considerable period after the cause has resolved (Nyland and Hager, 1985). In fact it has been calculated that, as a result of this loss of elasticity, the duct may never return to its original diameter following release of a complete obstruction (Raptopoulos *et al.*, 1985). Hence repeated examinations are required to identify an enlarging duct before obstruction can be reliably diagnosed.

Contraction of the gall bladder may be observed using ultrasonography after feeding a fatty meal. However, in normal dogs fed a standardized high-fat meal after fasting, the percentage emptying of the gall bladder is highly variable. Emptying is more rapid and consistent following intravenous injection of synthetic cholecystokinin, and therefore this is a more reliable method for measuring gall bladder contraction in clinical cases (Finn *et al.*, 1991). Cholecystokinin-induced emptying is more rapid and complete in normal dogs, or dogs with nonobstructive biliary disease, than in dogs with obstruction (Finn *et al.*, 1991). Use of this test may help overcome some of the existing difficulties with ultrasonographic diagnosis of biliary obstruction.

Spleen

As for the liver, ultrasonographic lesions of the spleen may be recognized as changes in size, shape, vascularity and parenchymal echotexture.

Size and shape

Abnormalities of splenic size and shape are diagnosed on the basis of subjective criteria. Common causes of splenomegaly (which cannot be reliably distinguished by ultrasonography) include congestion, lymphoid hyperplasia, extramedullary haematopoiesis, and infiltrative disease, principally lymphoma. When abnormal parenchymal echotexture is present this finding will support a

Fig. 2.8. The biliary tract. **(a)** Oblique sonogram showing echogenic material, producing an acoustic shadow (S), collected on the dependent aspect of the gall bladder. Multiple small calculi or sludge may produce this appearance. Single large calculi are uncommon. L = liver. **(b)** Oblique sonogram of an empty, contracted gall bladder in a cat (arrows). The wall is 1–2 mm thick with a well-defined mucosal surface. **(c)** Sagittal image of the gall bladder (GB) and tortuous, dilated cystic duct (arrow) of a dog with acute pancreatitis and secondary extrahepatic biliary obstruction. **(d)** Sagittal image in the same dog showing a dilated (4 mm diameter) common bile duct (arrow) parallel to the portal vein.

subjective assessment of enlarged or nodular spleen, and therefore provides a stronger indication for aspirate cytology or biopsy.

Vascularity

The splenic veins may be examined where they drain from the hilum. Enlargement (another subjective finding) and the ability to see large intrasplenic veins indicate congestion (Fig. 2.2b). In severe congestion (e.g. due to torsion) enlargement of splenic veins is accompanied by profound, diffuse hypoechogenicity of the parenchyma (Konde *et al.*, 1989).

Parenchymal abnormalities

These may be classified as focal or diffuse, hypo- or hyperechoic (Figs 2.2c and 2.2d; Table 2.2). Focal abnormalities are most often due to tumour or haematoma (Wrigley, 1991). Abscesses (Konde *et al.*, 1986a), infarcts (Schelling *et al.*, 1988), and hyperplastic nodules occur less frequently.

Table 2.2. Classification of splenic lesions identified by ultrasonography.

	Hypoechoic	Hyperechoic
Focal/multifocal lesions	Primary neoplasm, e.g. haemangiosarcoma Metastasis Lymphoma Lymphoid hyperplasia Haematoma Acute infarct Abscess	Fat around hilar vein Metastasis Chronic infarct
Diffuse lesions	Lymphoma Metastasis, e.g. mast cell tumour Histoplasmosis Severe congestion Necrosis	Cirrhosis

There is considerable overlap in the ultrasonographic appearance of neoplasms, haematomas and abscesses in the spleen, and fine needle aspirates often cannot distinguish these lesions (Wrigley, 1991). Therefore, when a splenic mass is identified, hepatic or cardiac metastasis should be ruled out using ultrasonography. Thoracic radiographs should be obtained to rule out pulmonary metastasis. If these studies are negative, splenectomy should be performed so that a histopathological diagnosis can be made from a large tissue sample.

Kidneys

Indications

The relative roles of intravenous urography (IVU) and ultrasonography have been discussed in detail (Konde *et al.*, 1986b; Feeney *et al.*, 1991). In general, the indications for renal ultrasonography are similar to those for IVU:

- to identify the kidneys if not visible on survey radiographs.
- normal survey radiographs in an animal with clinical signs of renal disease.
- abnormal renal size or shape.
- mass in the area of the kidney or ureter.
- renal haematuria or recurrent urinary tract infection.

Size

Renal ultrasonography provides specific diagnostic information less often when the kidneys are small than when they are enlarged. This is because chronic diseases, such as glomerulonephritis or pyelonephritis, cause fibrosis and contraction and ultimately produce a similar 'end-stage' lesion whatever the aetiology (Fig. 2.3c). Causes of enlarged kidneys in dogs and cats that may be reliably distinguished using ultrasonography include polycystic kidney disease (Fig. 2.9a), hydronephrosis (Fig. 2.9b), lymphoma (Fig. 2.9c), mass lesions (e.g. abscess, neoplasm) and subcapsular fluid or infiltration (Fig. 2.9d).

Focal lesions

Ultrasonography provides more specific information than IVU for differentiating renal lesions because it produces a more detailed image of the internal anatomy of the kidney. Ultrasonographic findings have been reported for renal masses, e.g. cyst (Walter *et al.*, 1988), tumour (Konde *et al.*, 1986b; Walter *et al.*, 1987b; Ackerman *et al.*, 1989), abscess (Konde *et al.*, 1986a), infarct (Biller *et al.*, 1991) and pararenal pseudocyst (Tidwell *et al.*, 1990).

Diffuse lesions

Although the normal variation in renal cortical echogenicity presents interpretive difficulties, certain kidney diseases are known to cause diffuse changes in cortical echogenicity. Increased echogenicity has been reported with acute nephrosis, nephritis, and hypercalcaemic nephropathy in dogs (Walter *et al.*, 1987b; Adams *et al.*, 1989; Barr *et al.*, 1989) and nephritis, feline infectious peritonitis and lymphoma in cats (Walter *et al.*, 1988). Decreased renal cortical echogenicity may also occur with lymphoma (Konde *et al.*, 1986b; Walter *et al.*, 1987b, 1988).

The medullary rim sign, described above as a potentially normal finding in cats, also occurs in some dogs and cats with metastatic calcification of the renal tubular basement membrane (Barr *et al.*, 1989; Biller *et al.*, 1992a). Underlying causes include acute tubular necrosis, oxalate nephrosis and hypercalcaemia.

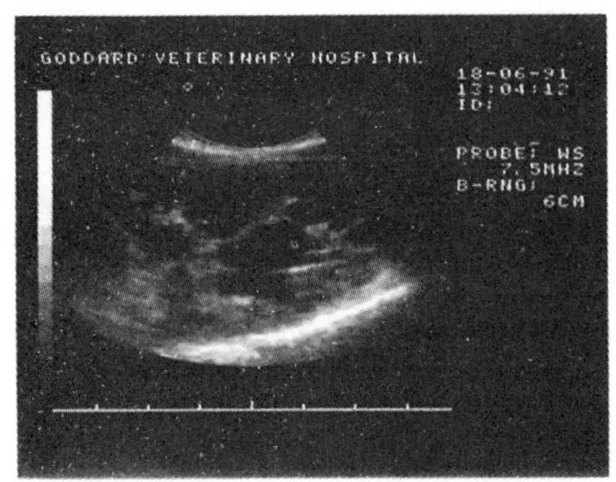
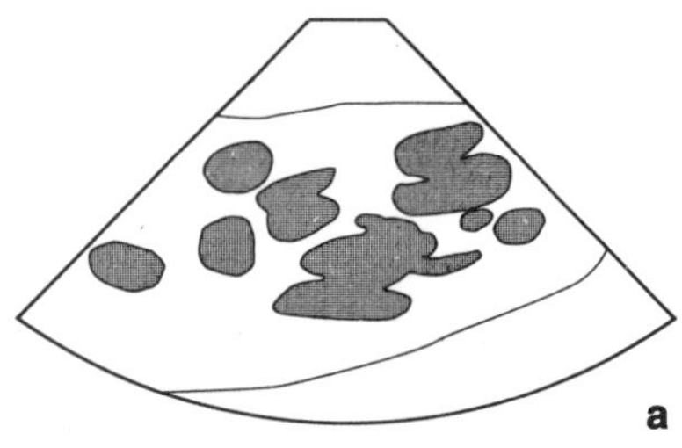

a

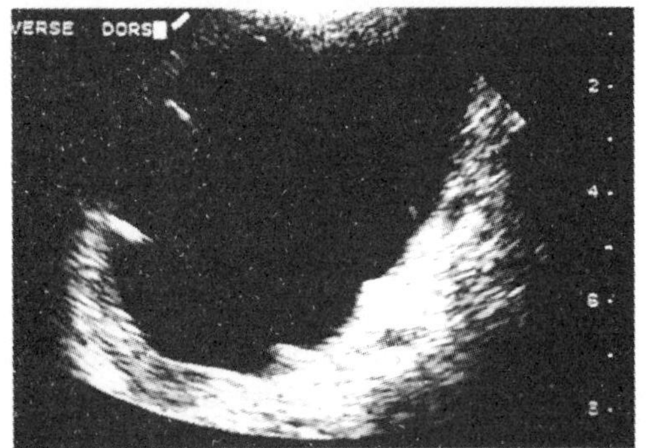
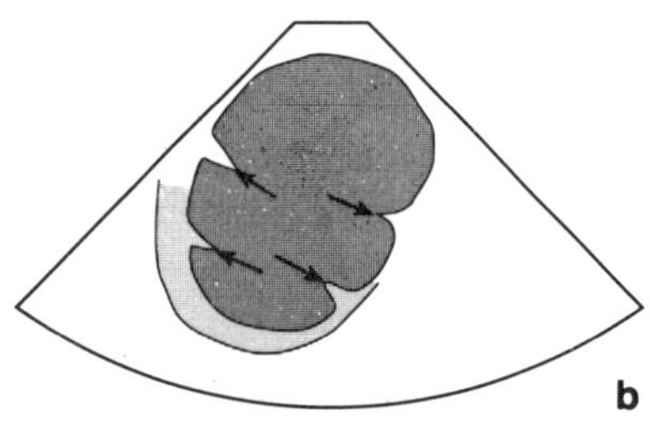

b

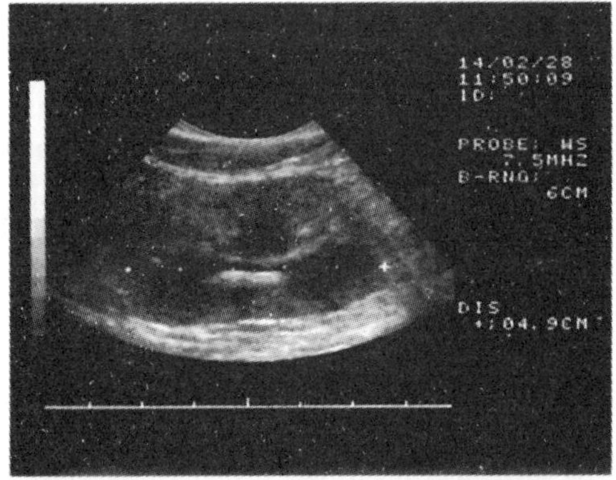
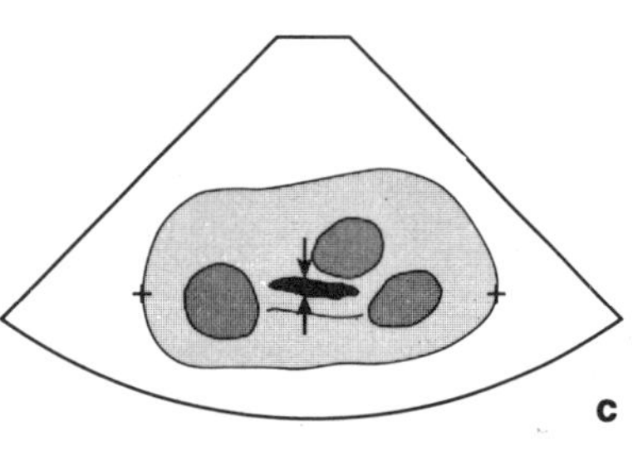

c

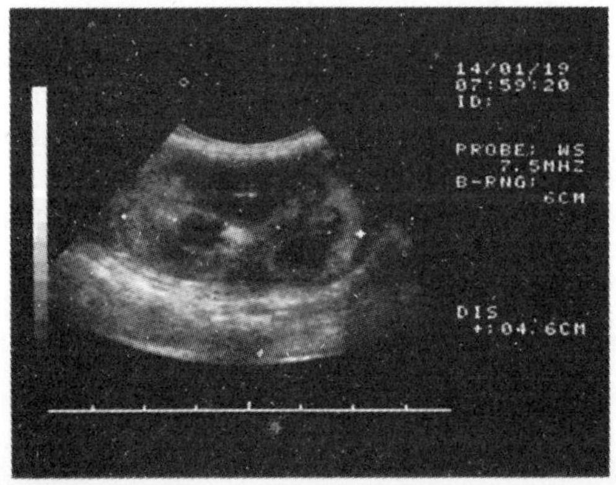
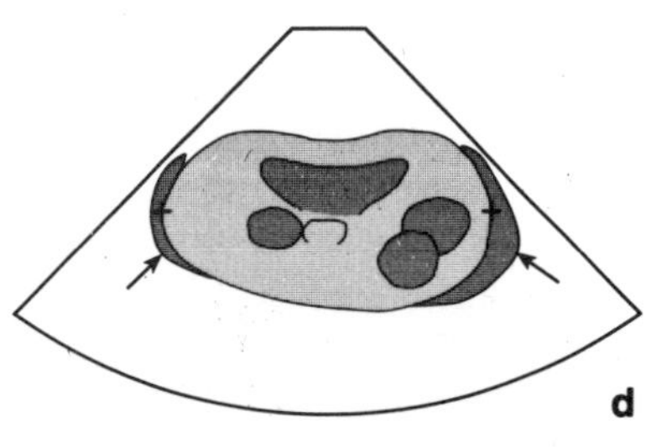

d

Ultrasonographic findings are variable in animals with naturally-occurring pyelonephritis. For example, dilatation of the renal pelvis by purulent material (pyonephrosis) is an inconsistent finding. Abnormalities that have been described in experimentally-induced pyelonephritis include hyperechoic mucosal line within the renal pelvis, dilated pelvis and proximal ureter, focal hyperechoic areas in the medulla, and focal hypo- or hyperechoic cortical lesions (Neuwirth *et al.*, 1993).

Adrenal glands

There are no established criteria for normal adrenal gland size, and hyperfunctional adrenal glands do not necessarily enlarge (Kelly *et al.*, 1971). Hence, ultrasonographic abnormalities of the adrenal glands may be more usefully divided into 'mass' and 'non-mass' lesions on the basis of their shape and echogenicity rather than size (Table 2.3) (Schelling, 1991).

Table 2.3. Classification of adrenal lesions by ultrasonography.

	Unilateral	Bilateral
Mass lesions	Functional adrenocortical tumour Non-functional adrenocortical tumour Phaeochromocytoma Aldosteronoma Nodular hyperplasia Metastasis Granuloma Haematoma Abscess Cyst	Nodular hyperplasia Metastasis
Non-mass lesions	Atrophy, i.e. contralateral functional adrenocortical tumour	Exogenous steroid-induced atrophy Hyperplasia, i.e. pituitary-dependent hyperadrenocorticism

Fig. 2.9. Renal diseases. **(a)** Sagittal sonogram of a kidney with severe polycystic disease characterised by the presence of multiple variously sized, anechoic cavities throughout the kidney parenchyma. The severity of the lesion is such that the kidney is barely recognizable. **(b)** Gross hydronephrosis secondary to obstructed ureter. The renal pelvis is severely dilated and has compressed the parenchyma into a thin rim of tissue. The pelvis is partially divided by regular septa (arrows) which are remnants of medullary connective tissue. The presence of these septa differentiates gross hydronephrosis from a large renal cyst. **(c)** Dorsal image of the left kidney of a cat with lymphoma. The kidney is enlarged. There is increased echogenicity affecting the medulla, and reduced clarity of internal architecture. Also, there is slight dilatation of the renal pelvis (arrows). **(d)** Dorsal image of the kidney in a cat with feline infectious peritonitis. There is subcapsular fluid visible at the poles of the kidney (arrows). Subcapsular cellular accumulations, e.g. due to haemorrhage or lymphoma, may produce a similar appearance. The kidney is enlarged.

Adrenal masses usually distort the shape of the gland, making it more rounded or irregular, and cause hypo- or hyperechogenicity (Fig. 2.4c). Irregular, echogenic foci, sometimes with acoustic shadowing, may be due to calcification and represent a common but non-specific sign of adrenocortical neoplasia (Kantrowitz *et al.*, 1986; Poffenbarger *et al.*, 1988; Voorhout *et al.*, 1990; Schelling, 1991). Invasion of the caudal vena cava by an adrenal mass is a sign of malignancy (Poffenbarger *et al.*, 1988; Voorhout *et al.*, 1990; Schelling, 1991). A gland that is subjectively considered large but which retains its normal shape (Fig. 2.4d) is better classified as 'non-mass' and is more likely to be hyperplastic than neoplastic (Schelling, 1991).

Due to the difficulties encountered examining the adrenal glands, inability to identify one or both does not rule out the possibility of disease. Also, the determination of unilateral versus bilateral disease is not possible in all cases (Kantrowitz *et al.*, 1986). This limits the diagnostic value of adrenal ultrasonography.

Pancreas

Pancreatitis in the dog and cat is a condition of varying severity, and the sensitivity of ultrasonography for this disease largely depends upon the experience of the ultrasonographer. Only an experienced veterinary ultrasonographer can be expected to consistently identify the normal gland and, therefore, relatively small lesions. Large lesions are more likely to be detected by less experienced ultrasonographers. Ultrasonographic findings in pancreatitis (Nyland *et al.*, 1983; Murtaugh *et al.*, 1985; Rutgers *et al.*, 1985; Salisbury *et al.*, 1988; Lamb, 1989; Edwards *et al.*, 1990; Saunders, 1991; Simpson *et al.*, 1994) include hypoechoic tissue in a position consistent with the pancreas (Fig. 2.5b), cavitary lesions (e.g. abscess, pseudocyst), dilated pancreatic duct (Fig. 2.5c), swollen, hypomotile duodenum (Fig. 2.5d), evidence of extrahepatic biliary obstruction, and peritoneal fluid.

Pancreatic neoplasia is less common than pancreatitis. Islet-cell tumours or adenocarcinomas are often small and difficult to detect using ultrasonography. Pancreatic neoplasms are often highly malignant, so metastasis to the liver and abdominal lymph nodes may be identified at a stage when the primary neoplasm is too small to be visible (Saunders, 1991).

Stomach and intestine

As described above, an optimal ultrasonographic examination of the stomach requires that it be filled with water, to distend the organ and to displace gas. Unless this is done, potential abnormalities must be interpreted with caution. Ultrasonography of the stomach may reveal foreign bodies (Tidwell and Penninck, 1992), chronic hypertrophic pyloric gastropathy (Biller *et al.*, 1994) and mural lesions such as neoplasia (Penninck *et al.*, 1990) or mucosal calcification due to uraemic gastropathy (Grooters *et al.*, 1994).

Under optimal conditions (fluid-filled stomach, drug-induced gastric hypomotility, and systematic examination using multiple positions of patient and transducer) ultrasonography of humans with gastric disease has a sensitivity of 82% (Worlicek *et al.*, 1989). However, under suboptimal conditions, ultrasonography of the stomach is a potentially misleading procedure. Physiological thickening of the contracted gastric wall and uneven echogenicity due to interference of ultrasound transmission by near-field structures, ingesta or gas may also contribute to interpretive difficulties (Lamb and Forster-van Hijfte, 1994).

Ultrasonography is now an established technique for detecting a variety of intestinal lesions, including dilatation and hypomotility (Fig. 2.6b), intussusception (Fig. 2.6c) (Flückiger and Arnold, 1986; Kantrowitz *et al.*, 1988), foreign body (Tidwell and Penninck, 1992), enteric duplication (Spaulding *et al.*, 1990), focal mural thickening (e.g. due to neoplasia) (Nyland and Kantrowitz, 1986; Penninck *et al.*, 1990; Saunders *et al.*, 1992), and diffuse intestinal mural thickening (e.g. due to lymphangiectasia).

Intestinal neoplasia tends to produce a consistent appearance on ultrasonography, i.e. localized, hypoechoic thickening of the intestinal wall and loss of the normal layered wall structure (Fig. 2.6d). This typically produces a doughnut- or horseshoe-shaped lesion when viewed in transverse section. Intestinal granulomas are uncommon, but may also produce this appearance, and hence biopsy is required for definite diagnosis. Ultrasound-guided fine needle aspiration and core biopsy techniques for the gastrointestinal tract in small animals have recently been described (Crystal *et al.*, 1993; Penninck *et al.*, 1993).

Mesentery and peritoneum

Ultrasonography may reveal mesenteric lymphadenopathy (Fig. 2.7b) (Saunders *et al.*, 1992), abscess (Konde *et al.*, 1986a), or diffusely thickened mesentery, for example in fat animals. Multiple small masses may be observed adherent to the mesentery and peritoneum in cats with infectious peritonitis (Fig. 2.7c).

Mesenteric and peritoneal lesions are most readily identified when a moderate amount of peritoneal fluid is present; however, a practical problem arises when evaluating the mesentery in the presence of a large volume of peritoneal fluid, because the mesentery and intestines tend to form an amorphous clump in the mid-abdomen which can obscure mesenteric lesions, including masses. Mesenteric masses may be recognized by their mid-abdominal location, irregular margins, heterogenous echotexture, and minimal attachment to the small intestine or other organs (Fig. 2.7d).

Urinary bladder

Abnormalities of the urinary bladder that may be visible on ultrasonography include mural thickening due to cystitis or neoplasia (Figs 2.10a and 2.10b) (Biller *et al.*, 1990; Leveille *et al.*, 1992) and abnormal contents such as calculi, echogenic sediment (Fig. 2.10c) or foreign body (Zanotti *et al.*, 1989). A large paraprostatic cyst (Stowater and Lamb, 1989) could be mistaken for the urinary bladder if the bladder is empty during the examination. Passing a urinary catheter and infusing water will help identify the bladder when doubt exists.

Dilated ureters may be visible ultrasonographically (Biller *et al.*, 1990; Leveille *et al.*, 1992). Ultrasonographic diagnosis of ectopic ureter is possible, based on absence of a ureteral jet and presence of a dilated ureter passing caudal to its normal site of insertion into the bladder (Fig. 2.10d) (Lamb and Gregory, 1994).

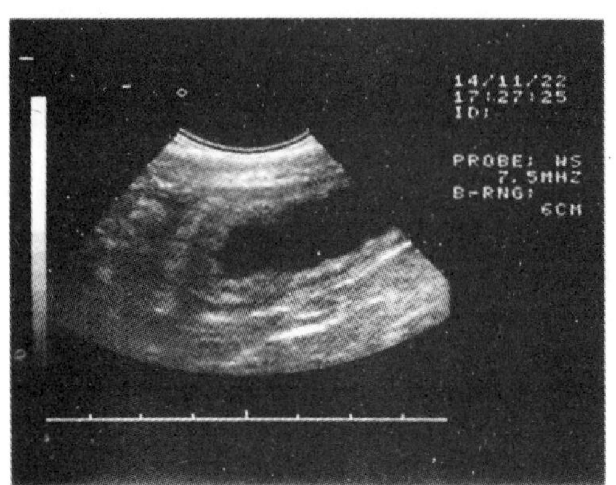
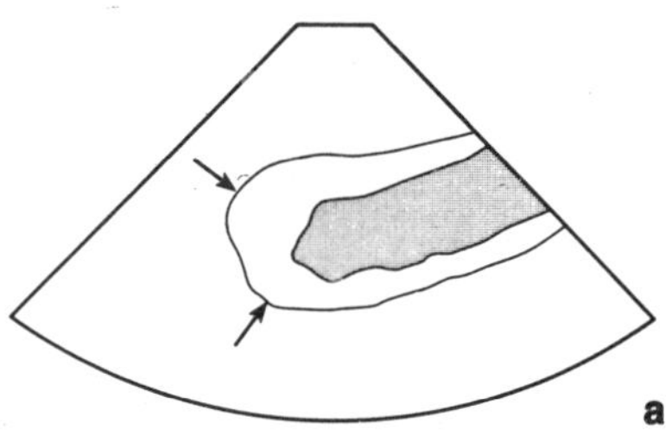

a

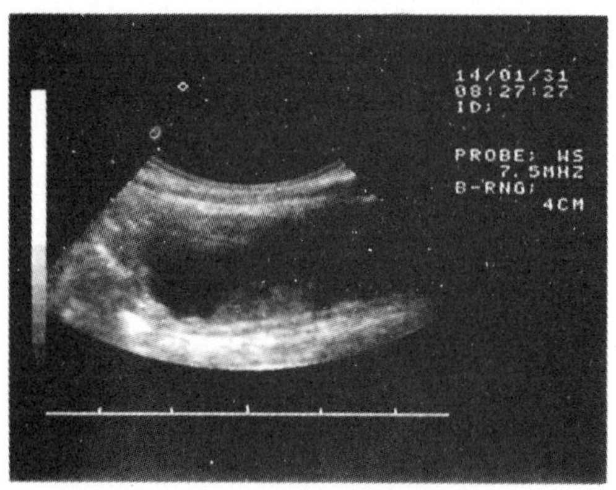
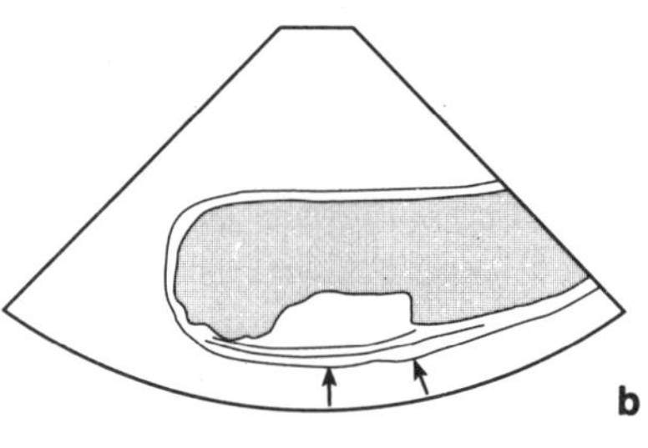

b

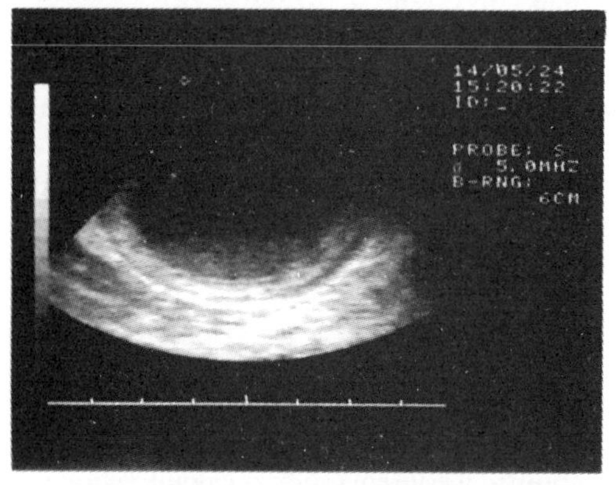
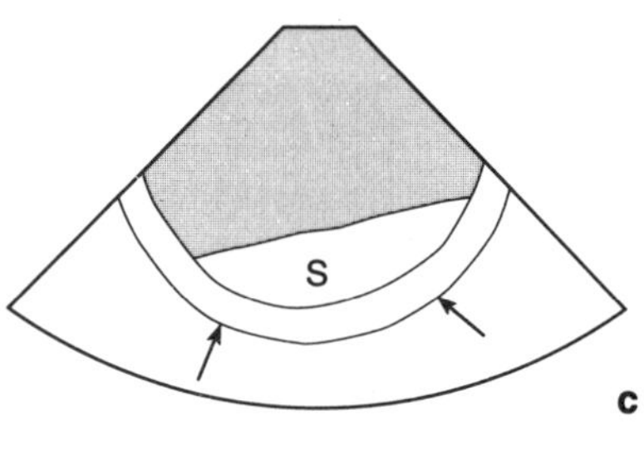

c

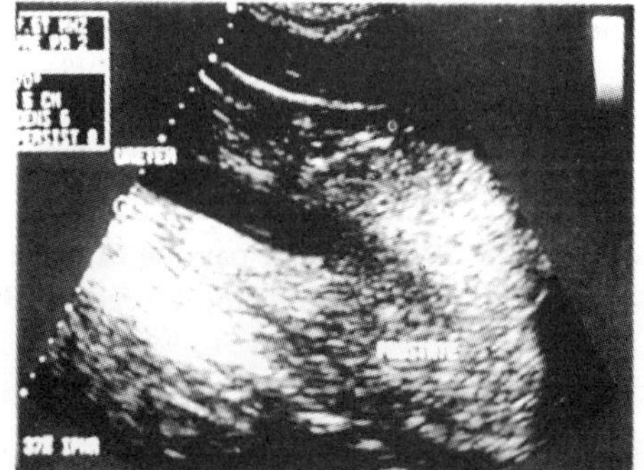

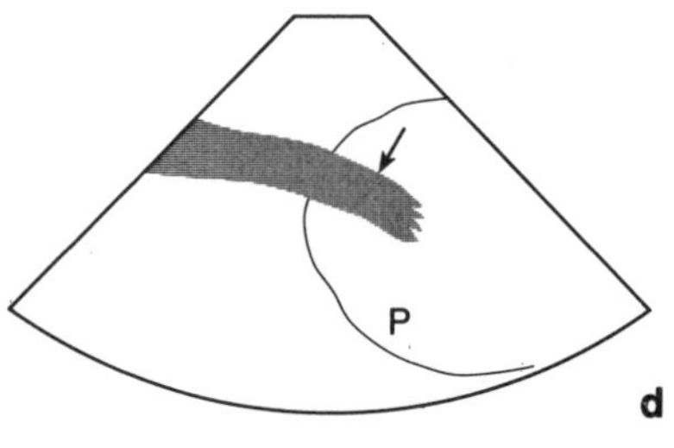

d

References

Ackerman, N., Hager, D.A. and Kaude, J.V. (1989) Ultrasound appearance and early detection of VX2 carcinoma in the rabbit kidney. *Veterinary Radiology*, 30, 88–96.

Adams, W.H., Toal, R.L., Walker, M.A. and Breider, M.A. (1989) Early renal ultrasonographic findings in dogs with experimentally induced ethylene glycol nephrosis. *American Journal of Veterinary Research*, 50, 1370–1376.

Afschrift, M., Cuvelier, C., Ringoir, S. and Barbire, F. (1987) Influence of pathological state on the acoustic attenuation coefficient slope of the liver. *Ultrasound in Medicine and Biology*, 13, 135–139.

Bailey, M.Q., Willard, M.D., McLoughlin, M.A., Gaber, C. and Hampton, J. (1988) Ultrasonographic findings associated with congenital hepatic arteriovenous fistula in three dogs. *Journal of the American Veterinary Medical Association*, 192, 1099–1101.

Barr, F.J. (1990) Evaluation of ultrasound as a method of assessing renal size in the dog. *Journal of Small Animal Practice*, 31, 174–179.

Barr, F.J. (1992a) Ultrasonographic assessment of liver size in the dog. *Journal of Small Animal Practice*, 33, 359–364.

Barr, F.J. (1992b) Normal hepatic measurements in dogs. *Journal of Small Animal Practice*, 33, 367–370.

Barr, F.J., Patteson, M.W., Lucke, V.M. and Gibbs, C. (1989) Hypercalcemic nephropathy in three dogs: sonographic appearance. *Veterinary Radiology*, 30, 169–173.

Barr, F.J., Holt, P.E. and Gibbs, C. (1990) Ultrasonographic measurement of normal renal parameters. *Journal of Small Animal Practice*, 31, 180–184.

Biller, D.S., Kantrowitz, B., Partington, B.P. and Miyabayashi, T. (1990) Diagnostic ultrasound of the urinary bladder. *Journal of the American Animal Hospital Association*, 26, 397–402.

Biller, D.S., Schenkman, D.I. and Bortnowski, H. (1991) Ultrasonographic appearance of renal infarcts in a dog. *Journal of the American Animal Hospital Association*, 27, 370–372.

Biller, D.S., Bradley, G.A. and Partington, B.P. (1992a) Renal medullary rim sign: ultrasonographic evidence of renal disease. *Veterinary Radiology and Ultrasound*, 33, 286–290.

Biller, D.S., Kantrowitz, B. and Miyabayashi, T. (1992b) Ultrasonography of diffuse liver disease: a review. *Journal of Veterinary Internal Medicine*, 6, 71–76.

Biller, D.S., Partington, B.P., Miayabayashi, T and Leveille, R. (1994) Ultrasonographic appearance of chronic hypertrophic gastropathy in the dog. *Veterinary Radiology and Ultrasound*, 35, 30–33.

Bondestam, S., Alanen, A. and Toikkanen, S. (1992) Correlations of liver echo intensity with cytology and chemical measurements of fat, water and protein content in live Burbots (*Lota lota*). *Ultrasound in Medicine and Biology*, 18, 75–80.

Fig. 2.10. The urinary bladder. **(a)** Sagittal image of a dog showing diffuse mucosal thickening principally on the cranial aspect (arrows). This appearance is typical of cystitis. **(b)** Sagittal image of the bladder showing a sessile mucosal mass protruding into the lumen. The outer layers of the bladder wall are visible (arrows) and apparently unaffected by the mass indicating that the lesion may be localized to the mucosa. The histological diagnosis was transitional cell carcinoma. **(c)** Transverse image of the urinary bladder of a dog with chronic cystitis showing a diffusely thickened wall (arrows) and echogenic sediment (S) which has settled on the dependent aspect. Inflammatory sediment or haemorrhage could produce this appearance. **(d)** Sagittal image of a male dog with ectopic ureter showing the dilated ureter (arrow) entering the prostate (P) rather than inserting normally into the bladder. The intraprostatic portion of the ureter was not visible on ultrasonography; however, ectopic ureter inserting into the prostatic urethra was confirmed by IVU.

Choi, B.I., Park, J.H., Kim, B.H., Kim, S.H., Han, M.C. and Kim, C.W. (1989) Small hepatocellular carcinoma: detection with sonography, computed tomography (CT), angiography and Lipiodol-CT. *British Journal of Radiology*, 62, 897–903.

Cloostermans, M.J.T.M., Mol, H., Verhoef, W.A., Thijssen, J.M. and Kubat, K. (1986) *In vitro* estimation of acoustic parameters of the liver and correlations with histology. *Ultrasound in Medicine and Biology*, 12, 39–51.

Crystal, M.A., Penninck, D.G., Matz, M.E., Pearson, S.H., Freden, G.O. and Jakowski, R.M. (1993) Use of ultrasound guided fine-needle aspiration biopsy and automated core biopsy for the diagnosis of gastrointestinal diseases in small animals. *Veterinary Radiology and Ultrasound*, 34, 438–444.

Douglass, J.P. (1993) Bladder wall mass effect caused by the intramural portion of the canine ureter. *Veterinary Radiology and Ultrasound*, 34, 107.

Edwards, D.F., Bauer, M.S., Walker, M.A., Pardo, A.D., McCracken, M.D. and Walker, T.L. (1990) Pancreatic masses in seven dogs following acute pancreatitis. *Journal of the American Animal Hospital Association*, 26, 189–198.

Feeney, D.A., Johnston, G.R. and Walter, P.A. (1991) Ultrasonography of the kidney and prostate gland. Has gray-scale ultrasonography replaced contrast radiography? In: Kaplan, P.M. (ed.) *Problems in Veterinary Medicine*, vol. 3. Saunders, Philadelphia, pp. 619–646.

Feleppa, E.J., Lizzi, F.L., Coleman, D.J. and Yaremko, M.M. (1986) Diagnostic spectrum analysis in ophthalmology: a physical perspective. *Ultrasound in Medicine and Biology*, 12, 623–631.

Finn, S.T., Park, R.D., Twedt, D.C. and Curtis, C.R. (1991) Ultrasonographic assessment of sincalide-induced canine gall bladder emptying: an aid to the diagnosis of biliary obstruction. *Veterinary Radiology*, 32, 269–276.

Finn-Bodner, S.T., Park, R.D., Tyler, J.W., Twedt, D.C. and Curtis, C.R. (1993) Ultrasonographic determination, in vitro and in vivo, of canine gall bladder volume, using four volumetric formulas and stepwise regression models. *American Journal of Veterinary Research*, 54, 832–835.

Flückiger, M. and Arnold, P. (1986) Die Darminvagination beim Hund – ihr sonographisces Bild. *Kleintierpraxis*, 31, 379–382.

Godshalk, C.P., Badertscher, R.R., Rippy, M.K. and Ghent, A.W. (1988) Quantitative ultrasonic assessment of liver size in the dog. *Veterinary Radiology*, 29, 162–167.

Goyal, A.K., Pokharna, D.S. and Sharma, S.K. (1990) Ultrasonic measurement of portal vasculature in the diagnosis of portal hypertension: a controversial subject reviewed. *Journal of Ultrasound in Medicine*, 9, 45–48.

Grooters, A.M., Miyabayashi, T., Biller, D.S. and Merryman, J. (1994) Sonographic appearance of uremic gastropathy in four dogs. *Veterinary Radiology and Ultrasound*, 35, 35–40.

Hager, D.A., Nyland, T.G. and Fisher, P.E. (1985) Ultrasound-guided biopsy of the canine liver, kidney, and prostate. *Veterinary Radiology*, 26, 82–88.

Hartzband, L.E., Tidwell, A.S. and Lamb, C.R. (1991) Relative echogenicity of the renal cortex and liver in normal dogs. *British Journal of Radiology* (abstract), 64, 654.

Kantrowitz, B.M., Nyland, T.G. and Feldman, E.C. (1986) Adrenal ultrasonography in the dog: detection of tumors and hyperplasia in hyperadrenocorticism. *Veterinary Radiology*, 27, 91–96.

Kantrowitz, B.M., Dimski, D., Swalec, K. and Biller, D.S. (1988) Ultrasonographic detection of jejunal intussusception and acute renal failure due to ethylene glycol toxicity in a dog. *Journal of the American Animal Hospital Association*, 24, 697–700.

Kelly, D.F., Siegel, E.T. and Berg, P. (1971) The adrenal gland in dogs with hyperadrenocorticism. A pathologic study. *Veterinary Pathology*, 8, 385–400.

Konde, L.J. (1985) Sonography of the kidney. In: Hering, D.S. (ed.) *Veterinary Clinics of North America: Small Animal Practice*, vol. 15. Saunders, Philadelphia, pp. 1149–1158.

Konde, L.J., Lebel, J.L., Park, R.D. and Wrigley, R.H. (1986a) Sonographic application in the diagnosis of intra-abdominal abscess in the dog. *Veterinary Radiology*, 27, 151–154.

Konde, L.J., Park, R.D., Wrigley, R.H. and Lebel, J.L. (1986b) Comparison of radiography and ultrasonography in the evaluation of renal lesions in the dog. *Journal of the American Veterinary Medical Association*, 188, 1420–1425.

Konde, L.J., Wrigley, R.H., Lebel, J.L, Park, R.D., Pugh, C. and Finn, S. (1989) Sonographic and radiographic changes associated with splenic torsion in dogs. *Veterinary Radiology*, 30, 41–45.

Kremkau, K.W. (1989) *Diagnostic Ultrasound – Principles, Instruments, Exercises*, 3rd edn. Saunders, Philadelphia.

Lamb, C.R. (1989) Dilatation of the pancreatic duct: an ultrasonographic finding in acute pancreatitis. *Journal of Small Animal Practice*, 30, 410–413.

Lamb, C.R. (1991) Ultrasonography of the liver and biliary tract. In: Kaplan, P.M. (ed.) *Problems in Veterinary Medicine*, vol. 3. Saunders, Philadelphia, pp. 555–573.

Lamb, C.R. (1994) Doppler ultrasonography of portosystemic shunts in dogs and cats: updated results of a prospective study. *Veterinary Radiology and Ultrasound*, 35, 258.

Lamb, C.R. and Forster-van Hijfte, M. (1994) Beware the gastric pseudomass. *Veterinary Radiology and Ultrasound*, 35, 398–399.

Lamb, C.R. and Gregory, S.P. (1994) Ultrasonography of the ureterovesicular junction in the dog: a preliminary report. *Veterinary Record*, 134, 36–38.

Lamb, C.R., Hartzband, L.E., Tidwell, A.S. and Pearson, S.H. (1991) Ultrasonographic findings in hepatic and splenic lymphosarcoma in dogs and cats. *Veterinary Radiology*, 32, 117–120.

Landini, L., Sarnelli, R., Salvadori, M. and Squartinin, F. (1987) Orientation and frequency dependence of backscatter coefficient in normal and pathological breast tissues. *Ultrasound in Medicine and Biology*, 13, 77–83.

Leveille, R., Biller, D.S., Partington, B.P. and Miyabayashi, T. (1992) Sonographic investigation of transitional cell carcinoma of the urinary bladder in small animals. *Veterinary Radiology and Ultrasound*, 33, 103–107.

Leveille, R., Partington, B.P. Biller, D.S. and Miyabayashi, T. (1993) Complications after ultrasound-guided biopsy of abdominal structures in dogs and cats: 246 cases (1984–1991). *Journal of the American Veterinary Medical Association*, 203, 413–415.

Lin, H.H., Changchien, C.S. and Lin, D.Y. (1989) Hepatic parenchymal calcifications – differentiation from intrahepatic stones. *Journal of Clinical Ultrasound*, 17, 411–415.

Marchal, G., Tshibwabwa-Tumba, E., Oyen, R., Pylyser, K. and Goddeeris, P. (1985) Correlation of sonographic patterns in liver metastases with histology and microangiography. *Investigative Radiology*, 20, 79–84.

Mills, P., Joseph, A.E.A. and Adam, E.J. (1989) Total abdominal and pelvic ultrasound: incidental findings and a comparison between outpatient and general practice referrals in 1000 cases. *British Journal of Radiology*, 62, 974–976.

Murray, F.E., Stinchcombe, S.J. and Hawkey, C.J. (1992) Development of biliary sludge in patients on intensive care unit: results of a prospective ultrasonographic study. *Gut*, 33, 1123–1125.

Murtaugh, R.J., Herring, D.S., Jacobs, R.M. and DeHoff, W.D. (1985) Pancreatic ultrasonography in dogs with experimentally induced acute pancreatitis. *Veterinary Radiology*, 26, 27–32.

Neuwirth, L., Mahaffey, M., Crowell, W., Selcer, B., Barsanti, J., Cooper, R. and Brown, J. (1993) Comparison of excretory urography and ultrasonography for detection of experimentally induced pyelonephritis in dogs. *American Journal of Veterinary Research*, 54, 660–669.

Nyland, T.G. and Fisher, P.E. (1990) Evaluation of experimentally induced canine hepatic cirrhosis using duplex Doppler ultrasound. *Veterinary Radiology*, 31, 189–194.

Nyland, T.G. and Hager, D.A. (1985) Sonography of the liver, gallbladder, and spleen. In: Herring, D.S. (ed.) *Veterinary Clinics of North America: Small Animal Practice*, vol. 15. Saunders, Philadelphia, pp. 1123–1147.

Nyland, T.G. and Kantrowitz, B.M. (1986) Ultrasound in the diagnosis and staging of abdominal neoplasia. In: Gorman, N.T. (ed.) *Contemporary Issues in Small Animal Practice*, vol. 6, Churchill Livingstone, New York, pp. 1–24.

Nyland, T.G., Mulvany, M.H. and Strombeck, D.R. (1983) Ultrasonic features of experimentally induced, acute pancreatitis in the dog. *Veterinary Radiology*, 24, 260–266.

Nyland, T.G., Kantrowitz, B.M., Fisher, P.E., Olander, H.J. and Hornof, W.J. (1989) Ultrasonic determination of kidney volume in the dog. *Veterinary Radiology*, 30, 174–180.

Penninck, D.G., Nyland, T.G., Fisher, P.E. and Kerr, L.Y. (1989) Ultrasonography of the normal canine gastrointestinal tract. *Veterinary Radiology*, 30, 272–276.

Penninck, D.G., Nyland, T.G., Kerr, L.Y. and Fisher, P.E. (1990). Ultrasonographic evaluation of gastrointestinal diseases in small animals. *Veterinary Radiology*, 31, 134–141.

Penninck, D.G., Crystal, M.A., Matz, M.E. and Pearson, S.H. (1993) The technique of percutaneous ultrasound guided fine-needle aspiration biopsy and automated microcore biopsy in small animal gastrointestinal disease. *Veterinary Radiology and Ultrasound*, 34, 433–436.

Platt, J.F., Rubin, J.M., Bowermann, R.A. and Marn, C.S. (1988) The inability to detect kidney disease on the basis of echogenicity. *American Journal of Roentgenology*, 151, 317–319.

Poffenbarger, E.M., Feeney, D.A. and Hayden, D.W. (1988) Gray-scale ultrasonography in the diagnosis of adrenal neoplasia in dogs: six cases (1981–1986). *Journal of the American Veterinary Medical Association*, 192, 228–232.

Pugh, C.H., Schelling, C.S., Moreau, R.E. and Golden, D. (1994) Iatrogenic renal pyelectasia in the dog. *Veterinary Radiology and Ultrasound*, 35, 50–51.

Raptopoulos, V., Fabian, T.M., Silva, W., D'Orsi, C.J., Karellas, A., Compton, C.C., Krolikowski, F.J., Doherty, P. and Smith, E.H. (1985) The effect of time and cholecystectomy on experimental biliary tree dilatation. *Investigative Radiology*, 20, 276–286.

Rubaltelli, L., Del Mashio, A., Canoliani, F. and Miotto, D. (1980) The role of vascularization in the formation of echogenic patterns of hepatic metastases: microangiographic and echography study. *British Journal of Radiology*, 53, 1166–1168.

Rutgers, C.H., Herring, D.S. and Orton, E.C. (1985) Pancreatic pseudocyst associated with acute pancreatitis in a dog: ultrasonographic diagnosis. *Journal of the American Animal Hospital Association*, 21, 411–416.

Salisbury, S.K., Lantz, G.C., Nelson, R.W. and Kazacos, E.A. (1988) Pancreatic abscess in dogs: six cases (1978–1986). *Journal of the American Veterinary Medical Association*, 193, 1104–1108.

Saunders, H.M. (1991) Ultrasonography of the pancreas. In: Kaplan, P.M. (ed.) *Problems in Veterinary Medicine*, vol. 3. Saunders, Philadelphia, pp. 583–603.

Saunders, H.M., Pugh, C.R. and Rhodes, W.H. (1992) Expanding applications of abdominal ultrasonography. *Journal of the American Animal Hospital Association*, 28, 369–374.

Schelling, C.G. (1991) Ultrasonography of the adrenal gland. In: Kaplan, P.M. (ed.) *Problems in Veterinary Medicine*, vol. 3. Saunders, Philadelphia, pp. 604–617.

Schelling, C.G., Wortman, J.A. and Saunders, H.M. (1988) Ultrasonographic detection of splenic necrosis in the dog. Three case reports of splenic necrosis secondary to infarction. *Veterinary Radiology*, 29, 227–233.

Schummer, A., Nickel, R. and Sack, W.O. (1979) *The Viscera of the Domestic Animals*, 2nd edn, Verlag Paul Parey, Berlin, pp. 291–293.

Simpson, K.W., Shiroma, J.T., Biller, D.S., Wicks, J., Johnson, S.E., Dimski, D. and Chew, D. (1994) Ante mortem diagnosis of pancreatitis in four cats. *Journal of Small Animal Practice*, 35, 93–99.

Spaulding, K.A., Cohn, L.A., Miller, R.T. and Hardie, E.M. (1990) Enteric duplication in two dogs. *Veterinary Radiology*, 31, 83–88.

Stowater, J.L. and Lamb, C.R. (1989) Ultrasonographic features of paraprostatic cysts in nine dogs. *Veterinary Radiology*, 30, 232–239.

Stowater, J.L., Lamb, C.R. and Schelling, S.H. (1990) Ultrasonographic features of canine hepatic nodular hyperplasia. *Veterinary Radiology*, 31, 268–272.

Tanaka, S., Kitamura, T., Imaoka, S, Sasaki, Y., Taniguchi, H. and Ishiguro, S. (1983) Hepatocellular carcinoma: sonographic and histologic correlation. *American Journal of Roentgenology*, 140, 701–707.

Taylor, K.J.W. and Wells, P.N.T. (1989) Tissue characterization. *Ultrasound in Medicine and Biology*, 15, 421–428.

Taylor, K.J.W., Riely, C.A., Hammers, L., Flax, S., Weltin, G., Garcia-Tsao, G., Conn, H.O., Kuc, R. and Barwick, K.W. (1986) Quantitative ultrasonography attenuation in normal liver and in patients with diffuse liver disease: importance of fat. *Radiology*, 160, 65–71.

Teefey, S.A., Baron, R.L. and Bigler, S.A. (1991) Sonography of the gallbladder: significance of striated (layered) thickening of the gallbladder wall. *American Journal of Roentgenology*, 156, 945–947.

Thijssen, J.M. and Oosterveld, B.J. (1990) Texture in tissue echograms: speckle or information? *Journal of Ultrasound in Medicine*, 9, 215–229.

Tidwell, A.S. and Penninck, D.G. (1992) Ultrasonography of gastrointestinal foreign bodies. *Veterinary Radiology and Ultrasound*, 33, 160–169.

Tidwell, A.S., Ullman, S.L. and Schelling, S.H. (1990) Urinoma (paraureteral pseudocyst) in a dog. *Veterinary Radiology*, 31, 203–206.

Voorhout, G. (1990) X-ray-computed tomography, nephrotomography, and ultrasonography of the adrenal glands of healthy dogs. *American Journal of Veterinary Research*, 51, 625–631.

Voorhout, G., Rijnberk, A., Sjollema, B.E. and van den Ingh, T.S.G.A.M. (1990) Nephrotomography and ultrasonography for localization of hyperfunctioning adrenocortical tumors in dogs. *American Journal of Veterinary Research*, 51, 1280–1285.

Walter, P.A., Feeney, D.A., Johnston, G.R. and Fletcher, T. (1987a) Feline renal ultrasonography: quantitative analyses of imaged anatomy. *American Journal of Veterinary Research*, 48, 596–599.

Walter, P.A., Feeney, D.A., Johnston, G.R. and O'Leary, T.P. (1987b) Ultrasonographic evaluation of renal parenchymal diseases in dogs: 32 cases (1981–1986). *Journal of the American Veterinary Medical Association*, 191, 999–1007.

Walter, P.A., Johnston, G.R., Feeney, D.A. and O'Brien, T.D. (1987c) Renal ultrasonography in healthy cats. *American Journal of Veterinary Research*, 48, 600–607.

Walter, P.A., Johnston, G.R., Feeney, D.A. and O'Brien, T.D. (1988) Applications of ultrasonography in the diagnosis of parenchymal kidney disease in cats: 24 cases (1981–1986). *Journal of the American Veterinary Medical Association*, 192, 92–98.

Wegener, N., Borsch, G., Schneider, J., Wedmann, B., Winter, R. and Zacharias, J. (1987) Gallbladder wall thickening: a frequent finding in various non-biliary disorders. *Journal of Clinical Ultrasound*, 15, 307–312.

Wernecke, K., Vassallo, P., Bick, U., Diederich, S. and Peters, P.E. (1992a) The distinction between benign and malignant liver tumors on sonography: value of a hypoechoic halo. *American Journal of Roentgenology*, 159, 1005–1009.

Wernecke, K., Henke, L., Vassallo, P., von Bassewitz, D.B., Diederich, S., Peters, P.E. and Edel, G. (1992b) Pathological explanation for hypoechoic halo seen on sonograms of malignant livers: an in vitro correlative study. *American Journal of Roentgenology*, 159, 1010–1016.

Whiteley, M.B., Feeney, D.A., Whiteley, L.O. and Hardy, R.M. (1989) Ultrasonographic appearance of primary and metastatic canine hepatic tumors: a review of 48 cases. *Journal of Ultrasound in Medicine*, 8, 621–630.

Worlicek, H., Dunz, D. and Engelhard, K. (1989) Ultrasonic examination of the fluid-filled stomach. *Journal of Clinical Ultrasound*, 17, 5–14.

Wrigley, R.H. (1991) Ultrasonography of the spleen: life-threatening splenic disorders. In: Kaplan, P.M. (ed.), *Problems in Veterinary Medicine*, vol. 3. Saunders, Philadelphia, pp. 574–581.

Wrigley, R.H., Konde, L.J., Park, R.D. and Lebel, J.L. (1987) Ultrasonographic diagnosis of portacaval shunts in young dogs. *Journal of the American Veterinary Medical Association*, 191, 421–424.

Yeager, A.E. and Anderson, W.I. (1989) Study of association between histologic features and echogenicity of architecturally normal cat kidneys. *American Journal of Veterinary Research*, 50, 860–863.

Zanotti, S.W., Kaplan, P.M., Garlick, D.S. and Lamb, C.R. (1989) Endocarditis associated with a urinary bladder foreign body in a dog. *Journal of the American Animal Hospital Association*, 25, 557–561.

Zeman, R.K., Taylor, K.J.W., Rosenfield, A.T., Schwartz, A. and Gold, J.A. (1981) Acute experimental biliary obstruction in the dog: sonographic findings and clinical implications. *American Journal of Roentgenology*, 136, 965–967.

Zeman, R.K., Pauschter, D.M., Schiebler, M.L., Choyke, P.L., Jaffe, M.H. and Clark, L.R. (1985) Hepatic imaging: current status. *Radiologic Clinics of North America*, 23, 473–487.

3 Small Animal Reproductive Ultrasonography

G.C.W. England

Department of Farm Animal and Equine Medicine and Surgery, Royal Veterinary College, University of London, Hawkshead Lane, North Mymms, Hatfield, Hertfordshire AL9 7TA, UK

Introduction

The use of diagnostic real-time B-mode ultrasound for medical imaging has increased considerably over the past ten years. Ultrasonography has had a particular impact in the field of reproduction. Not only has it proved to be extremely valuable as a tool in obstetrics, but its use in research has allowed improved understanding of normal reproductive physiology.

This chapter addresses the use of diagnostic ultrasound in small animal reproduction, and aims to highlight both normal variations and pathological conditions that may be met in clinical practice. There have been limited studies with ultrasound in the cat; attention will be drawn to those areas where species differences are relevant.

The Female Reproductive Tract

The uterus

The uterus lies dorsal to the bladder, but its position may vary with the extent of bladder filling, and the size of the uterus and the stage of the reproductive cycle. Imaging is most conveniently performed with the bitch in the standing position after clipping the hair of the ventral abdomen. However, dorsal and lateral recumbent positions are preferred by some ultrasonographers.

The normal non-pregnant uterus

The uterine body of the pre-pubertal and non-pregnant bitch during anoestrus may be less than 1 cm in transverse diameter; imaging the uterus at this time can therefore be difficult (Bondestam *et al.*, 1983; England and Allen, 1989a; Stowater *et al.*, 1989). The uterus may be identified dorsal or dorso-lateral to the bladder, and can be shown to be tubular by imaging in two perpendicular planes. The uterus may be more readily imaged in older, pluriparous bitches, when the uterine bifurcation can be detected in approximately 40% of cases. Similarly, the distal portions of the two uterine horns can also be imaged. These and the uterine body are composed of two distinct layers: a central homogeneous, relatively hypoechoic region surrounded by a peripheral hyperechoic layer (England and Yeager, 1993). These layers are likely to be endometrium and myometrium with uterine serosa, respectively.

During oestrus, the uterus becomes increasingly hypoechoic but develops central radiating hyperechoic lines, a change which can be induced by the administration of oestrogen to ovariectomized bitches (England and Allen, 1989a). It is likely that this ultrasonographic appearance is the result of oedematous endometrial folds similar to those seen in the mare during oestrus (Ginther, 1986). Indeed, histological examination has confirmed the presence of extracelluar fluid within the stratum spongiosum during oestrus (England, 1990). The changes in uterine echotexture are associated with an increase in uterine diameter, and central uterine fluid may be identified in mated bitches (England and Yeager, 1993). Similar endometrial changes have been identified in mares and in women, and attempts have been made to relate these findings to the timing of ovulation and the likelihood of conception (Allen, 1989; Nowroozi *et al.*, 1991). In the bitch, however, the changes in uterine size and echogenicity are not sufficiently specific to allow the prediction of ovulation time.

Uterine transverse sectional diameter continues to increase during early metoestrus (dioestrus), although the appearance of the uterus is similar to that seen during proestrus (England and Yeager, 1993). This increase in diameter occurs in both pregnant and non-pregnant bitches, which is contrary to the claim of Cartee and Rowles (1984) that the uterine enlargement of pregnancy can be detected from seven days after mating.

The uterus of the cat has a similar ultrasonographic appearance to that of the dog, although since the cat is an induced ovulator, changes during the luteal phase are only noted after mating or, occasionally, spontaneous ovulation.

Abnormalities of the non-pregnant uterus

Cystic endometrial hyperplasia

Endometrial hyperplasia occurs during metoestrus of the bitch and appears to be a direct effect of the hormone progesterone upon the endometrium; it is not noted in the queen. During metoestrus there are characteristic gross changes in the appearance of the uterus, which becomes tightly coiled. This appearance is not often detected by ultrasound, when the uterus appears relatively homogeneous and hypoechoic.

In some older bitches the endometrium may become markedly thickened and cystic during the luteal phase. Affected animals may show vague clinical signs of lethargy and anorexia, although frequently the condition is not diagnosed unless it develops into pyometra. It has been suggested that sub-clinical cystic endometrial hyperplasia may be responsible for the failure of conception and may cause embryonic resorption. Therefore, ultrasound examination of middle-aged infertile bitches may be rewarding. In certain cases the cystic lesions may be microscopic and not identifiable with ultrasound, although the uterine diameter may be larger than anticipated for the animal's age, parity and breed. Ultrasound examination may demonstrate multiple small (up to 5 mm diameter) fluid-filled, anechoic cysts scattered throughout the endometrium. Cystic lesions are most easily identified in the uterine body, which is conveniently imaged when the bladder is filled with urine. Several lesions may coalesce to give the appearance of larger anechoic zones within the uterus. Uterine cysts have no well-defined border, and are frequently asymmetrically positioned, since they are not lumenal structures. However, uterine fluid may also be noted (Fig. 3.1).

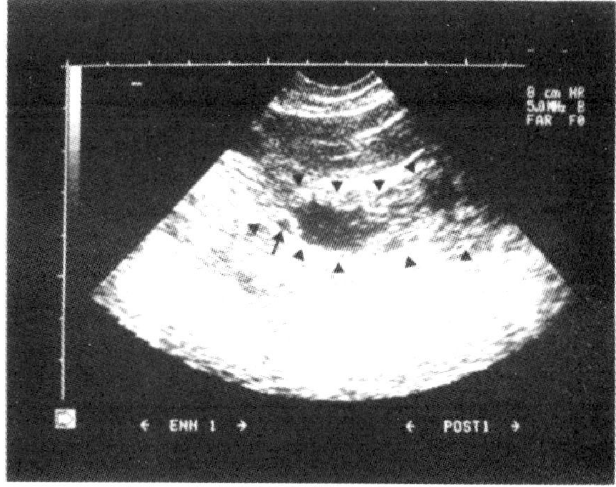

Fig. 3.1. Ultrasound image of the uterus (arrowheads) of a bitch with cystic endometrial hyperplasia. Small circular anechoic cystic lesions may be identified within the uterine wall (arrow), and free anechoic lumenal fluid with scant echogenic particles is present centrally.

Pyometra

Pyometra may follow the development of cystic endometrial hyperplasia unless it is the result of exogenous oestrogen or progesterone therapy. Pyometra may occur during the same metoestrus in which cystic endometrial hyperplasia is diagnosed, but it is likely that bacteria colonize the uterus during oestrus when the cervix is patent, with clinical pyometra developing during the following metoestrus. Pyometra in the cat may follow mating or spontaneous ovulation.

The early ultrasonographic diagnosis of pyometra, before the onset of clinical signs, has been reported (Fayrer-Hosken *et al.*, 1991). In most cases, however, ultrasound examination is performed because of the clinical signs of vaginal discharge and anorexia, although both may occur normally in the pregnant bitch (England and Allen, 1990a).

Ultrasonographically, the uterus has an increased diameter and may be folded upon itself so that two or more sections of each horn are imaged in a single plane. The uterine diameter may vary, depending on whether the pyometra is 'open' or 'closed'. The wall of the uterus is commonly increased in thickness (up to 2 mm) and is relatively hyperechoic with respect to the surrounding tissue. The uterine lumen is frequently grossly dilated by anechoic fluid (Fig. 3.2). Small echogenic particles and mass lesions may be identified, which probably represent inflammatory debris or haemorrhage, although mucus may have a similar ultrasonographic appearance. Poffenbarger and Feeney (1986) noted that when the uterus was imaged at its proximal (ovarian) end, the transverse image had a target-like appearance. These authors noted an outer echogenic area, an inner hypoechoic to anechoic ring and a central hyperechoic zone. They suggested that the hypoechoic region was the result of vascular engorgement and secretory gland activity.

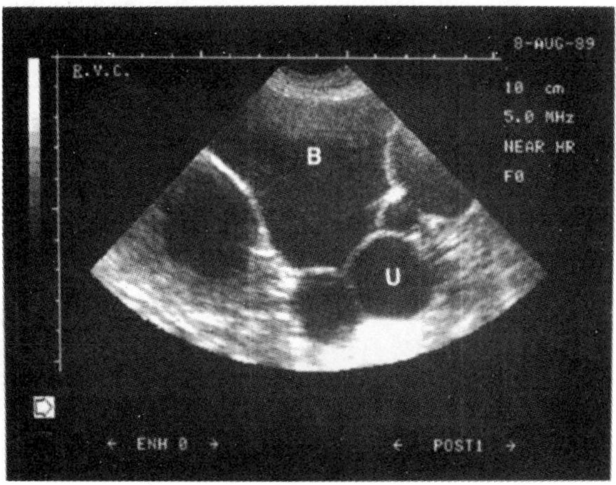

Fig. 3.2. Ultrasound image of the uterus of a bitch with pyometra. Several portions of the anechoic fluid-dilated uterus (U) have been imaged, since the organ is coiled upon itself. The uterus has a thin echogenic wall, and is positioned dorsal and lateral to the bladder (B).

If distention is not marked, the fluid-filled uterus may be mistaken for loops of intestine. However, the uterus lacks peristalsis, does not contain gas and can be traced to a position dorsal to the bladder and ventral to the colon at the pelvic inlet. Diagnosis is more simple when the diameter of the uterus is greater than that of the small intestine. With larger volumes of fluid there is usually a far enhancement of the ultrasound image (Feeney and Johnston, 1986b). Cases of unilateral pyometra, as a result of stenosis or segmental aplasia of the uterine horns, may give a confusing appearance, since only a portion of the uterus is involved and the fluid-filled swelling is often not tubular.

It is not possible, using ultrasound, to distinguish other causes of uterine fluid accumulation (mucometra and hydrometra) from cases of pyometra.

Recently, Renton *et al.* (1993) suggested that ultrasonography could be used both to diagnose pyometra and to monitor bitches during treatment with exogenous prostaglandins.

Uterine mass lesions

Uterine neoplasms have been diagnosed using ultrasound (Feeney and Johnston, 1986b; Poffenbarger and Feeney, 1986). These lesions are uncommon in the bitch and queen, and since ultrasound cannot readily differentiate neoplastic from granulomatous tissue, it should not be relied upon as the sole diagnostic tool. Characteristically, uterine neoplasms are homogeneous mass lesions attached to the uterine wall which project into the lumen and may produce uterine fluid accumulation (Poffenbarger and Feeney, 1986). Uterine neoplasms may be echogenic or have a complex mixed echogenicity if they are necrotic or fibrotic (Feeney and Johnston, 1986b). Ultrasound-guided needle biopsy may be useful to establish the nature of these lesions.

Uterine stump granuloma

It is extremely difficult to differentiate uterine neoplasia and granulomata using ultrasound alone. However, ultrasound examination may provide diagnostic information when investigating bitches with chronic draining flank fistulae, or chronic, purulent vaginal discharges following ovariohysterectomy.

Granulomata or abscesses usually comprise irregular, mixed-echogenicity tissue, which arises dorsal to the bladder and ventral to the colon. The presence of discrete, fluid-filled zones within the mass may indicate uterine stump abscessation. Failure to identify a stump lesion does not eliminate this as a diagnosis. The infusion of saline into the vagina, using a Foley catheter, will allow a more accurate identification of the proximal portion of the stump.

Pregnancy

Doppler and A-mode ultrasonography have been used to diagnose pregnancy in the bitch for some time (Allen and Meredith, 1981). More recently, real-time B-mode ultrasound has been found to be reliable and accurate (Bondestam *et al.*, 1983; Cartee and Rowles, 1984; Inaba *et al.*, 1984; Toal *et al.*, 1986). However, several studies using ultrasound have been confused by the authors' assumption that pregnancy commenced on the first day of mating. This has resulted in a wide time range over which the features of pregnancy are said to be detected. Parturition in the dog occurs, however, over a narrow spread of three days when considered in relation to the pre-ovulatory surge of plasma luteinizing hormone (LH) (Concannon *et al.*, 1983; Concannon and Rendano, 1983). The LH surge precedes ovulation by approximately two days (Smith and McDonald, 1971; Concannon *et al.*, 1977) and oocytes are not fertilizable for a further two days. Matings which occur before the LH peak are only fertile if spermatozoa reside within the reproductive tract, 'waiting' for ovulation and for oocytes to become fertilizable. An 'early' mating therefore results in an apparently long gestation period. Conversely, oocytes may remain fertilizable for at least five days after ovulation; a 'late' mating results in an apparently short pregnancy length (England *et al.*, 1989). This information is relevant since ultrasound examination of bitches during early pregnancy in relation to an 'early' mating, may result in a false negative diagnosis. Pregnancy may be confirmed from 17 days after the LH surge (Yeager and Concannon, 1990a; England and Yeager, 1993). However, in practice the time of the LH surge is not known and ultrasound examination is commonly performed one month after the last mating.

Diagnosis of early pregnancy

Gestational sacs may first be imaged from 17 days after the LH surge as noted above, at which time they appear as spherical, anechoic structures, approximately 2 mm in diameter. The dorsal and ventral margins of the conceptus produce characteristic bright specular echoes, similar to those observed 14 days after ovulation in the mare (Ginther, 1986). The uterine wall surrounding the gestational sacs is generally more echogenic than the uterine wall between the conceptual swellings.

The anechoic fluid is that of the yolk sac which has completely filled the chorionic cavity. The accumulation of sufficient yolk sac fluid is the determinant of when pregnancy can first be imaged. At this time the embryo is located adjacent to the uterine wall and is not imaged; placentation is considered to be choriovitelline. The conceptus rapidly increases in size and may lose its spherical outline, becoming oblate in appearance. From day 22 after the LH surge the conceptus is approximately 7 mm in diameter and 15 mm in length, and the embryo may be imaged (Yeager and Concannon, 1990a; England and Yeager, 1993). The embryo appears as a homogeneous, oblong-shaped, hyperechoic structure, which becomes increasingly separated from the uterine wall and protrudes into the anechoic yolk sac. The presence of the embryo's heart-beat can be detected from approximately day 24 after the LH surge. It appears as a rapid flickering in the centre of the embryonic mass. From this time onward the embryo appears to have two poles, although this development has actually occurred some time previously.

The formation of the fetal membranes is complicated and may be confusing ultrasonographically, since a three-dimensional structure is imaged in only a two-dimensional slice (Fig. 3.3). From 24 days after the LH surge it is possible to identify a second fluid-filled region adjacent to the embryo; this is the developing allantois. The allantois, a diverticulum of the hind-gut, appears initially as a nearly spherical structure within the conceptual swelling. The allantois increases in volume and becomes intercalated between the chorion and yolk sac. It has a greater volume than the yolk sac 28 days after the LH surge. The allantoic membrane is less echogenic than that of the yolk sac, and the latter develops an extensively folded appearance when it is surrounded by the allantois (Fig. 3.4). The yolk sac cavity may be almost obliterated by the extensive folding of its membrane. When examined in the longitudinal plane, the collapsing yolk sac can be identified as a tubular structure when completely surrounded by the allantois (Fig. 3.5), although it subsequently assumes a more spherical outline. From 30 days after the LH surge, allantoic fluid predominates within the gestational sac, surrounding the fetus. Several fine fetal membranes are often identified at this time; those directed towards the periphery are fused portions of the allantois, whilst the amnion is positioned centrally, surrounding the fetus. The amnion may be noted from 25 days after the LH surge and increases in volume to become a sizeable structure during mid- and late pregnancy.

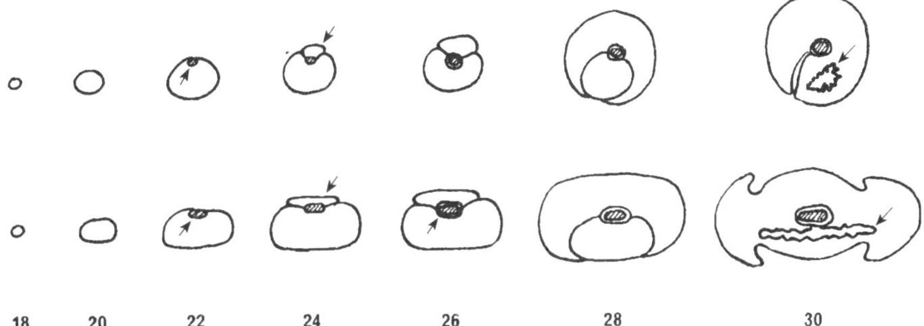

Fig. 3.3. Schematic representation of the ultrasonographic development of the dog conceptus from 18 to 30 days after the LH surge when imaged in the transverse (top) and sagittal (bottom) planes.

18 days: The fluid-filled yolk sac can be imaged and appears as a spherical anechoic structure with specular echoes produced by the dorsal and ventral surface of the conceptus. No embryonic tissue can be imaged.

20 days: The conceptus is similar to day 18, although it is larger and may be oblate in outline.

22 days: Embryonic tissue (arrow) can be imaged adjacent to the uterine wall. This is visible due to the enlarging allantois which pushes the embryo centrally.

24 days: The almost spherical fluid-filled allantois (arrow) is imaged adjacent to the embryo.

26 days: The allantois has increased in volume and is becoming intercalated between the chorion and the yolk sac. The amnion is visible as a fine hypoechoic membrane surrounding the embryo (arrow).

28 days: The allantois has increased in size and partially surrounds the yolk sac. The yolk sac is oblate in appearance and smaller in volume than the allantois.

30 days: The allantoic membranes have surrounded the yolk sac and joined together. The tubular yolk sac (arrow) is easily identified since its membrane is more echogenic than the allantois and it has an extensively folded appearance. The embryo has increased in size.

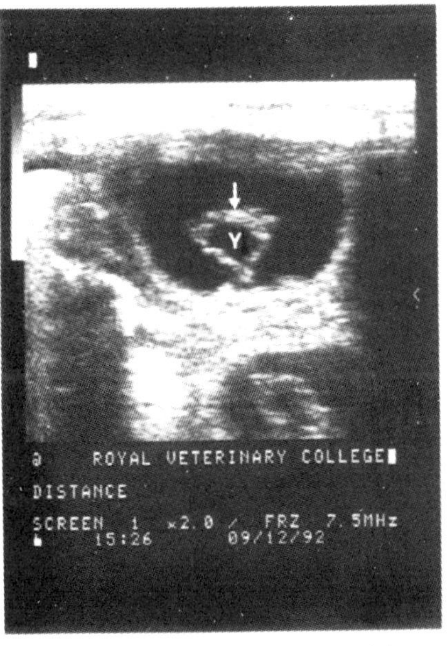

a

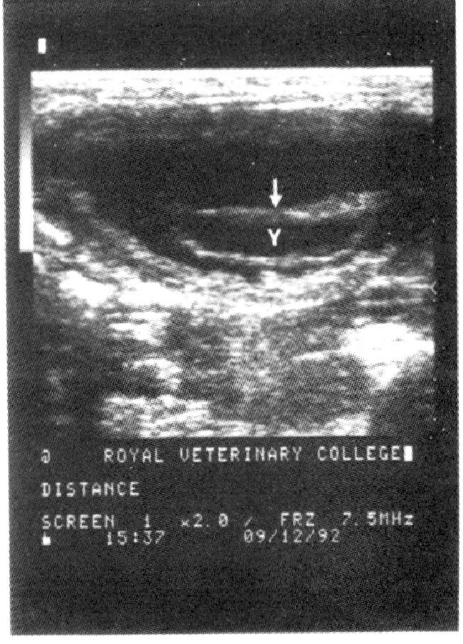

b

Fig. 3.4. Transverse **(a)** and sagittal **(b)** ultrasound images of a dog pregnancy 32 days after the LH surge. The folded and echogenic yolk sac membrane (arrow) is prominent surrounding the yolk sac (Y). The embryo is not present in this imaging plane.

The dog's zonary placenta wraps around the central portion of the conceptus like a waistband. When imaging in the longitudinal plane the curved and thickened edge of the placenta is seen; this represents the region of the marginal haematoma (Fig. 3.5).

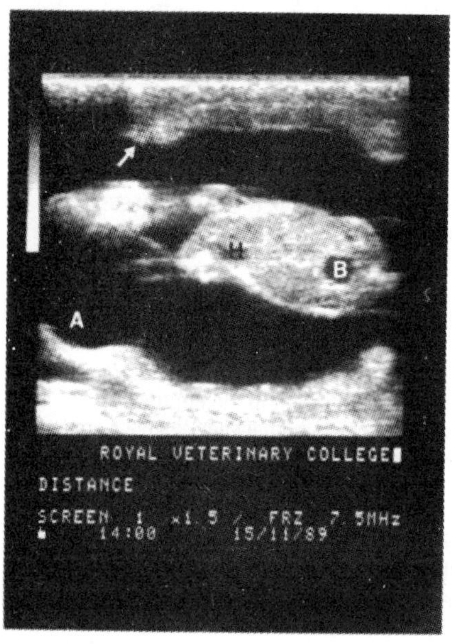

Fig. 3.5. Sagittal ultrasound image of a dog pregnancy 55 days after the LH surge. The fetus lies within the margins of the zonary placenta, the head extending partially beyond the marginal haematoma (arrow). The fetal heart (H) and bladder (B) are clearly defined, as are portions of the fore- and hindlimbs. The predominant fluid surrounding the fetus is allantoic (A).

Diagnosis of mid-pregnancy

The most rapid growth of the fetus occurs between days 32 and 55. Before this time, only the heart and a focal anechoic region within the cranial pole (Yeager *et al.*, 1992) may be identified. However, from 32 days after the LH surge, limb buds and the choroidal plexus of the brain may be imaged (Yeager *et al.*, 1992), and from day 35, clear differentiation into head, trunk and abdomen is detectable (England *et al.*, 1990b). The fetal skeleton becomes evident from 40 days onwards when fetal bone appears hyperechoic, and casts acoustic shadows. At this stage the hyperechoic heart valves can be imaged and are seen to be moving. The great vessels can be traced cranially and caudally. Generally, from 40 days onwards the trunk diameter exceeds the head diameter (Yeager *et al.*, 1992). Pulmonary tissue surrounding the heart is hyperechoic with respect to the liver, and the line of their separation (the region of the forming diaphragm) can easily be identified. From 45 days onwards it is possible to identify the anechoic stomach caudal to the liver in more than 90% of fetuses, and a few days later the bladder is identifiable in the caudal abdomen; with careful examination the urachus may be imaged.

Diagnosis of late pregnancy

The appearance of the fetal skeleton becomes enhanced during late pregnancy; the head, spinal column and ribs produce intense reflections that are easily identifiable. All structures previously described become larger and more easy to identify (Fig. 3.5). In the last 20 days of pregnancy the kidneys can be imaged; these are frequently more echogenic than observed in the adult animal. Fetal vasculature becomes obvious, and the umbilical vessels may be traced from the liver to the umbilicus. In late pregnancy intestine may be detected (Yeager *et al.*, 1992).

Pregnancy diagnosis in the cat

The cat is an induced ovulator, and therefore in most cases pregnancy length can be estimated from the mating date. Uterine enlargement of pregnancy is claimed to be evident from four days after mating (Davidson *et al.*, 1986). However, these authors did not examine ovulating non-pregnant queens for comparison. The accurate imaging of a gestational sac is possible from 11 days after mating, when the conceptus appears similar to that of the dog. Embryonic tissue can be imaged from day 14, and cardiac motion is often detected one day later. Fetal structures appear similar to those described for the dog. Whilst embryonic and fetal development may appear to occur earlier in the queen than the bitch, when events are related to the fertilization period they are similar.

Determination of gestational age

In many cases pregnancy diagnosis is undertaken for the interest of the owner. However, in bitches with multiple or uncertain mating times, the ability to determine gestational age and to predict the time of expected parturition is a considerable advantage.

The ultrasonographic appearance of certain organs may be useful for the prediction of gestational age, e.g. the fetal bladder is usually only imaged during the last 20 days of gestation. Many studies which examined ultrasonographic changes during pregnancy were flawed since they did not accurately identify gestational age (Bondestam *et al.*, 1983; Cartee and Rowles, 1984).

England *et al.* (1990b) made assessments of the diameter of the conceptus, the combined thickness of the uterus and the placenta, the fetal occipito-sacral length, the biparietal head diameter, the trunk diameter, and the diameter of the fetal stomach and bladder in a group of 50 bitches. They showed that for a single breed, certain measures had a linear relation to the gestational age during mid- and late pregnancy. Yeager *et al.*, (1992) made similar estimates of fetal size during pregnancy and found that the best correlation was between fetal head diameter and gestational age. These results were similar to those of England *et al.* (1990b), although the latter authors suggested that the most important aspect of an analysis of fetal aging was an estimate of the variability associated with a given prediction, rather than a simple correlation. They showed that the variability for single parameter estimates was in the range of 3.8–4.7 days, and that this could be significantly reduced when multiple regression analysis was performed.

In the cat, Davidson *et al.* (1986) suggested that fetal crown–rump length was not an accurate predictor of gestational age; the difficulties of assessing this parameter have been described for the dog (England *et al.*, 1990b). Other studies have found that measures of head and body diameter have a high accuracy for the estimation of gestational age and the prediction of parturition (Beck *et al.*, 1990).

Accuracy of pregnancy diagnosis with ultrasound

It is unlikely that bitches or queens in late pregnancy would be incorrectly diagnosed as pregnant or non-pregnant. However, earlier examinations may produce inaccuracies, particularly in the bitch. The greatest problem is determining the actual gestational age, since bitches mated early in the oestrous cycle may be presented for examination before ultrasonographic evidence of pregnancy can be detected (England and Allen, 1990b). False negative diagnoses may also be produced by overlooking a conceptus, or because of acoustic artifacts produced by gas or faecal material 'hiding' a conceptus. False positive diagnoses (Shille and Gontarek, 1985) may be the result of confusion of empty loops of small intestine with early pregnancy, although intestine can be shown to be tubular by imaging in two planes. Fetal resorption may also produce a disparity between the number of conceptuses imaged and the number of offspring born.

Estimation of fetal number

The accuracy of detecting absolute fetal number is poor (Toal *et al.*, 1986; England and Allen, 1990b). Recently, England (1992) suggested that, for the bitch, the greatest accuracy was before day 30 after the LH surge, when 38% of examinations were successful in predicting fetal number. Generally the number of fetuses is underestimated; the error being associated with overlooking fetuses, or mistaking them as already counted or due to acoustic artifacts. The accuracy is reduced for larger litters (Shille and Gontarek, 1985; England, 1990), and so England (1992) classified bitches as having either five pups or more, or four pups or fewer, and found the efficiency of prediction to be 97%. The accuracy of predicting actual fetal number is low in later pregnancy (Shille and Gontarek, 1985; England *et al.*, 1990b). For examinations between 30 and 50 days of pregnancy England (1992) found the accuracy to be 18%, and after 50 days of pregnancy to be 8%.

Abnormalities of pregnancy

There have been limited ultrasonographic studies of pregnancy in the queen and there is little information available concerning abnormalities of this period. The following discussion is relevant primarily to the bitch.

Embryonic resorption
Should embryonic death occur before 25 days after ovulation, there is usually complete resorption of the conceptus (Evans, 1979). The incidence of embryonic death followed by resorption is not known, although Andersen and Simpson (1973) reported the frequency in the bitch to be approximately 11% in relation to the number of corpora lutea. Resorption of multiple conceptuses with continuation of a pregnancy in the absence of clinical disease has been reported (Allen, 1982). England (1992) recently demonstrated that five of 100 bitches suffered isolated spontaneous embryonic resorption with continuation of the pregnancy, and a second study demonstrated an incidence of 13% in 31 bitches (Muller and

Arbeiter, 1993). There appears to be no difference between those bitches which have previously had reproductive disease, and those which have previously been normal (England, 1992). The ultrasonographic components of embryonic resorption are: reduced volume and changes in echogenicity of the embryonic fluid, loss of the embryonic mass and heartbeat, collapse of the conceptus with thickening and inward bulging of the uterine wall, and reduced size in comparison with adjacent conceptuses. Following resorption, the uterus appears homogeneous and moderately hypoechoic (Fig. 3.6), having a similar ultrasonographic appearance to the post-partum uterus (England and Allen, 1989c; Yeager and Concannon, 1990a).

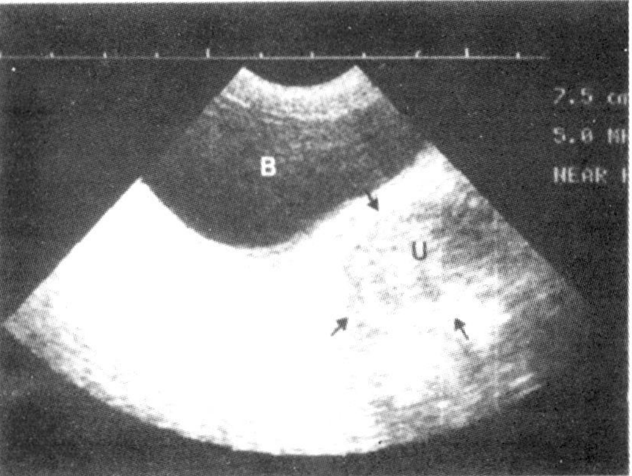

Fig. 3.6. Ultrasound image of the uterus (U) of a bitch following embryonic resorption. The uterus is positioned adjacent to the bladder (B) and appears similar to that seen after parturition.

Fetal abortion

Abortion of fetuses has been demonstrated in the bitch 'by use of ultrasound (Taverne *et al.*, 1989; England, 1992). Abortion is associated with the passage of large quantities of mucohaemorrhagic material, and may be noted from 35 days of pregnancy onwards. Initial findings are an increased echogenicity of the fetal fluid and thickening of the uterine wall. Fetal tissue may be difficult to identify and heart-beats are absent. Later the fetal fluid may become speckled in appearance due to breakdown of fetal tissue. These changes are similar to those seen in other species during abortion (Simpson *et al.*, 1982; Ginther *et al.*, 1985). Following abortion, the uterus assumes an ultrasonographic appearance similar to that seen after parturition.

Fetal abnormalities

Ultrasound examination of the fetus has been used for some time in man for the diagnosis of abnormalities, and common imaging regimes claim to have a high success rate for detecting normal and abnormal fetuses (Sabbagha *et al.*, 1985). However, human fetuses are large and are frequently single, while in the dog, multiple fetuses are present, and it is not possible to reliably image each one during late pregnancy, which is the time when most anomalies are evident. Fetal abnormalities are therefore not commonly detected by ultrasound in the dog. Enlargement of the gestational sac and herniation of the small intestine was reported in a single pup (Poffenbarger and Feeney, 1986), and a case of hydrops fetalis was diagnosed by Allen *et al.* (1989). In the latter case fluid was identified within the fetal thorax, pericardial sac, and subcutaneously. Fetal pathology was noted in a cat with ethylene glycol poisoning (Adams *et al.*, 1991).

Dystocia and fetal death

Ultrasound is of particular value for assessing fetal viability. Heart-beats can be detected from 23 days after the LH surge, and generalized fetal movements are apparent from day 28 (Barr, 1988). It has been suggested that ultrasound may be useful for the detection of fetal distress by detecting changes in heart rate at the time of parturition (Barr, 1988). In dog fetuses, assessments of heart rate are often inaccurate (Verstegen *et al.*, 1993). These workers found rates to be greater than previously reported (up to 230 beats per minute), and showed a normal increase during pregnancy and a significant decrease at parturition. Poffenbarger and Feeney (1986) proposed that detection of a heart rate less than twice that of the maternal rate suggested significant fetal distress, although Taverne *et al.* (1989) found transient bradycardia and tachycardia in normal fetuses and suggested that such assessments were of little value.

Signs of fetal death detected by ultrasound include: absence of heart-beat, lack of fetal movement, reduced volume and increased echogenicity of fetal fluid and accumulation of gas within the fetal stomach, fetus or uterus. The latter should not be confused with artifacts produced by overlying intestine.

Post-partum uterine involution

Following parturition, the uterine body and horns are easily imaged. The horns remain enlarged and fluid-filled for a variable time after parturition (England and Allen, 1989a). Central lumenal fluid is not invariably anechoic and may have echogenic material within it. Uterine diameter decreases during the first two days after parturition and assumes a characteristic ultrasonographic appearance. In the first week the horns are composed of multiple layers of varying echogenicity and have multiple discrete enlargements with hypoechoic centres at placental sites (Yeager and Concannon, 1990b). Large variations are noted in uterine diameter between placental sites and interplacental zones (Pharr and Post, 1992). The uterus may return to the size noted during anoestrus within 4 to 6 weeks (England, 1990; Pharr and Post, 1992); however, uterine involution is not complete ultrasonographically until 15 weeks post-partum.

Post-partum abnormalities

Retained fetus

The presence of retained fetuses may be diagnosed clinically by the animal's behaviour and a persistent vulval discharge. Fetuses may be readily diagnosed with ultrasound by the presence of echogenic skeletons. Fetal viability may be assessed as previously discussed.

Retained placentae

The retention of placental tissue in the bitch and queen is not common. It may be characterized clinically by a persistent green-coloured vaginal discharge. The diagnosis of placental retention with ultrasound has not been reported. This may be complicated, since soft tissue debris or blood clots may persist normally within the uterus after parturition (Pharr and Post, 1992), and may be indistinguishable from remnants of placental tissue.

Metritis

Uterine infection after parturition is rare. It occurs most commonly secondary to dystocia or fetal or placental retention. The diagnosis is commonly made on the clinical signs of a persistent vaginal discharge and systemic illness. However, ultrasound may be of value in these cases since imaging should allow the elimination of retained fetal or placental material as causal factors. Ultrasound may be used to monitor uterine wall thickness as well as the success of treatment in reducing uterine fluid accumulation.

Sub-involution of placental sites

It is not uncommon for one or more placental sites to fail to involute normally after parturition. In these cases there is a haemorrhagic vaginal discharge which persists until the subsequent oestrus. It may be possible to use ultrasound to identify those placental sites which do not reduce in size after parturition. These areas may have a similar ultrasonographic appearance to normal involution, but are larger in diameter and may have persistent mixed-echogenicity lumenal fluid.

The ovary

The ovaries of the dog are difficult to examine with ultrasound, due to their small size and superficial location. During anoestrus the ovaries are located adjacent to the caudal pole of the kidney, level with the fifth lumbar vertebrae. They are positioned mid-abdominally in the standing bitch, close to the lateral abdominal wall. Imaging of the ovary is therefore best achieved with the bitch either in the standing position after clipping the hair from the lateral abdominal wall, or with the bitch in dorsal recumbency, with the transducer placed over the ventro-lateral abdomen. During oestrus the position of the ovaries may vary slightly and they are often located more caudally and ventrally (England and Allen, 1989a).

Ovarian cyclical events

There has been controversy concerning the ability to image the ovaries of the bitch and, while early studies claimed to have detected ovulation (Inaba *et al.*, 1984; Wilson and Hayward, 1985), these have been challenged (Allen and Davies, 1984). Ovarian follicular development has since been monitored (England and Allen, 1989a; Wallace *et al.*, 1989). More recent studies have characterized the changes occurring around the time of ovulation in the bitch (Wallace *et al.*, 1992; Boyd *et al.*, 1993; England and Yeager, 1993; Hayer *et al.*, 1993). During anoestrus, the ovaries of the bitch are less than 1.5 × 1.0 × 0.8 cm in size, and are relatively homogeneous in their echotexture. They appear hypoechoic with respect to the surrounding small intestine and are frequently less echogenic than the adjacent renal cortex. When examined in a water bath, small anechoic follicles may be identified (England and Allen, 1989b), although these are not usually imaged *in vivo*.

During the onset of proestrus, small fluid-filled anechoic follicles may be detected within the ovarian stroma, becoming obvious in all bitches between six to eight days before the plasma LH surge. When first imaged, the internal diameter of follicles is 1–2 mm. Follicles enlarge during proestrus, and become less spherical in outline, with their margins being somewhat triangular in appearance (Fig. 3.7a). At this stage ovarian volume has increased, although the outline of the

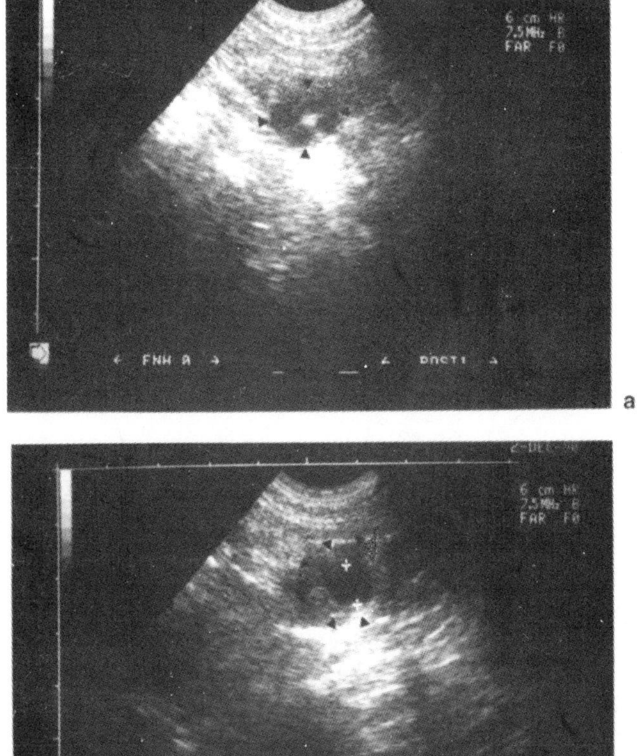

Fig. 3.7. Ultrasound image of the ovary of a bitch during oestrus. **(a)** One day before the LH surge, demonstrating ovary (arrowheads) containing four slightly triangular anechoic follicles which do not protrude above the ovarian margin. **(b)** Four days after the LH surge, demonstrating ovary (arrowheads) containing a single, thick, hypoechoic-walled and centrally-anechoic corpus luteum (white crosses). Other luteal tissue is not present in this plane.

ovary remains smooth. The maximum follicular diameter (4–6 mm) is usually attained one day after the plasma LH surge, i.e. the day before ovulation. At this stage the ovaries appear to be somewhat nodular (blackberry-like) in outline, and their hypoechoic wall, which may be up to 1 mm in thickness, can now be imaged.

There have been differing interpretations of the follicular changes at the time of ovulation, which may be attributed to the use of different quality imaging equipment (Boyd *et al.*, 1993). Recent studies (England and Yeager, 1993) show that anechoic follicles are replaced by hypoechoic structures (presumably early corpora lutea) between one and three days after the LH surge which is the anticipated time of ovulation. These structures are present only transiently, persisting for up to 16 hours before being replaced by anechoic structures with hypoechoic walls 2 mm thick (Fig. 3.7b). England and Yeager (1993) did not identify collapsed follicles, and the presence of initially hypoechoic and subsequently cavitated luteal structures was considered normal. The fact that luteal structures are normally cavitated in the bitch has been known for some time (Evans and Cole, 1931), and the finding of centrally anechoic luteal tissue has been reported in an ultrasonographic and histological study (England and Allen, 1989b).

The time of ovulation appears to be difficult to demonstrate without repeated examination of the bitch, and it is possible that even daily examinations may fail to identify the early hypoechoic luteal structures. This is potentially a serious problem since the preovulatory follicles and early cavitated corpora lutea have a similar ultrasonographic appearance (England and Allen, 1989a; Wallace *et al.*, 1992; England and Yeager, 1993). This difficulty in discrimination is not surprising, since grossly and histologically these structures appear similar (Concannon, 1986), and the changes after ovulation are gradual, with luteinization of post-ovulatory follicles occurring over two weeks (Wildt *et al.*, 1977). Corpora lutea do not reach maximum compactness until much later (Evans and Cole, 1931). The fact that luteal structures tend to partially protrude above the follicular margin, giving the ovary an irregular appearance, and the increased thickness of the wall of the corpora lutea compared with the follicle, may allow differentiation (Fig. 3.8).

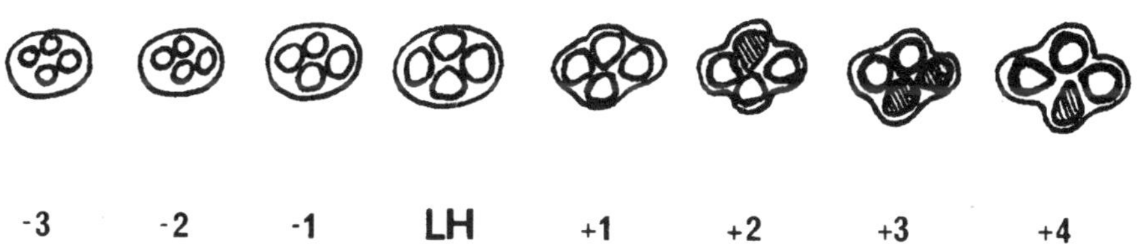

Fig. 3.8. Schematic representation of the ultrasonographic development of the canine ovary, between three days before (−3) and four days after (+4) the LH surge (LH). Follicles become enlarged and triangular in outline one day before the LH surge and reach maximum diameter one day after the LH surge. At ovulation, follicles are replaced by early hypoechoic corpora lutea, which subsequently cavitate and appear centrally anechoic with a thick hypoechoic wall. The ovary assumes a nodular appearance after the LH surge, as follicles and corpora lutea protrude above its surface.

At present, the detection of ovulation with ultrasound has limited value, especially when compared with more simple techniques such as vaginal cytology (Wright, 1990; England, 1992), measurement of plasma progesterone concentration (England *et al.*, 1989), and vaginoscopy (Lindsay, 1983; Jeffcoate and Lindsay, 1989). Should ultrasound be used to detect ovulation, the fertilization period is probably between two and four days after this event since ova are released as primary oocytes and do not mature until two to three days later (Andersen and Simpson, 1973; Phemister *et al.*, 1973).

There are no reports of the use of ultrasound to image the ovary of the cat. Ultrasonography may in any case only be of limited value (except for the confirmation of ovulation), since the queen is induced to ovulate by coitus.

Abnormalities of the ovary

The ultrasonographic detection of abnormalities of the ovary has been reported in the bitch (Feeney and Johnston, 1986a; Poffenbarger and Feeney, 1986; Wrigley and Finn, 1989; Rivers and Johnston, 1991). Lesions are infrequent but are often suggested by the clinical signs, with ultrasound being used to confirm the diagnosis.

Ovarian cysts

Ovarian cysts may frequently be imaged in the older bitch. The majority of these structures are endocrinologically inactive and have no consequence for fertility. Many structures thought to be ovarian cysts originate from the ovarian bursa, and are not significant findings.

Cystic structures are of variable appearance and size, although most commonly they contain anechoic fluid and have a thin hypoechoic wall. Careful attention should be given to the position of these structures in relation to the ovarian stroma. Lesions which are adjacent to the ovary are not usually significant, whilst those originating from the ovary may be follicular or luteal cysts. True ovarian cysts have been identified in up to 10% of bitches (Dow, 1960). Follicular cysts may be associated with persistent or prolonged oestrus, whilst luteal cysts are more commonly found in older bitches and may be associated with persistent haemorrhagic vulvar discharge. Luteal cysts may also be identified in bitches with pyometra. Should there be doubt over the significance of ovarian cystic lesions, ultrasound-guided needle aspiration may be attempted, allowing measurement of hormone concentration within the cyst fluid.

The occurrence of polycystic ovaries has been documented in the dog by the use of ultrasound (Barr, 1990). The significance of these lesions is uncertain, although they are more commonly found at the first oestrus, or after an oestrus-induction regime using exogenous gonadotrophins.

It should be remembered that certain ovarian tumours may have a cystic component.

Ovarian neoplasia

Ovarian neoplasia is uncommon in the bitch. The commonest neoplasms include granulosa cell tumours (which may become large and cystic), papillary adenomata, and papillary adenocarcinomata. The clinical signs of these tumours may include persistent oestrus or cystic endometrial hyperplasia, if they secrete oestrogen or progesterone, respectively. Clinical signs may not be noticed until the tumour is advanced. Many ovarian tumours are associated with ascites, which is easily detected with ultrasound. The ultrasonographic appearance of ovarian tumours is variable. The ovaries are frequently grossly enlarged and consist of mixed echogenicity tissue. This is often characterized by hyperechoic fibrous tissue, heterogeneous neoplastic tissue, and anechoic cystic regions (Wrigley and Finn, 1989). Bilateral ovarian adenocarcinoma was recently reported in the bitch (Goodwin *et al.*, 1990) and was characterizedby large ovaries containing multiple irregular cystic structures.

Absence of the ovaries

It may be be useful in bitches of uncertain history to determine whether ovariohysterectomy has been performed, without the need for laparotomy or the requirement to wait for the occurrence of oestrus. It is difficult to examine the ovaries of the bitch with ultrasound, and therefore this method cannot be recommended for confirmation of absence of ovarian tissue. Recently Boyd *et al.* (1993) found that it was possible in a proportion of cases. A more reliable method is the gonodotrophin-releasing hormone (GnRH) challenge test, which relies upon the stimulation of ovarian tissue to produce oestrogen (Jeffcoate, 1993).

The Male Reproductive Tract

Diagnostic imaging of the reproductive tract of the male may be useful for both scrotal and abdominal structures. Ultrasonography has been increasingly used over the past five years although there are no reports of its use in the tom. Data available for the dog is, however, likely to be relevant, although, in addition to a prostate gland, the tom has paired bulbourethral glands which are not present in the dog.

The testes and epididymides

The testes and epididymides are located within the scrotum and may be easily palpated. However, the ability of ultrasound to allow imaging of the internal architecture of these organs is extremely valuable. Examination is most conveniently performed with the animal in the standing position, and while it is not usually necessary to clip the hair, copious amounts of water-soluble coupling gel should be applied to the scrotum. Several imaging planes have been suggested for examination of the testes. For complete data collection the transverse, sagittal and dorsal imaging planes, together with the pre-scrotal position should be used (England, 1991a).

The normal testes and epididymides

The testicular parenchyma appears relatively hypoechoic in echotexture, with regular diffuse echogenic stippling scattered evenly throughout the organ (Pugh *et al.*, 1990). The stippling represents an extension of the fibrous mediastinum which is responsible for supporting the parenchymal tissue. The mediastinum testis, a fibrous invagination from the tunica albuginea, is located centrally within the testis. In a sagittal plane this structure appears as an echogenic line approximately 2 mm wide, extending from the cranial to the caudal pole, whilst in the transverse plane it appears as a central echogenic circular structure (Fig. 3.9). Acoustic shadowing is often noted distal to the mediastinum testis. Surrounding the testis the hyperechoic summed testicular and vaginal tunics are clearly defined.

The head and body of the epididymis are often difficult to identify, arising cranio-medially and lying on the dorso-lateral border of the testis. However, with slightly oblique imaging planes, these can be traced to the characteristic tri-

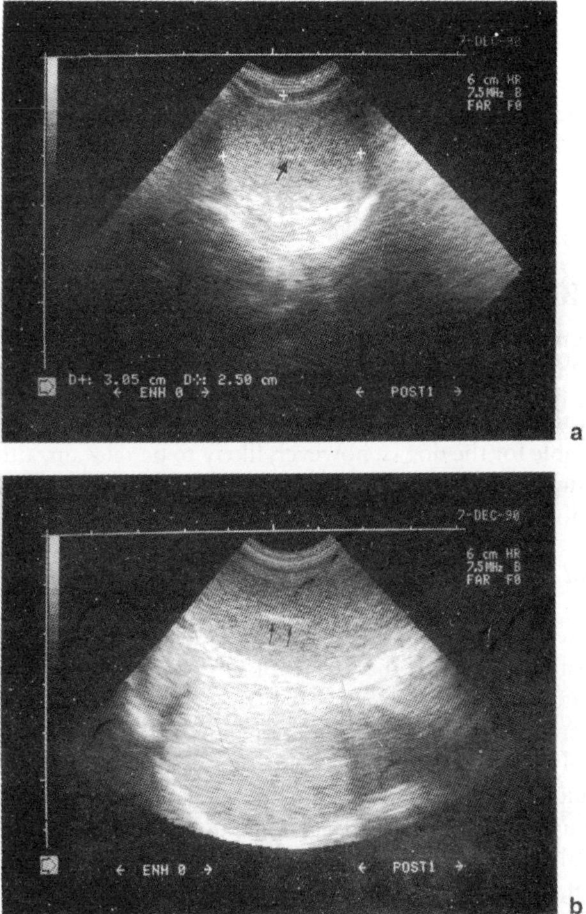

Fig. 3.9. Ultrasound image of the testes of a dog in transverse **(a)** and sagittal **(b)** planes. The testicular parenchyma appears relatively hypoechoic with diffuse regular echogenic stippling. The mediastinum testis appears as a central echogenic circular structure in the transverse plane, and an echogenic line in the sagittal plane (arrows).

angular-shaped tail of the epididymis, on the caudal border of the testis. The epididymis appears hypoechoic with respect to testicular parenchyma when imaged *in vivo*, and is closely applied to the testicular tunic. Normally a line of separation cannot be distinguished between these structures.

The relationship between testicular size and semen quality

Measurements of testicular size have been used in the bull for the prediction of sperm output (Ott, 1986). Similar measurements have been suggested as being of value in the dog (Olar *et al.*, 1983; Mialot *et al.*, 1985). Recently however, despite the accuracy of ultrasound in calculating testicular volume, these relationships have not been confirmed (England, 1991a), specifically because azoospermic dogs and dogs with severe sperm abnormalities may have a normal testicular volume.

Imaging non-scrotal testes

In the dog, the absence of one testis from the scrotum is not uncommon. Ultrasound may be of value in locating the position of ectopic testes, which are commonly inguinal or abdominal. In man, the accuracy of detection of non-descended testes is high (Wolverson *et al.*, 1983).

Ultrasound may be useful for demonstrating the architecture of these gonads (which are initially atrophic but may become neoplastic), to allow differentiation from other abdominal mass lesions (Miyabayashi *et al.*, 1990).

Diffuse abnormalities of the testes and epididymides

Whilst focal testicular and epididymal lesions may be readily imaged, diffuse changes may be difficult to appreciate. In most cases comparison with the adjacent testis is all that is required. When lesions are bilateral, comparison with the splenic parenchyma may be useful, since these organs have similar echogenicity when examined with high frequency (7.5 MHz) transducers. Alternatively, imaging of a known normal dog or reliance on the experience of the operator may be necessary. Measurements of testicular size may be compared with body weight as these have been shown to be isometrically related (Woodall and Johnstone, 1988). A simple technique to assess changes in the size of the testis or epididymis is to compare transverse image diameters, since at the mid-testes position the epididymal diameter is approximately 20% of the testis diameter (England, 1991a).

Diffuse testicular neoplasms

Testicular tumours in the dog have a variable gross appearance (Cotchin, 1960). Large tumours cause disruption of the normal ultrasonographic testicular architecture and compression of normal tissue to a peripheral position; often the mediastinum testis cannot be imaged. Large tumours are more likely to be either seminomas or Sertoli cell tumours and generally have a mixed, complicated echotexture (Johnston *et al.*, 1991a). Areas of haemorrhage and necrosis may produce focal zones of relatively hypoechoic or anechoic tissue (Johnston *et al.*, 1991a). England (1991a) and Pugh and Konde (1991) noted that testicular seminomas were generally hypoechoic with respect to normal testicular parenchyma, although this relationship is unlikely to be true in all cases.

Orchitis and epididymitis

Dogs with infectious orchitis frequently have diffuse patchy hypoechoic regions within the testicular parenchyma (Pugh and Konde, 1991). Commonly the gonad and the epididymis are enlarged and painful.

Testicular atrophy

Reduced size of the testis can often be assessed by palpation. Ultrasound imaging provides a rapid and accurate method of measuring testicular volume. Testicular parenchymal atrophy is usually characterized by reduced echogenicity. The assessment of epididymal and testicular width may allow the accurate assessment of testicular atrophy in marginal cases, since epididymal diameter may remain unchanged.

Torsion of the spermatic cord

Torsion of the spermatic cord (frequently referred to as testicular torsion) may be evaluated using ultrasound (Hricak *et al.*, 1983). The characteristic appearance is of a uniformly echogenic testis with an irregular contour, and thickening and increased echogenicity of the spermatic cord. Thickening of the testicular capsule and accumulation of fluid surrounding the testis have also been reported (Pugh and Konde, 1991), as has enlargement of the epididymis (Johnston *et al.*, 1991b). Ultrasound only offers limited diagnostic value, since it may be difficult to differentiate torsion from other causes of orchitis.

Abnormal semen quality

Ultrasonography may be useful for the examination of infertile dogs with abnormal testicular histology. Changes, including prominent hyperechoic parenchymal stippling, despite normal testicular and epididymal dimensions, have been identified (England, 1991a).

Focal abnormalities of the testes and epididymides

The great advantage of ultrasound in the evaluation of testicular abnormalities is the ability to detect those lesions which do not produce gross changes of testicular size and cannot be palpated (Moudy and Makhija, 1983).

Focal testicular neoplasms

The ultrasonographic appearance of focal testicular neoplasia varies, depending upon the tumour type, size and age. Tumours are often not difficult to diagnose since they are well circumscribed, and cause distortion of or compress the normal testicular parenchyma. The tumour margins may be well-defined and appear hyperechoic, due to calcification of their capsule (Fig. 3.10).

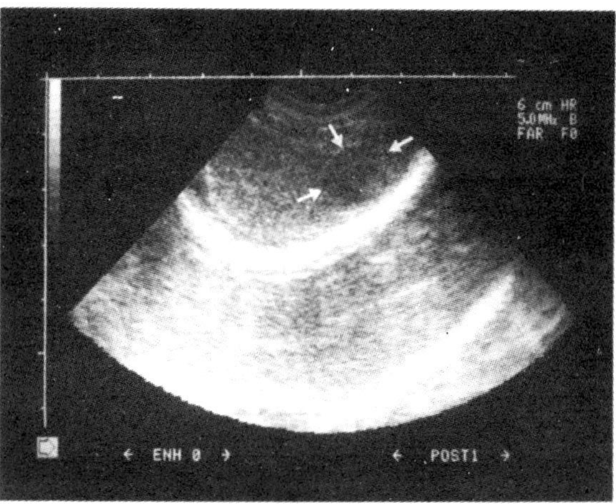

Fig. 3.10. Sagittal plane ultrasound image of the testes of a dog with a testicular tumour. A hypoechoic interstitial cell adenoma which has a well-defined calcified echogenic margin is present within the cranial pole of the testis (arrows).

Small solid mass lesions are most likely to be interstitial cell adenomas (Johnston *et al.*, 1991a), although the presence of central haemorrhage and necrosis is not uncommon, occurring more frequently as tumour size increases (Cotchin, 1960). Sertoli cell tumours tend to have a more mixed echogenicity and no particular pattern predominates (Johnston *et al.*, 1991b). Seminomas have a variable appearance and may involve the entire testis. They may be focal hypoechoic or hyperechoic in nature.

Testicular calcification

The presence of calcification within the testicular parenchyma is not common in the dog, unlike the ram, where it occurs secondary to a range of testicular insults (N. Ahmad, pers. comm.). In the dog, calcification is often limited to the capsule of slowly growing neoplasms.

Testicular cysts

Spherical fluid-filled cystic lesions have been identified within the testicular parenchyma of dogs (England, 1991a). The fluid within these lesions does not contain spermatozoa, and it is unlikely that they have any significance for fertility unless blockage of the seminiferous tubules or epididymis occurs due to a mass effect. Small cystic lesions in human testes are considered normal (Leung *et al.*, 1984). Cystic structures may rarely occur within the epididymis, but no convincing ultrasonographic evidence of these lesions has been presented.

Spermatocoele/granuloma

The incidence of testicular spermatocoele in the dog is unknown. They have been identified infrequently with ultrasound, having a similar appearance to testicular cysts, although the cyst fluid may produce patchy echoes due to the presence of spermatozoa.

Sperm granulomata may develop secondary to spermatocoeles. These lesions appear hypoechoic with ultrasound and commonly have a well-defined capsule. Sperm granulomata have not been reported in the dog.

The scrotum

The scrotum contains the testes, epididymides, testicular and vaginal tunics, and cremaster muscle. The structures surrounding the testes are not separately identifiable in the absence of pathological changes. The scrotal surface distal to the transducer is more readily imaged than that in contact with it. Multiple oblique imaging planes may be required for adequate examination.

The normal scrotum

The summed testicular and vaginal tunics, the cremaster muscle (where present), and the scrotal skin appear as a well-defined hyperechoic line surrounding the testicle.

Diseases of the scrotum

Inflammation/oedema

The presence of fluid around the testis (hydrocoele) has been infrequently identified in the dog. The ultrasonographic appearance is that of anechoic fluid accumulation with far enhancement (Johnston *et al.*, 1991b). Hydrocoeles may occur secondary to neoplasia, traumatic injury, or inflammatory disease of the testes or scrotum. A small volume of fluid has been identified and is considered a normal finding in the vaginal cavity of bulls (Pechman and Eilts, 1987), and while this has not been reported in the dog, pathological change should not be assumed in the absence of evidence of thickening of the scrotal skin or testicular or vaginal tunics.

Scrotal haematoma

Haemorrhage into the scrotum may occur secondary to trauma or following castration with inadequate haemostasis. Initially haematoma appear as anechoic cavities with thickening of the scrotal wall (Johnston *et al.*,1991b). Later organization of the clot produces a homogeneous, hypoechoic appearance.

Scrotal hernia

The presence of herniated material within the scrotum can be diagnosed clinically. Loops of gas-filled intestine may produce a zone of complete ultrasound attenuation, whilst omental fat may appear hyperechoic with respect to the adjacent testis.

The prostate gland

Examination of the prostate gland is facilitated by the presence of fluid within the bladder. This can be achieved by preventing urination, or the infusion of sterile isotonic saline via a catheter. Saline infusion may, however, introduce gas into the urethra, which can hinder imaging of the prostate. Imaging is achieved by placing the ultrasound transducer on the caudo-ventral abdomen adjacent to the prepuce, after clipping the hair and positioning the animal in dorsal or lateral recumbency. Imaging may be difficult if the gland lies entirely within the pelvis. However, the transducer may be placed into the dog's rectum (England, 1991b) and directed ventrally to allow adequate imaging of the caudal prostate (Fig. 3.11). This technique, although it requires sedation or anaesthesia, is particularly useful, since it allows examination of the disseminated portion of the prostate gland (England *et al.*, 1990a) which cannot be examined trans-abdominally, and is frequently disregarded clinically.

The normal prostate gland

The prostate gland is located at the neck of the bladder, encircling the urethra; its position may be confirmed by rectal palpation during transabdominal imaging. Variations in the size of the prostate gland have been established (Cartee and Rowles, 1983) although these studies used few animals. Recently, Forbes (1992) found that there was a positive correlation between body weight and prostatic volume, although in proportion to body weight, prostatic volume was less in heavier dogs.

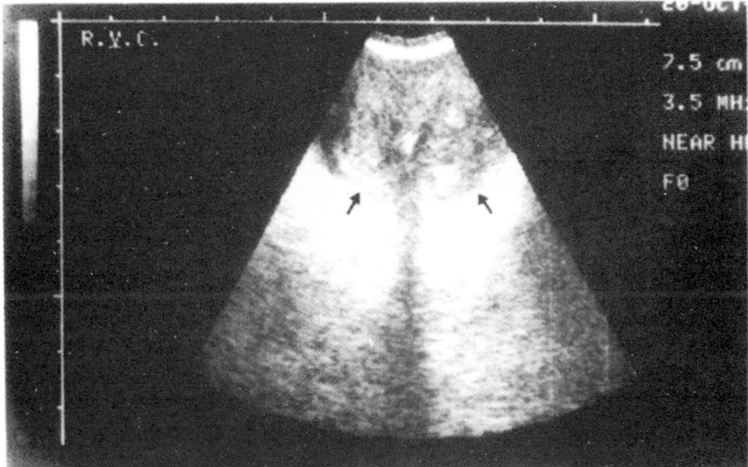

Fig. 3.11. Ultrasound image of the caudal portion of the prostate gland of a dog examined by placing the transducer into the dog's rectum. Small focal hyperechoic zones are present within this portion of the prostate gland; these could not be imaged trans-abdominally. Gas has been introduced into the urethra, and appears as a central echogenic area with distal acoustic shadowing.

The normal prostate gland is well circumscribed, although frequently the prostatic capsule is difficult to identify since its specular echo is sensitive to the direction of the ultrasound beam. The gland usually has a symmetrical, bi-lobed outline, with a midline furrow dorsal to the prostatic urethra. The prostatic parenchyma is moderately echogenic, and there is coarse stippling present evenly throughout the gland (Fig. 3.12). In the hilar region, the prostate has linear echogenic streaks associated with peri-urethral tissue. The prostatic urethra is not normally visible, although during sedation or anaesthesia this may be urine-filled, and appears as an anechoic line in longitudinal section. It is not possible to demonstrate the position of the vas deferens using ultrasound, although these paired structures enter the prostate gland dorsally in the cranial portion.

In the castrated male, the prostate is small and hypoechoic, the smallest size occurring in dogs castrated before puberty.

Abnormalities of the prostate gland

There are several disease processes of the prostate gland which lend themselves to diagnosis with ultrasound. Several abnormalities, however, do not generate specific ultrasonographic findings.

Cavitated focal parenchymal lesions

The commonest variation of the normal prostatic architecture is the presence of anechoic cysts. These may be single or multiple and are generally regular in outline, well defined, and less than 1 cm in diameter. Small cysts represent accumu-

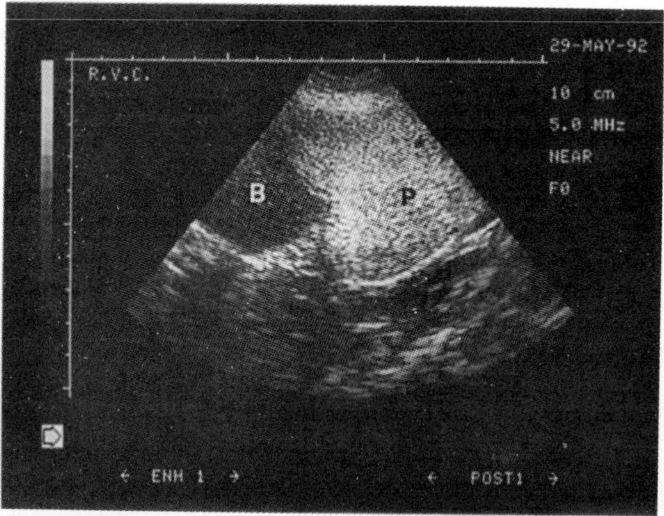

Fig. 3.12. Ultrasound image of the cranial portion of the prostate gland (P) of a dog examined with the transducer placed on the ventral abdomen. The prostate gland encircles the urethra at the caudal border of the bladder (B). The parenchyma appears moderately echogenic with coarse stippling present evenly throughout.

lations of prostatic secretion and may be found both within the prostate gland and its disseminate portion. These findings usually have no clinical significance.

Larger prostatic anechoic lesions may be found in cases of prostatic fluid retention cysts, prostatic abscessation, bacterial and non-bacterial prostatitis (Feeney *et al.*, 1987), haematomata, haematocysts, cavitating neoplasms, and cystic prostatic hyperplasia. Large cystic lesions may produce an irregular prostatic outline, increased parenchymal echogenicity, and asymmetrical prostatic enlargement, and are usually associated with far enhancement. The size, margination and appearance of large cystic lesions do not, however, allow differentiation of lesion type. For example, prostatic retention cysts, abscesses and cavitated neoplasms may all have a thick echogenic wall, be septate, and contain irregular anechoic to hypoechoic fluid. Therefore further diagnostic aids such as ultrasound-guided needle aspiration (Hager *et al.*, 1985; Finn and Wrigley, 1989), bacterial culture and cytology of semen and prostatic washings, and haematological investigations are often required (Barsanti and Finco, 1984).

Focal parenchymal mass lesions

Patchy focal echogenic regions may be identified, associated with a generalized increase in parenchymal echogenicity, in cases of bacterial prostatitis (Johnston *et al.*, 1991b). Fine echogenic speckles associated with calcification may be noted within the parenchyma.

Similar changes can also be identified in early cases of prostatic neoplasia and benign prostatic hyperplasia. These cases are best differentiated by bacteriological examination of semen, or ultrasound-guided needle aspiration of the gland. It is unusual to image discrete nodular neoplasia in the dog, since cases are often presented later than those seen in man. Prostatic neoplasia often presents as a diffuse parenchymal change with a mixed ultrasonographic pattern and increased gland size (see below).

Diffuse parenchymal lesions

The commonest diffuse abnormality of the dog prostate is benign prostatic hyperplasia, which is characterized by enlargement of the gland and slightly increased echogenicity. This change may mask the normal appearance of the hilar echo. The gland usually maintains a smooth outline and normal shape. If the condition progresses to cystic hyperplasia (see above) then the gland margin may become irregular.

Acute bacterial prostatitis may also produce a similar ultrasonographic appearance, although prostatic echogenicity may initially be decreased and later tends to develop a hyperechoic patchy distribution.

Cases of prostatic neoplasia are infrequently examined in the early stages of disease. Commonly they appear as increased prostatic size, with an indistinct margin containing disorganized focal or multifocal areas of increased echogenicity. These echogenic zones may coalesce, while there may also be areas of necrosis and haemorrhage characterized by regions of reduced echogenicity; it is not common for these to cavitate. Focal mineralization is not uncommon.

Paraprostatic lesions

Thin- or thick-walled cystic lesions may develop adjacent to the prostate gland, and are often attached by small stalk-like adhesions. The aetiology of these lesions is poorly understood but they may be enlarged prostatic retention cysts or remnants of the uterus masculinus (vestigial Müllerian ducts), or formed subsequent to prostatic haematoma (Weaver, 1978; Atilola and Pennock, 1986; Stowater and Lamb, 1989).

Paraprostatic cysts are frequently large anechoic structures positioned cranial or dorso-cranial to the bladder. The removal of urine or injection of small volumes of air into the bladder may allow differentiation from the paraprostatic cyst in cases of doubt. The cyst wall can be of variable thickness and may be echogenic due to calcification. The cyst fluid may contain echogenic material which often sediments to the dependent portion. Many cysts have echogenic internal septae and a connection to the prostate gland may sometimes be imaged (Stowater and Lamb, 1989). It is not uncommon for cystic lesions also to be identified within the prostate gland.

Conclusions

To date there has been limited use of diagnostic ultrasound when studying the reproductive tracts of small animals, compared to the situation in humans. However, recent studies have attempted to use this imaging modality to improve the understanding of reproductive physiology and diseases of reproduction, and in both cases ultrasonography has facilitated major advances.

There is no doubt that diagnostic ultrasound has an integral role to play in the process of evaluating both normal reproductive function and diseases of the reproductive tract of small animals.

References

Adams, W.H., Toal, R.L. and Breider, M.A. (1991) Ultrasonographic findings in ethylene glycol (antifreeze) poisoning in a pregnant queen and 4 fetal kittens. *Veterinary Radiology*, 32, 60–62.

Allen, W.E. (1982) Attempted oestrus induction in four bitches using pregnant mare serum gonadotrophin. *Journal of Small Animal Practice*, 23, 223–231.

Allen, W.E. (1989) Variation in the intensity of oedema in the mare's uterus and its relationship to ovulation. *British Journal of Radiology*, 62, 642.

Allen, W.E. and Davies, J.V. (1984) Use of echography in bitches. *Veterinary Record*, 115, 447.

Allen, W.E. and Meredith, M.J. (1981) Detection of pregnancy in the bitch; a study of abdominal palpation, A-mode ultrasound and Doppler ultrasound techniques. *Journal of Small Animal Practice*, 22, 609–622.

Allen, W.E., England, G.C.W. and White, K.B. (1989) Hydrops fetalis diagnosed by real time ultrasonography in a bichon frise bitch. *Journal of Small Animal Practice*, 30, 465–467.

Andersen, A.C. and Simpson, M.E. (1973) *The Ovary and Reproductive Cycle of the Dog (Beagle)*. Geron-X Inc., Los Altos, California.

Atilola, M.A.O. and Pennock, P.W. (1986) Cystic uterus masculinus in the dog. *Veterinary Radiology*, 27, 8–14.

Barr, F.J. (1988) Pregnancy diagnosis and assessment of fetal viability in the dog: A review. *Journal of Small Animal Practice*, 29, 647–656.

Barr, F. (1990) *Diagnostic Ultrasound in the Dog and Cat.* Blackwell Scientific Publications, London.

Barsanti, J.A. and Finco, D.R. (1984) Evaluation of techniques for diagnosis of canine prostatic disease. *Journal of the American Veterinary Medical Association*, 185, 198–200.

Beck, K.A., Baldwin, C.J. and Bosu, W.T.K. (1990) Ultrasound prediction of parturition in queens. *Veterinary Radiology*, 31, 32–35.

Bondestam, S., Alitalo, I. and Karkkainen, M. (1983) Real time ultrasound pregnancy diagnosis in the bitch. *Journal of Small Animal Practice*, 24, 145–151.

Boyd, J.S., Renton, J.P., Harvey, M.J., Nixon, D., Eckersall, P.D. and Ferguson, J.M. (1993) Problems associated with ultrasonography of the canine ovary around the time of ovulation. *Journal of Reproduction and Fertility* (supplement), 47, 101–105.

Cartee, R.E. and Rowles, T. (1983) Transabdominal sonographic evaluation of the canine prostate. *Veterinary Radiology*, 24, 156-164.

Cartee, R.E. and Rowles, T. (1984) Preliminary study of the ultrasonographic diagnosis of pregnancy and fetal development in the dog. *American Journal of Veterinary Research*, 45, 1259–1265.

Concannon, P.W. (1986) Canine physiology of reproduction. In: Burke, T. (ed.) *Small Animal Reproduction and Infertility; A Clinical Approach to Diagnosis and Treatment.* Lea and Febiger, Philadelphia, pp. 23–77.

Concannon, P.W. and Rendano, V. (1983) Radiographic diagnosis of canine pregnancy: onset of fetal skeletal radiopacity in relation to times of breeding, preovulatory luteinizing hormone release, and parturition. *American Journal of Veterinary Research*, 44, 1506–1511.

Concannon, P.W., Hansel, W. and McEntee, K. (1977) Changes in LH, progesterone and sexual behaviour associated with preovulatory luteinization in the bitch. *Biology of Reproduction*, 17, 604–613.

Concannon, P.W., Whaley, S., Lein, D. and Wissler, R. (1983) Canine gestation length: variation related to time of mating and fertile life of sperm. *American Journal of Veterinary Research*, 44, 1819–1821.

Cotchin, E. (1960) Testicular neoplasms in dogs. *Journal of Comparative Pathology*, 70, 232–247.

Davidson, A.P., Nyland, T.G. and Tsutsui, T. (1986) Pregnancy diagnosis with ultrasound in the domestic cat. *Veterinary Radiology*, 27, 109–114.

Dow, C. (1960) Ovarian abnormalities in the bitch. *Journal of Comparative Pathology and Therapeutics*, 70, 59–69.

England, G.C.W. (1990) Optimising canine fertility; an anatomical, physiological and pharmacological study. PhD thesis, University of London, p. 87.

England, G.C.W. (1991a) Relationship between ultrasonographic appearance, testicular size, spermatozoal output and testicular lesions in the dog. *Journal of Small Animal Practice*, 32, 306–311.

England, G.C.W. (1991b) Ultrasonography of the reproductive tract of the dog. *British Journal of Radiology*, 64, 653.

England, G.C.W. (1992) Ultrasound evaluation of pregnancy and spontaneous embryonic resorption in the bitch. *Journal of Small Animal Practice*, 33, 430–436.

England, G.C.W. and Allen, W.E. (1989a) Real time ultrasonic imaging of the canine ovary and uterus. *Journal of Reproduction and Fertility* (supplement), 39, 91–100.

England, G.C.W. and Allen, W.E. (1989b) The ultrasonographic and histological appearance of the canine ovary. *Veterinary Record*, 125, 555–556.

England, G.C.W. and Allen, W.E. (1989c) Ultrasound imaging of the reproductive tract of the bitch. *British Journal of Radiology*, 62, 642.

England, G.C.W. and Allen, W.E. (1990a) Diagnosis of pregnancy and pyometra in the bitch using real-time ultrasonography. *Veterinary Annual*, 30, 217–222.

England, G.C.W. and Allen, W.E. (1990b) Studies on canine pregnancy using B-mode ultrasound; Diagnosis of early pregnancy and the number of conceptuses. *Journal of Small Animal Practice*, 31, 321–323.

England, G.C.W. and Yeager, A.E. (1993) Ultrasonographic appearance of the ovary and uterus of the bitch during oestrus, ovulation and early pregnancy. *Journal of Reproduction and Fertility* (supplement), 47, 107–117.

England, G.C.W., Allen, W.E. and Porter, D.J. (1989) A comparison of radioimmunoassay with quantitative and qualitative enzyme-linked immunoassay for plasma progestogen detection in bitches. *Veterinary Record*, 125, 107–108.

England, G.C.W., Allen, W.E. and Middleton, D.J. (1990a) An investigation into the origin of the first fraction of the canine ejaculate. *Research in Veterinary Science*, 49, 66–70.

England, G.C.W., Allen, W.E. and Porter, D.J. (1990b) Studies on canine pregnancy using B-mode ultrasound; development of the conceptus and determination of gestational age. *Journal of Small Animal Practice*, 31, 324–329.

Evans, H.E. (1979) Reproduction and prenatal development. In: Miller, M.E. (ed.) *Miller's Anatomy of the Dog*. Saunders, Philadelphia, pp. 13–77.

Evans, H.M. and Cole, H.H. (1931) An introduction to the study of the oestrous cycle in the dog. *Memoirs of the University of California*, 9, 65–103.

Fayrer-Hosken, R.A., Mahaffey, M., Miller-Liebl, D. and Caudle, A.B. (1991) Early diagnosis of canine pyometra using ultrasonography. *Veterinary Radiology*, 32, 287–289.

Feeney, D.A. and Johnston, G.J. (1986a) The ovaries and testes. In: Thrall, D. (ed.) *Textbook of Veterinary Diagnostic Radiology*. Saunders, Philadelphia, pp. 467–472.

Feeney, D.A. and Johnston, G.J. (1986b) The uterus. In: Thrall, D. (ed.) *Textbook of Veterinary Diagnostic Radiology*. Saunders, Philadelphia, pp. 458–466.

Feeney, D.A., Johnston, G.J., Klausner, J.S., Perman, V., Leininger, J.R. and Tomlinson, M.J. (1987) Canine prostatic disease – comparison of ultrasonographic appearance with morphologic and microbiologic findings: 30 cases (1981–1985). *Journal of the American Veterinary Medical Association*, 190, 1027–1034.

Finn, S.T. and Wrigley, R.H. (1989) Ultrasonography and ultrasound-guided biopsy of the canine prostate. In: Kirk, R.W. (ed.) *Current Veterinary Therapy*. Saunders, Philadelphia, pp. 1232–1238.

Forbes, L. (1992) An ultrasonographic study of the effects of age, bodyweight and castration on the size of the canine prostate gland. Dissertation submitted for the 5th B.Vet.Med. examination, University of London, pp. 12–18.

Ginther, O.J. (1986) *Ultrasonic Imaging and Reproductive Events in the Mare*, 2nd edn. Equiservices, Cross Plains, USA.

Ginther, O.J., Bergfelt, D.R., Leith, G.S. and Scraba, S.T. (1985) Embryonic loss in mares: incidence and ultrasonic morphology. *Theriogenology*, 24, 73–86.

Goodwin, J-K., Hager, D., Phillips, L. and Lyman, R. (1990) Bilateral ovarian adenocarcinoma in a dog: ultrasonographic-aided diagnosis. *Veterinary Radiology*, 31, 265–267.

Hager, D.A., Nyland, T.G. and Fisher, P. (1985) Ultrasound-guided biopsy of the canine liver, kidney and prostate. *Veterinary Radiology*, 26, 82–88.

Hayer, P., Günzel-Apel, A.-R., Lüerssen, D. and Hoppen, H.-O. (1993) Ultrasonographic monitoring of follicular development, ovulation and the early luteal phase in the bitch. *Journal of Reproduction and Fertility* (supplement), 47, 93–100.

Hricak, H., Lue, T., Filly, R.A., Alpers, C.E., Zeineh, S.J. and Tanagho, E.A. (1983) Experimental study of the sonographic diagnosis of testicular torsion. *Journal of Ultrasound in Medicine*, 2, 349–356.

Inaba, T., Matsui, N., Shimizu, R. and Imori, T. (1984) The use of echography in bitches for detection of ovulation and pregnancy. *Veterinary Record*, 115, 267–277.

Jeffcoate, I.A. (1993) Gonadotrophin-releasing hormone challenge to test for the presence of ovaries in the bitch. *Journal of Reproduction and Fertility* (supplement), 47, 536–538.

Jeffcoate, I.A. and Lindsay, F.E.F. (1989) Ovulation detection and timing of insemination based on hormone concentrations, vaginal cytology and the endoscopic appearance of the vagina of domestic bitches. *Journal of Reproduction and Fertility* (supplement), 39, 277–287.

Johnston, G.R., Feeney, D.A., Johnston, S.D. and O'Brien, T.D. (1991a) Ultrasonographic features of testicular neoplasia in dogs: 16 cases (1980–1988). *Journal of the American Veterinary Medical Association*, 198, 1779–1784.

Johnston, G.R., Feeney, D.A., Rivers, B. and Walter, P.A. (1991b) Diagnostic imaging of the male canine reproductive organs. *Veterinary Clinics of North America: Small Animal Practice*, 21, 553–589.

Leung, M.L., Gooding, G.A.W. and Williams, R.D. (1984) High-resolution sonography of scrotal contents in asymptomatic subjects. *American Journal of Radiology*, 143, 161–164.

Lindsay, F.E.F. (1983) The normal endoscopic appearance of the caudal reproductive tract of the cyclic and non-cyclic bitch; post uterine endoscopy. *Journal of Small Animal Practice*, 24, 1–5.

Mialot, J.P., Guerin, Ch, and Begon, D. (1985) Growth, testicular development and sperm output in the dog from birth to post pubertal period. *Andrologia*, 17, 450–460.

Miyabayashi, T., Biller, D.S. and Cooley, A.J. (1990) Ultrasonographic appearance of torsion of a testicular seminoma in a cryptorchid dog. *Journal of Small Animal Practice*, 31, 401–403.

Moudy, P.C. and Makhija, J.S. (1983) Ultrasonic demonstration of a non-palpable testicular tumour. *Journal of Clinical Ultrasound*, 11, 54–55.

Muller, K. and Arbeiter, K. (1993) Ultrasonographic and clinical signs of fetal resorption in the bitch. *Journal of Reproduction and Fertility* (supplement), 47, 558–559.

Nowroozi, K., Check, J.H., Choe, J., Dietterich, C. and Goldsmith, G. (1991) Increased endometrial thickness at the time of hCG is associated with an increased pregnancy rate following IVF-ET and a leuprolide-acetate-hMG hyperstimulation protocol. *Assisted Reproductive Technology and Andrology*, 2, 223.

Olar, T.T., Amann, R.P. and Pickett, B.W. (1983) Relationships among testicular size, daily production and output of spermatozoa, and extragonadal spermatozoal reserves of the dog. *Biology of Reproduction*, 29, 1114–1120.

Ott, R.S. (1986) Breeding Soundness Examination of Bulls. In: Morrow, D.A. (ed.) *Current Therapy in Theriogenology II*. Saunders, Philadelphia, pp. 130–132.

Pechman, R.D. and Eilts, B.E. (1987) B-mode ultrasonography of the bull testicle. *Theriogenology*, 27, 431–441.

Pharr, J.W. and Post, K. (1992) Ultrasonography and radiography of the canine postpartum uterus. *Veterinary Radiology and Ultrasound*, 33, 35–40.

Phemister, R.D., Holst, P.A., Spano, J.S. and Hopwood, M.L. (1973) Time of ovulation in the beagle bitch. *Biology of Reproduction*, 8, 74–82.

Poffenbarger, E.M. and Feeney, D.A. (1986) Use of gray-scale ultrasonography in the diagnosis of reproductive disease in the bitch: 18 cases (1981–1984). *Journal of the American Veterinary Medical Association*, 189, 90–95.

Pugh, C.R. and Konde, L.J. (1991) Sonographic evaluation of canine testicular and scrotal abnormalities: a review of 26 case histories. *Veterinary Radiology*, 32, 243–250.

Pugh, C.R., Konde, L.J. and Park, R.D. (1990) Testicular ultrasound in the normal dog. *Veterinary Radiology*, 31, 195–199.

Renton, J.P., Boyd, J. and Harvey, M.J.A. (1993) Observations on the treatment and diagnosis of open pyometra in the bitch (*Canis familiaris*). *Journal of Reproduction and Fertility* (supplement), 47, 465–469.

Rivers, B. and Johnston, G.J. (1991) Diagnostic imaging of the reproductive organs of the bitch. *Veterinary Clinics of North America: Small Animal Practice*, 21, 437–466.

Sabbagha, R.E., Sheikh, Z. and Tamura, R.K. (1985) Predictive value, sensitivity and specificity of targeted imaging for fetal anomalies in gravid women at high risk for birth defects. *American Journal of Obstetrics and Gynaecology*, 152, 822–836.

Shille, V.M. and Gontarek, J. (1985) The use of ultrasonography for pregnancy diagnosis in the bitch. *Journal of the American Veterinary Medical Association*, 187, 1021–1025.

Simpson, D.J., Greenwood, R.E.S., Ricketts, S.W., Rossdale, P.D., Sanderson, M. and Allen, W.R. (1982) Use of ultrasound echography for early diagnosis of single and twin pregnancy in the mare. *Journal of Reproduction and Fertility* (supplement), 32, 431–439.

Smith, M.S. and McDonald, L.E. (1971) Serum levels of luteinizing hormone and progesterone during the estrous cycle, pseudopregnancy and pregnancy in the dog. *Endocrinology*, 94, 404–412.

Stowater, J.L. and Lamb, C.R. (1989) Ultrasonographic features of paraprostatic cysts in nine dogs. *Veterinary Radiology*, 30, 232–239.

Stowater, J.L., Memon, M.A., Hartzband, L.E. and Tidewell, A.S. (1989) Ultrasonic features of the dog uterus and fetus. *Journal of Reproduction and Fertility* (supplement), 39, 329.

Taverne, M.A.M., van der Weyden, G.C. and van Oord, H.A. (1989) Pregnancy and parturition in dogs: approached from some diagnostic, pathophysiological and therapeutic points of view. In: Christiansen, D.J. (ed.) *Symposium on Reproduction in the Dog*, Copenhagen, pp. 71–88.

Toal, R.L., Walker, M.A. and Henry, G.A. (1986) A comparison of real-time ultrasound, palpation and radiography in pregnancy detection and litter size determination in the bitch. *Veterinary Radiology*, 27, 102–108.

Verstegen, J., Silva, L.D.M., Onclin, K. and Donnay, I. (1993) Echocardiographic study of heart rate in dog and cat fetuses *in utero*. *Journal of Reproduction and Fertility* (supplement), 47, 175–180.

Wallace, S.S., Mahaffey, M.B., Miller, D.M. and Thompson, F.N. (1989) Ultrasonography of the dog ovary during follicular and early luteal phases. *Journal of Reproduction and Fertility* (supplement), 39, 331.

Wallace, S.S., Mahaffey, M.B., Miller, D.M., Thompson, F.N., and Chakraborty, P.K. (1992) Ultrasonographic appearance of the ovaries of dogs during the follicular and luteal phases of the estrous cycle. *American Journal of Veterinary Research*, 53, 209–215.

Weaver, A.D. (1978) Discreet prostatic (paraprostatic) cysts in the dog. *Veterinary Record*, 102, 435–440.

Wildt, D.E., Levinson, C.J. and Seager, S.W.J. (1977) Laparoscopic exposure and sequential observation of the ovary of the cycling bitch. *Anatomical Record*, 189, 443–450.

Wilson, J. and Hayward, J. (1985) Real-time ultrasound scanning of bitches. *Veterinary Record*, 116, 698–699.

Wolverson, M.K., Houttinum, E. and Heilberg, E. (1983) Comparison of computer tomography with high resolution real-time ultrasound for localization of the impalpable testis. *Radiology*, 146, 133–136.

Woodall, P.F. and Johnstone, I.P. (1988) Dimensions and allometry of testes, epididymides and spermatozoa in the domestic dog (*Canis familiaris*). *Journal of Reproduction and Fertility*, 82, 603–609.

Wright, P.J. (1990) Application of vaginal cytology and plasma progesterone determinations to the management of reproduction in the bitch. *Journal of Small Animal Practice*, 31, 335–340.

Wrigley, R.H. and Finn, S.T. (1989) Ultrasonography of the canine uterus and ovary. In: Kirk, R.W. (ed.) *Current Veterinary Therapy*. Saunders, Philadelphia, pp. 1239–1242.

Yeager, A.E. and Concannon, P.W. (1990a) Association between the preovulatory luteinizing hormone surge and the early ultrasonographic detection of pregnancy and fetal heartbeats in beagle dogs. *Theriogenology*, 34, 655–665.

Yeager, A.E. and Concannon, P.W. (1990b) Serial ultrasonographic appearance of postpartum uterine involution in beagle dogs. *Theriogenology*, 34, 523–535.

Yeager, A.E., Mohammed, H.O., Meyers-Wallen, V., Vannerson, L. and Concannon, P.W. (1992). Ultrasonographic appearance of the uterus, placenta, fetus, and fetal membranes throughout accurately timed pregnancy in beagles. *American Journal of Veterinary Research*, 53, 342–351.

4 Ocular Ultrasonography

P. Boydell
*The Animal Medical Centre, 511 Wilbraham Road, Chorlton,
Manchester M21 1UF, UK*

Introduction

The first application of ultrasound to ophthalmology was reported by Mundt and Hughes in 1956, with clinical applications shortly afterwards (Oksala and Lehtinen, 1957; Baum and Greenwood, 1958). Veterinary applications were first described in 1968 by Rubin and Koch. Advances have paralleled the development of improved machinery and computers.

The eye is the perfect organ for ultrasonographic examination. It is made up of several tissues delineated by distinct interfaces. Some of these interfaces are curved, producing specular reflections, enabling the ultrasonographer to obtain an image of the eye which is easily recognizable when using B-mode. There is direct access to the superficially-located eye, permitting the use of high-frequency probes allowing greater resolution. Fisher (1989) stated that ultrasound was the only method for obtaining architectural and real-time information in opaque media or obstructed view situations prior to surgical intervention, and Coleman (1972) indicated that ultrasound was essential for evaluation of all eyes with opaque media and all suspected ocular tumours. The technique is safe and permits easy re-examination.

B-mode is used most frequently in ocular examination, but there are other techniques which may assist diagnosis. A-mode can give detailed information regarding the amplitude of the returning echo and the distance travelled by the sound wave. It may be used to obtain precise data concerning the nature of the tissue being scanned, although the development of good grey-scale and colour enhanced B-mode has largely superseded A-mode in this respect. However, the measurement of the length of the ocular axis (biometry) is of great importance in the calculation of intra-ocular lens power in humans, and many A-mode devices are available for this purpose. Corneal pachymetry is the determination of corneal thickness and this also requires accurate and precise measurements achievable with A-mode systems.

C-mode (coronal modulation) permits visualization of the orbit in the coronal plane to demonstrate lesions of the orbit and optic nerve (Restori and Wright, 1977). D-mode (deflection modulation) superimposes the amplitude data onto the vertical axis of the B-mode image to make up a pseudo-three-dimensional display (Coleman *et al.*, 1975). Colour encoding can be used to enhance the recognition of subtle grey-scale differences (Coleman and Katz, 1974), although this technique can create confusing 'false' interfaces. Holographic ultrasound images have been produced to provide a three-dimensional image (Restori, 1978).

M-mode may be used to study dynamic changes in ocular tissues which vary in thickness and in the assessment of vascular orbital abnormalities (Coleman and Weininger, 1969) although Doppler techniques now allow detailed investigation of the orbital vasculature (Erickson *et al.*, 1989).

High-frequency acoustic microscopes have been shown to achieve resolution and magnification comparable to that of a light microscope (Marmor *et al.*, 1977), and similar devices can produce images to assist in the assessment of anterior segment disease and to permit quantitative gonioscopy in intact eyes (Pavlin *et al.*, 1991).

Echoes produced by the surfaces and the internal tissues of diseased ocular structures may be compared with known standards to permit quantitative ultrasonography (Bronson and Southampton, 1969; Ossoinig, 1974). Computer data analysis of sonograms may aid the identification of tumour masses (Coleman and Lizzi, 1983; Paunksnis *et al.*, 1989).

As with other forms of energy, ultrasound has the potential to damage tissues. This is particularly important when dealing with the fragile structures within the globe. Fortunately diagnostic ultrasound causes no significant pathological changes (Torchia *et al.*, 1967; Ziskin *et al.*, 1974).

This chapter will be largely restricted to the use of real-time B-mode techniques. At the time of writing there are a number of machines available to the veterinarian: their frequencies range up to 13 MHz although most ophthalmologists use a probe with a frequency of either 7.5 or 10 MHz.

Technique

Most examinations involve scanning across the cornea with the eyelids held open. This avoids the necessity of clipping the hair from the eyelids and eliminates any attenuation of the sound waves by eyelid tissue. Also, the eye itself can be observed during scanning, facilitating the correlation of the ultrasonographic image with the orientation of the globe. In large animals, particularly the horse, there is less hair on the eyelids, and scanning may be performed with the eyelids closed in many cases.

The procedure is generally well-tolerated, and manual restraint by an assistant is usually all that is required. Following the instillation of local anaesthetic eye drops, a mound of contact gel is placed upon the cornea. This gel must be viscous to maintain its shape for as long as possible so that it can act as a stand-off despite the action of gravity. Probes with built-in stand-offs can be used, but the gel mound has the added advantage that the probe need not contact the eye, thereby avoiding the deformation of ocular structures and potential ocular damage, particularly in the traumatized globe. A stand-off of some form is required when imaging anterior ocular structures, to avoid the reverberation artifact adjacent to the transducer head. Immersion techniques have been described in humans (Coleman *et al.*, 1969) but these are impractical in veterinary patients.

The eye should be scanned in both horizontal and vertical planes at a fairly high gain setting for maximum sensitivity. Following this screening manoeuvre, a more detailed assessment of any tissues is made at a lower amplification level to reduce acoustic artifact. When scanning longitudinally along the ocular axis it is easy to obtain an anatomically recognizable picture, as the lens capsules permit orientation of the image. Transverse scans through the sclera may be a little more difficult to interpret unless the direction of gaze relative to the ultrasound beam is known. In carnivores there is an incomplete lateral bony wall to the orbit and a coronal image of the eye and anterior orbit, may be obtained by scanning across the lateral orbital ligament.

Adjustment of the gain settings may be important in the identification of tissues. Compression of the globe by the probe may also assist the evaluation of cystic or solid components of ocular or orbital lesions.

Real-time scanning permits kinetic studies so that the behaviour of intra-ocular structures may be observed during rotation of the globe, and particularly following cessation of this rotation (the aftermovement). The animal must be distracted so that it alters the direction of gaze without moving the head, so that the probe can remain in position. A certain amount of luck is necessary, particularly with an uncooperative patient, but the technique can provide a considerable amount of information and should be a routine part of any vitreous assessment.

Biometry may be performed using a dedicated A-mode unit. A B-mode device may permit reasonably precise measurements, although not to the same level of accuracy. For routine clinical use this is generally adequate in veterinary practice. A B-mode image is obtained so that the reflections from the ocular interfaces are at maximum amplitude and may therefore be considered to be perpendicular to the sound beam. The positioning of cursors on the anterior cornea and the vitreo-retinal interface will then allow measurement. The procedure should be repeated until a consistent length is achieved. Fixation of gaze is necessary if the length of the visual axis of the globe is desired. There must be no distortion of the eye and a stand-off of some form may assist recognition of the anterior corneal echo.

The orbit may be considered as an extension of the globe as far as methods of examination are concerned, although the anatomy of the orbit may be less easy to recognize and evaluate. Greater depth of penetration is required, so that it may be necessary to use a transducer of lower frequency.

Indications for Ocular and Orbital Ultrasonography

Ophthalmology is a clinical discipline highly dependent on direct visual assessment of the eye, and the majority of clinical examination techniques involve optical devices of some form. The main role of ultrasonography is in the evaluation of eyes where opacity precludes a visual inspection of posterior structures. Thus opacity of the cornea, anterior chamber and lens may require ultrasonographic investigation to permit a diagnosis of their aetiology. More commonly, posterior structures are assessed when intraocular surgery is contemplated (Boydell, 1993a). In the author's ophthalmology department, the commonest use of ultrasound is in the assessment of cataract patients, where the condition of the retina and vitreous is of considerable importance: 10% of canine cataract patients have been shown to have significant unsuspected abnormalities of the posterior segment (Boydell, 1990). These would not have been detectable prior to surgery using other conventional noninvasive techniques. Using ultrasonography, the surgeon can plan appropriate measures in an elective procedure (Boydell 1993b, 1994). Ultrasound inspection may be augmented in such cases by electroretinographic examination to assess retinal function. Intraocular masses may include tumours and accumulations of exudate or organizing haemorrhage, and these may require differentiation.

Biometry may be performed to obtain the ocular axis length to calculate intraocular lens power for implantation following cataract removal (Gaiddon *et al.*, 1989), although this appears to be of minimal importance compared to the situation in humans. More commonly, the technique may quantify a diagnosis of microphthalmos in breeds where the condition may have an inherited component (Gelatt *et al.*, 1983).

Pachymetry is used to measure the corneal thickness and thereby evaluate the corneal endothelium, which is the tissue responsible for controlling the state of hydration (and therefore thickness) of the cornea. This might be valuable following ocular trauma and surgery, in the diagnosis of primary corneal endothelial disease or when considering corneal surgery (Gilger *et al.*, 1990).

Disease of the orbit may be more simply classified, usually leading to diagnoses of enophthalmos or exophthalmos, and here ultrasonography assumes a major role in the standard examination protocol.

At this point the phrase 'the eye is the mirror of the soul' should be remembered, since many ocular signs may reflect disease involving other body systems where ultrasonography is indicated.

Normal Structure

Figure 4.1 illustrates the images obtained by scanning along the ocular axis in a normal eye. The concave interfaces of the posterior lens capsule and the posterior wall of the eye provide an image which is readily identifiable, whereas the convex interfaces of the cornea and anterior lens capsule are not well depicted.

The anterior chamber is poorly imaged without a stand-off, but one should be able to detect anterior and posterior corneal surfaces and the anterior lens capsule, together with the iris and ciliary body. Otherwise the anterior chamber should be clear. The normal lens also has no internal reflections between the anterior and posterior lens capsules.

The lateral wall of the eye is poorly imaged as the reflective surfaces are paral-

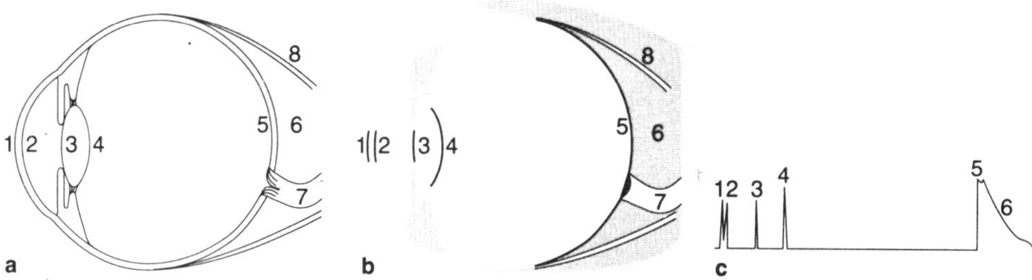

Fig. 4.1. Ultrasonography along the ocular axis. **(a)** Longitudinal cross-section of globe. 1 = anterior corneal surface, 2 = posterior corneal surface, 3 = anterior lens capsule, 4 = posterior lens capsule, 5 = retina, 6 = retrobulbar fat, 7 = optic nerve, 8 = rectus muscle. **(b)** B-mode image of globe and **(c)** A-mode image of globe. 1 = cornea–stand-off interface, 2 = cornea–aqueous interface, 3 = aqueous–anterior lens capsule interface, 4 = posterior lens capsule–vitreous interface, 5 = vitreo–retinal interface, 6 = retrobulbar fat pattern.

lel to the sound beam, but as the vitreo-retinal interface curves to become perpendicular to the beam a bright line is seen. The normal vitreous is acoustically clear.

Posterior to the retinal reflection the choroid and sclera may be identified, behind which retrobulbar fat is the most obvious structure. A uniform echogenic fat pattern results from the acoustic discontinuities between cell membranes and loose connective tissue, and even between intracellular lipid tissue and cell membranes. This pattern may be interrupted by the optic nerve, which is rarely seen as a well-delineated structure and the poorly echogenic optic nerve shadows must be interpreted with a degree of caution. In humans, the gap in the orbital fat is V-shaped when the eye is in the anterior gaze position, the posterior enlargement of the notch being an acoustic artifact created by the shadowing effect of the bends of the optic nerve. Echolucent lines may represent the extraocular musculature where the organized tissue planes run roughly parallel to the sound beam. A regular pulsation in the orbit indicates the location of blood vessels. Orbital musculature may be identified and the bony wall of the orbit may be seen anteriorly, although the echoes from the funnel shape of the orbit can confuse the posterior region of the sonogram.

Conditions of the Anterior Chamber

Corneal oedema results from damage to the corneal endothelium and is seen as a thickening of the cornea with some intrastromal echoes. This may be a primary dystrophy, or may be secondary to congenital defects, uveitis, glaucoma, lens luxation or neoplasia. In addition, corneal epithelial abnormalities may lead to similar signs. If visual inspection cannot confirm the aetiology, ultrasound may be used to assess the anterior chamber and may reveal an anteriorly displaced lens, accumulations of blood or exudate, or a neoplastic mass. A luxated lens appears as an oval structure (Fig. 4.2), although often the entire outline will not be visible.

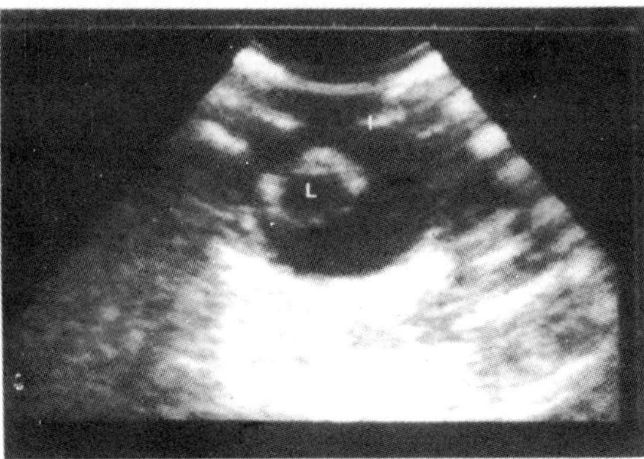

Fig. 4.2. Posterior lens luxation. I = iris, L = luxated lens displaced posteriorly. The entire outline of the lens is visible due to cataractous changes.

The appearance of hypopyon and haemorrhage depends greatly on the degree of organization. Fresh blood and pus may not be seen, as they are composed of many small cells which are individually too small to cause a detectable reflection. As the material coagulates the membranous structures produce reflections which impart a meshwork-like appearance to the image, although a dense exudate may appear as a highly echogenic mass. Blood or pus may be detected ventrally rather than throughout the entire anterior chamber.

Neoplasms also have a varied ultrasonographic representation dependent on the nature of the tissue. Masses with a dense cell and membrane population may appear as highly reflective regions (Fig. 4.3) or, if the cells are very tightly packed together, there may be a highly echogenic anterior surface with an echolucent body to the mass (Fig. 4.4).

The state of pupillary dilation may be revealed as the iris is easily seen, and if there are posterior synechiae causing pupillary block glaucoma the anterior bowing of iris bombe may be detected.

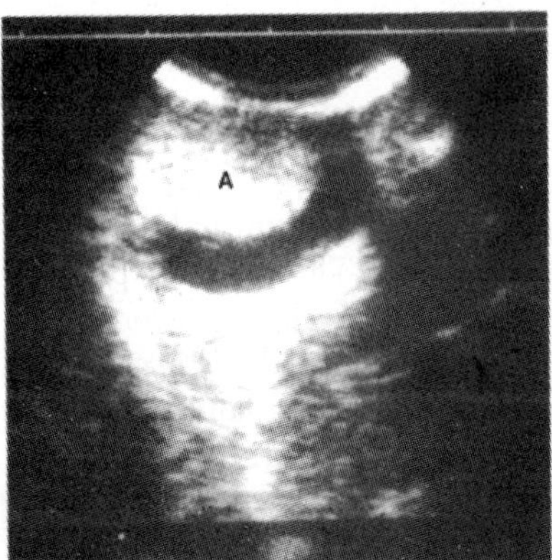

Fig. 4.3. Ocular neoplasm. A = ciliary body mass. This was not evident on visual examination due to secondary corneal inflammatory changes. Fine needle aspiration biopsy (FNAB) permitted a diagnosis of ciliary body adenocarcinoma.

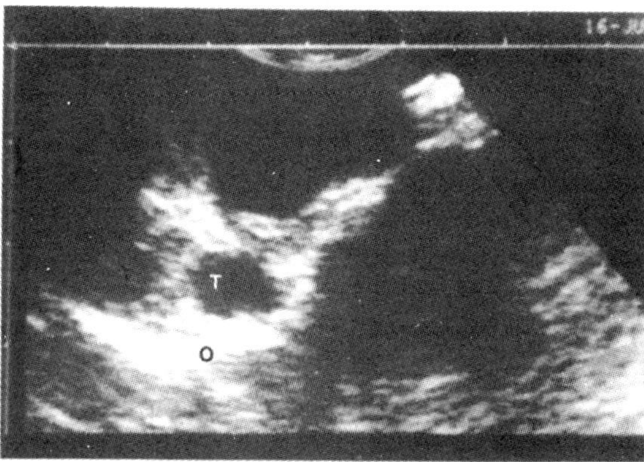

Fig. 4.4. Orbital tumour. O = postero-medial wall of orbit, T = orbital tumour. This mass was diagnosed as an adenocarcinoma of the nictitans by fine needle aspiration biopsy. Dense packing of the tumour cells eliminates interfaces within the body of the tumour, producing an acoustically clear region.

Where corneal opacity prevents adequate inspection of intraocular structures and corneal surgery is contemplated, ultrasound might be indicated to exclude other conditions. Unsuspected cataract may be revealed and its presence radically change the proposed therapeutic approach. Cataract may be diagnosed if the normally clear lens is seen to include some reflections.

Reflections from within the lens substance and thickening of the lens capsules are indicative of cataract. Subluxation of the lens may lead to a reduction of depth in the anterior chamber or slight tilting of the normal capsular echoes. If the lens is displaced anteriorly or posteriorly its position is easily seen (Fig. 4.2).

Conditions of the Posterior Segment

Any abnormalities of the vitreous may be immediately obvious. These may include haemorrhage and exudate, membrane formation and retinal detachment, neoplasia, luxated lenses, or lens material and foreign bodies, in addition to congenital defects. Vitreous degenerative changes such as asteroid hyalosis may also be easily seen as a large number of high-amplitude echoes, but other disease processes may be much more subtle, necessitating a more detailed examination.

In many cases of vitreous disease visual methods cannot provide adequate information. As veterinary ophthalmologists become more adept at vitreous and retinal surgery, the ability to accurately diagnose and classify the extent of posterior segment disease becomes much more important, both in planning a suitable approach and in facilitating a prognosis (Coleman and Franzen, 1974). The surgeon should perform, or at least be present during, the scanning as the real-time information is of much greater use than static pictures (Jack *et al.*, 1974).

The appearance of blood and exudate again depends upon the extent of coagulation. Fresh haemorrhage gives rise to very low amplitude echoes and is not detectable until there has been some clotting, and the echogenicity of the resulting mass may vary considerably. Ultimately there may remain a meshwork of organized fibrin and collagen with possibly some cellular proliferation, although the majority of the blood components will have been resorbed. The result is a membranous mass which is easily seen sonographically but can be optically clear and may not interfere with vision (Fig. 4.5). The organized membranes may remain attached to the posterior wall of the globe (Fig. 4.6), although

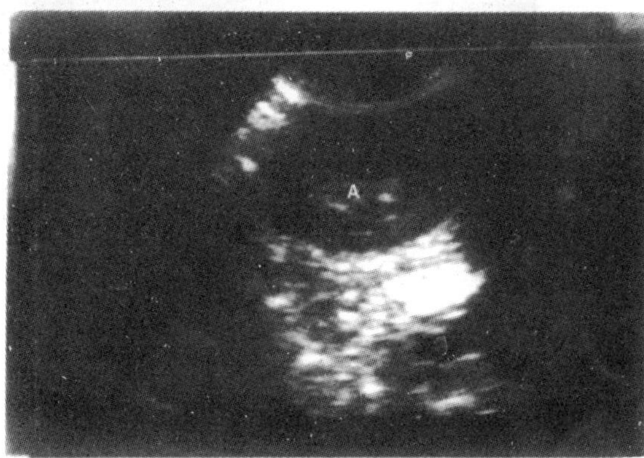

Fig. 4.5. Long-standing vitreous haemorrhage. A = meshwork of organized vitreous membranes. This lesion was noted as an incidental finding. The membranes were optically clear and the retina was easily examined ophthalmoscopically. There was no evidence of other ocular disease, and vision appeared normal.

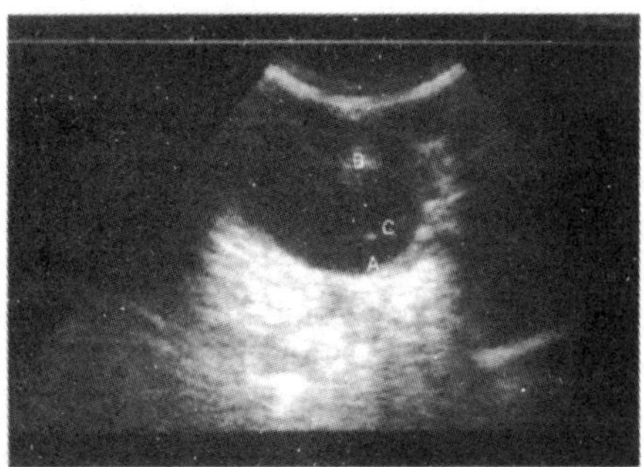

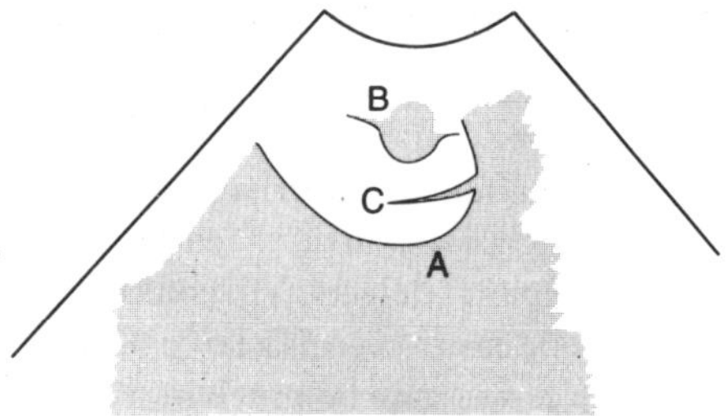

Fig. 4.6. Vitreous membrane attached to posterior globe. A = vitreo–retinal interface, B = cataractous lens, C = high-amplitude vitreous membrane. This structure exhibited no aftermovement on kinetic studies. This patient, a diabetic dog, was presented for lentectomy. Initially there was a brisk complete pupillary light reflex and a good dazzle response, but this reaction to light was lost over a three-month period. The aetiology of the membrane remains uncertain but it might be related to haemorrhage, possibly associated with diabetic vascular changes in the retina.

one end may stop abruptly within the vitreous compartment. Adhesion to the retina can lead to further problems, as contraction of the membranes may lead to retinal tears and subsequent traction retinal detachment (Fig. 4.7). Regular ultrasonographic assessment is necessary with a view to arranging vitrectomy. In humans, vitreous haemorrhage is a not infrequent complication of diabetic retinopathy and is a common indication for ultrasonography.

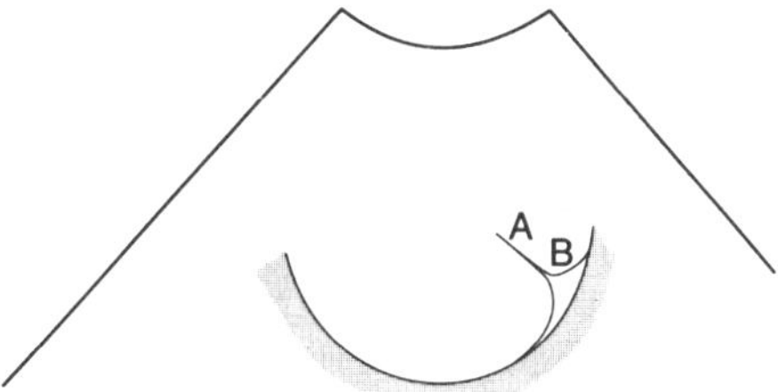

Fig. 4.7. Traction retinal detachment. A = contracting vitreous membrane, B = 'Tenting' of the retina under traction from the membrane. This will lead to a tear and possible detachment.

Many vitreous membranes are poorly reflective and fairly high gain settings are required to pick them up, although long-standing membranes may be well organized with a proliferating cellular component, resulting in a greater amount of sound reflection.

The appearance of a vitreous membrane may also depend upon the condition of the vitreous gel. As normal vitreous ages it degenerates and undergoes liquefaction as the collagen skeleton condenses. Collagen fibres organize with the fibrin strands from the blood and, with cellular material, form the membrane. If the surrounding vitreous remains gel-like, the membrane will appear 'stiff' and will exhibit characteristic 'shimmering' as an aftermovement. If the surrounding vitreous is liquified, then the membrane aftermovement may be a sinuous waveform, although a well-organized membrane may remain fixed within a liquid medium.

Vitreous degeneration may be detected in the absence of other disease, although the interfaces between gel and liquid phases are very poorly reflective. At high-amplification settings fluid-filled lacunae may be seen, and kinetic studies can reveal the swirling motion of solid vitreous surrounded by liquid. An interface may be seen between anterior solid vitreous and posterior liquified vitreous, indicating a posterior vitreous detachment (PVD), separation of the vitreous body from the internal limiting membrane of the retina. The PVD may be more apparent if it is accompanied by the organization of blood components. Some haemorrhage can often accompany the detachment. The posterior vitreous face may remain attached at the optic disc and the condition may, therefore, resemble retinal detachment, particularly if the membrane is fibrotic and gives rise to a higher amplitude echo. The posterior hyaloid interface usually inserts onto the retina just anterior to the equator. This can have implications if intraocular surgery is to be performed (Boydell, 1992, 1993b).

Vitreous membranes must be distinguished from retinal detachment. The ultrasonographic appearance of this latter condition may be similar to that of a vitreous membrane, but the two can generally be differentiated by varying the sensitivity and by kinetic studies (Boydell, 1991b). Detachments may range from a small bullous elevation from the underlying tissues, through to a complete detachment with massive preretinal retraction. The progression of one case is illustrated in Fig. 4.8.

Retinal detachment may be classified by aetiology into rhegmatogenous, traction, and exudative. Rhegmatogenous detachment results from the leakage of liquefied vitreous through a break to lift the neuroretina away from the retinal pigment epithelium. Traction detachment may occur when a contracting vitreous membrane causes the tear in the retina. Retinal holes are not easily demonstrable sonographically, but the probable location at the insertion of the vitreous membrane may be demonstrable (Fig. 4.7). Exudative detachment may occur as a result of material produced by the choroid accumulating beneath the retina in instances of inflammatory disease or neoplasia involving the posterior wall of the eye and this may be easily apparent on imaging. Rhegmatogenous detachment is often associated with posterior vitreous detachment and invasion of the vitreous cavity by blood cells and pigment cells which may produce low amplitude echoes. Traction detachment will follow vitreous membrane formation. Retinal detachment is a reported complication of cataract surgery (Hendrix *et al.*, 1991), and the surgeon should be aware of any predisposition to detachment prior to lentectomy.

The retina will always remain connected to the posterior wall of the eye. A totally detached retina will be attached at the ora serrata and the optic nerve head, although disinsertion from the anterior attachment may be seen.

The retina is a much more echogenic tissue than most vitreous membranes, and the ultrasonic image will persist even at low gain levels and approximates to the brightness/amplitude of scleral echoes, although atrophic retinal leaves may produce echoes of much lower amplitude. Conversely, a long-standing detachment may organize with vitreous collagen and pigment epithelial cells, to thicken and produce a very high amplitude echo. An anterior bridging membrane lying along the detached posterior vitreous face may connect the retinal leaves (Fig. 4.8c). The behaviour of the retina on kinetic studies may also assist the clinician, in the same way that the aftermovement of vitreous membranes may provide useful information. A mobile sinuous retinal leaf is suggestive of a rhegmatogenous detachment, possibly amenable to reattachment with appropriate treatment, whereas if the retinal movements are damped or absent there may be a long-standing detachment with proliferation and organization of other vitreoretinal components, indicative of a poor visual prognosis.

The condition of persistent hyperplastic primary vitreous is rare in veterinary patients, although it is an inherited defect in certain breeds of dog. It can cause a visual deficit itself or lead to cataract development. Sonographically, a highly echogenic retrolenticular plaque may be detected, possibly with a strand of tissue extending posteriorly to the optic disc. Doppler examination may reveal patency of a blood vessel in this hyaloid remnant.

The posterior wall of the globe may be thickened in inflammatory conditions such as scleritis. The thickened sclera has high internal reflectivity and there may

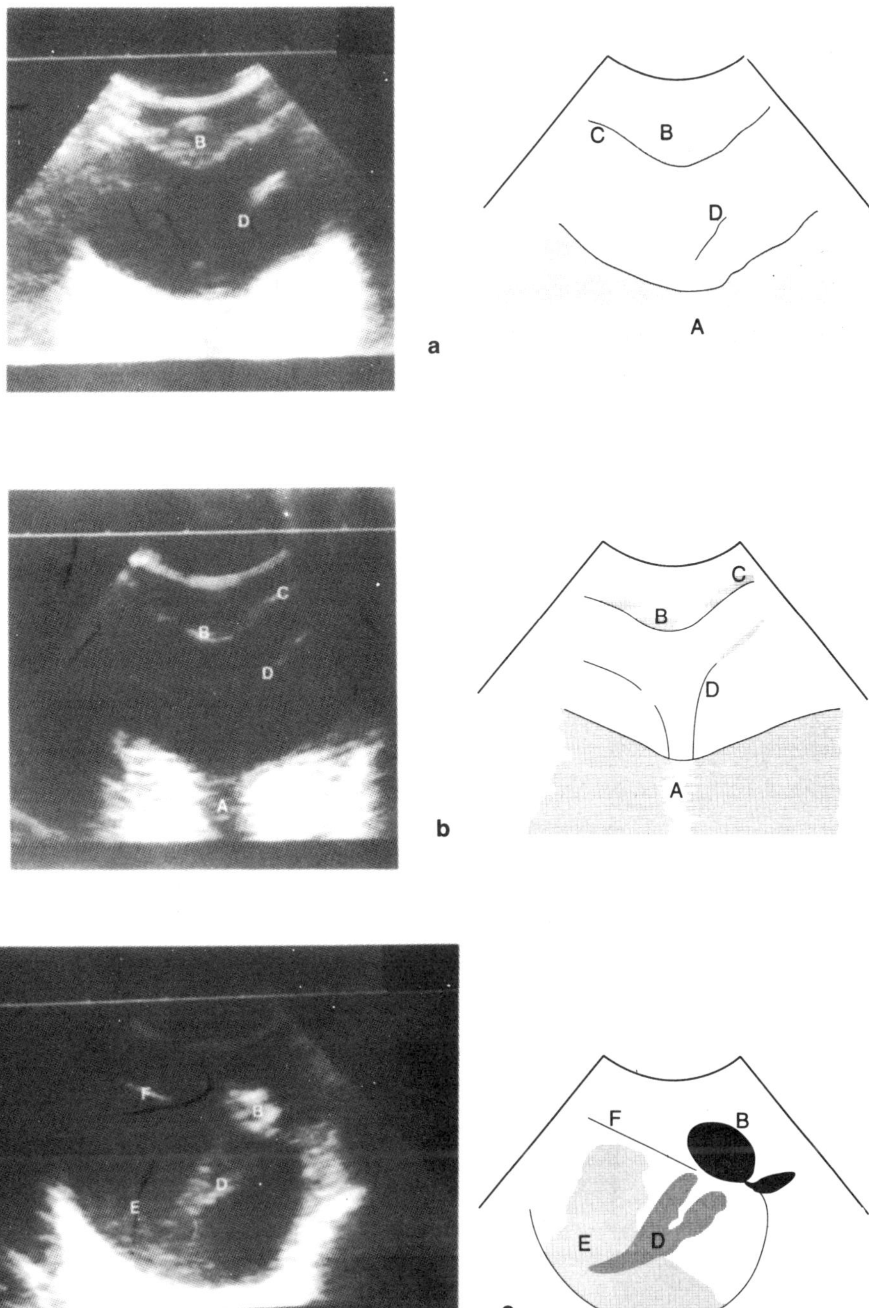

Fig. 4.8. The progression of retinal detachment in a dog with cataract. **(a)** Early detachment, and **(b)** complete detachment 2 months later. A = optic nerve shadow, B = cataract, C = lens zonules and ciliary body, D = detached retina. **(c)** 8 months later, a long-standing retinal detachment. B = cataract, D = organized, thickened retinal folds with proliferating cellular deposits, E = haemorrhage and cellular infiltration into the vitreous, F = cyclitic membrane composed of organized material along the posterior vitreous face.

be adjacent retrobulbar oedema. There may be associated exudative retinal detachment.

The optic disc may be swollen in cases of increased intracranial pressure, vitamin A deficiency in cattle, and some instances of optic neuritis. This swelling may be obvious sonographically as a solid enlargement of the optic nerve head. Conversely, there may be a depression in the optic disc as with colobomata, or there may be cupping following glaucoma. Large defects may be detected by ultrasonography and may be of importance in preoperative prognostication of eyes with opaque media (Darnley-Fisch *et al.*, 1990), provided a strongly focused transducer with a narrow beam width is used (Cohen *et al.*, 1976).

Conditions of the Orbit

The commonest sign of orbital disease in domestic animals is exophthalmos caused by a retrobulbar space-occupying lesion, and many of these lesions may be detected and, to some extent, characterized sonographically. The aetiology will usually involve inflammation, neoplasia, cystic structures, proliferative disease, trauma or vascular anomalies. Accurate diagnosis is important prior to the traumatic procedure of exploratory orbitotomy, which is only indicated for treatment in 20% of cases (Boydell, 1991a).

Cellulitis of the orbit leads to an area of mottling where the echoes from the retrobulbar fat become dispersed (Fig. 4.9) as the interfaces are separated by

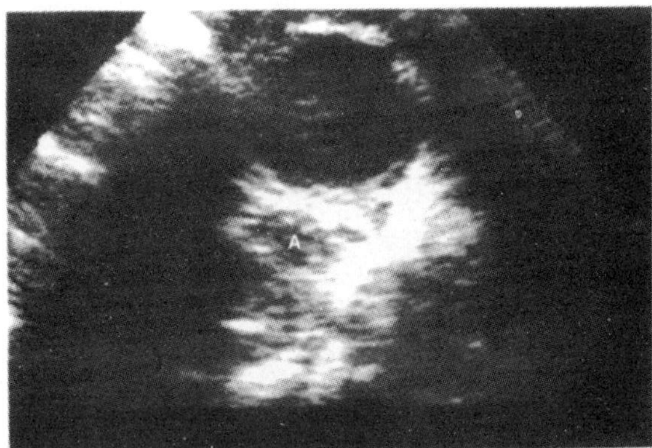

Fig. 4.9. Retrobulbar cellulitis. A = retrobulbar cellulitis. Material for microbiological investigation was obtained by fine needle aspiration biopsy.

oedema and exudate. Orbital haemorrhage may have a similar appearance. Abscessation may develop, with the walling off of the exudate from the surrounding tissues, to permit the typical ultrasonographic picture of an abscess (Fig. 4.10) with an echogenic capsule and a cystic cavity with many low-amplitude echoes, and sometimes echogenic membranes, indicative of fibrous strands.

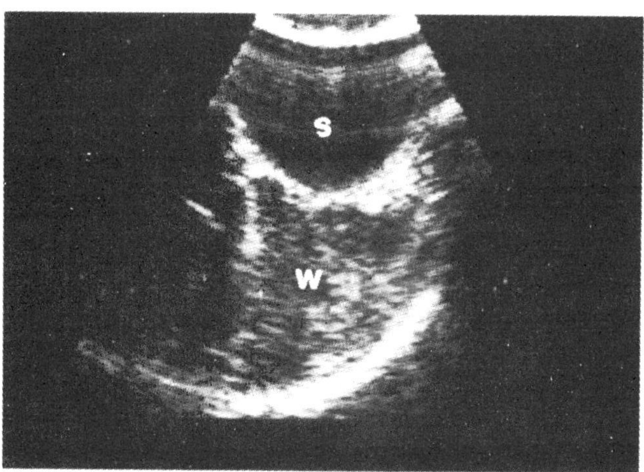

Fig. 4.10. Orbital abscess. S = globe, W = abscess.

It may be difficult to differentiate abscesses from other cystic-type lesions, although the history and clinical signs associated with inflammation are usually characteristic. Some species, particularly birds, suffer from solid inspissated abscess formation and these may appear as solid masses sonographically. Orbital foreign bodies such as lead shot produce a typical echogenic reflection with a posterior stream of reverberations.

Inflammatory disease of the periorbital musculature may affect any or all of this group of muscles, but may be restricted to the medial pterygoid muscle within the orbit. Ultrasound may suggest swelling by revealing an increase in the sonolucent space in the medial orbit, but further definition is difficult and diagnosis might be confirmed by electromyography or biopsy. Disease of the extraocular musculature is very rare in veterinary practice but the sonographic picture is diagnostic with a V-shaped echolucent area. The condition may respond to corticosteroid therapy (Fig. 4.11).

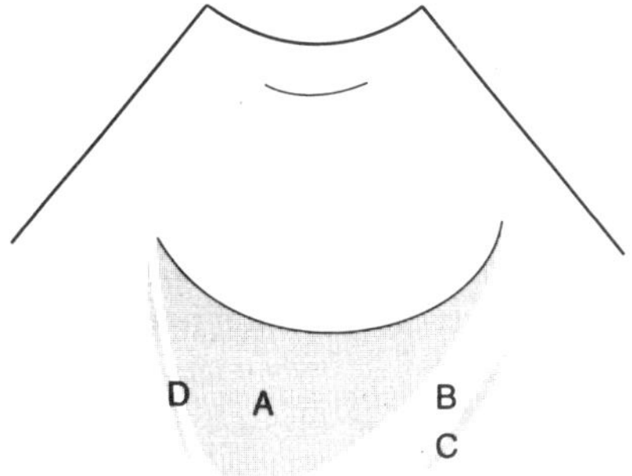

Fig. 4.11. Myositis of the medial rectus muscle. A = retrobulbar fat, B = swollen medial rectus muscle – fine needle aspiration biopsy demonstrated numbers of eosinophils. The size of the muscle diminished following the administration of corticosteroids. C = medial wall of orbit, D = normal lateral rectus muscle.

Neoplastic lesions may be broadly classified into three types: cystic, solid or infiltrative. Their position relative to the orbital cone is also important, though the majority seem to be outside this structure. Cystic tumours have a well-differentiated anterior and posterior capsule and poor internal echogenicity, and are thus often similar in appearance to abscesses. Other tumours also have an obvious outline on the near interface, but the internal characteristics may vary between poorly to highly echogenic. Low-amplitude echoes within the tumour substance indicate tissue interfaces typical of a solid, homogeneous mass. There may be sufficient attenuation within the mass to prevent imaging of the far wall. Infiltrative masses are poorly defined and may appear as a slight alteration in the normal echo pattern. Any of these may displace other normal orbital contents (Fig. 4.12).

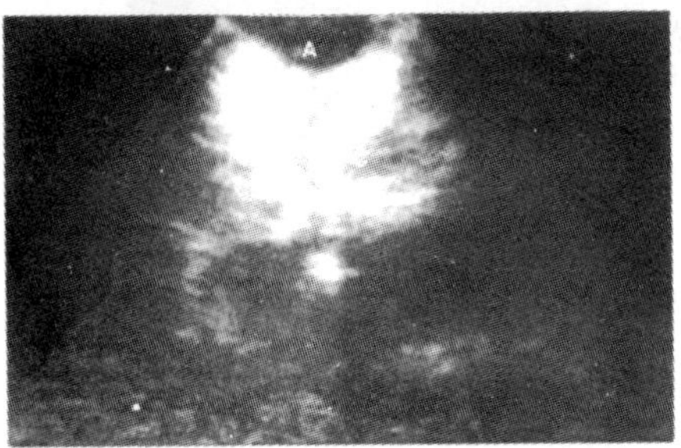
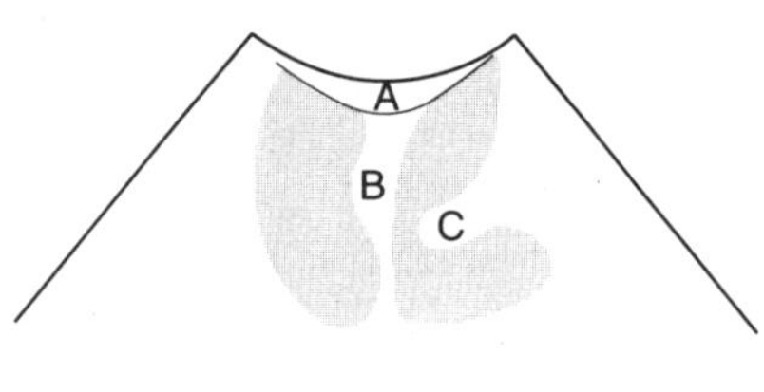

Fig. 4.12. Orbit of a cat distorted by neoplasia. A = globe, B = optic nerve shadow, C = infiltrative tumour (squamous cell carcinoma).

A comparative evaluation of the contralateral orbit may be performed to aid the differentiation of subtle pathological changes.

Cysts are generally derived from glandular tissues within the orbit, commonly the zygomatic salivary gland. These have the typical appearance of a well-encapsulated echolucent mass. Cysts may be produced by the accumulation of lacrimal fluid, particularly when any glandular tissue remains in the orbit following enucleation.

A sample of the orbital lesion may be obtained by fine needle aspiration biopsy (FNAB). The needle may be guided by ultrasound (Spoor *et al.*, 1980). FNAB has a reported accuracy of 92% in humans (Kennerdell *et al.*, 1985) and 97% in veterinary patients (Boydell, 1991a). Needle aspiration of the orbital mass may be used therapeutically in the case of certain cystic lesions (Skalka, 1981) and abscesses.

Vascular anomalies of the orbit are rare. They may be seen as an abnormal pulsation on real-time scanning but can be better defined with Doppler studies.

The limitations of orbital ultrasonography are a result of the shape of the area. The narrowing of the bony walls into a cone shape can give rise to multidirectional reverberations which can confuse the image, and lesions contiguous with the orbital walls may be missed. Bony lesions are not well demonstrated. Ultrasound energy is rapidly absorbed by orbital fat and detail of the orbital apex is poor. The diagnosis of orbital disease may be significantly improved by using additional imaging techniques (Dallow *et al.*, 1976).

Conditions of the Optic Nerve

The distal optic nerve is seen as an echolucent notch posterior to the globe wall. Few echoes are produced by the nerve, as the interfaces run roughly parallel to the direction of the sound waves, but there may be a visible interface between the orbital fat and the dura. There is also some acoustic shadowing immediately behind the optic disc. The proximal nerve is rarely distinctive on echography, due to the multiple reverberations in the apex of the cone-shaped orbit. While ultrasonography is reported to be useful for the evaluation of the distal region of the nerve in humans, other imaging techniques are superior as the orbital apex is approached (Skalka and Kline, 1984).

Optic neuritis may appear as irregular enlargement of the optic nerve (Fig. 4.13) which generally decreases following the administration of anti-inflammatory agents. Tumours of the distal optic nerve may have a similar appearance but will remain unaffected by such treatment. In cross-sectional ultrasonography of the optic nerve, echoes are produced by the dura. The dural diameter is increased in cases of optic neuritis, and it has been shown that this increase in diameter can parallel the severity of the visual deficit (Schroeder and Guthoff, 1981). There may be accentuation of the optic nerve sheath echo or echoes from within the nerve itself (Kerlen, 1981).

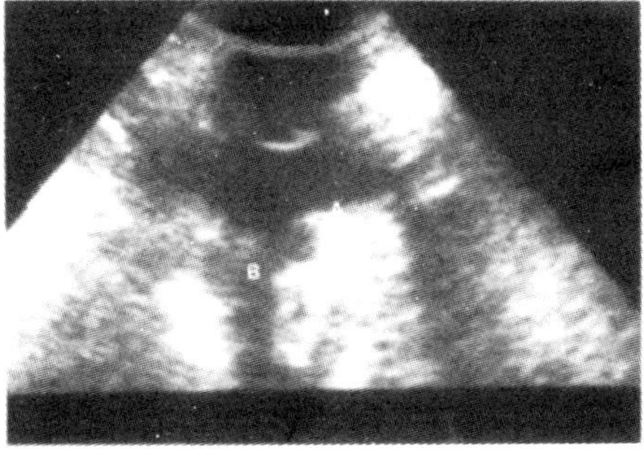

Fig. 4.13. Optic neuritis. A = vitreo-retinal interface, B = swollen irregular optic nerve shadow.

Therapeutic Applications of Ultrasound

Ultrasound can be involved in the treatment of certain ocular conditions, when it is applied at higher frequencies and uses considerably more energy than for scanning.

In cataract surgery the electrical energy converted to mechanical energy by an ultrasonic vibrator in the probe is used to fragment lens material so that it can be aspirated through the probe. This process of phacoemulsification and aspiration permits lentectomy through a small incision. Concurrent irrigation maintains the depth of the anterior chamber.

The basic principles described by Kelman in 1967 remain virtually unchanged, but the technique has been modified to reduce the amount of postoperative inflammatory response (Krohne and Lindley, 1991) and thus the risk of complications, so that the short-term success rate in the dog may be as high as 95% (Miller *et al.*, 1987; Moore and Fischer, 1990). This improved success also applies to cataract surgery in other species such as horses (Dziezyc *et al.*, 1991) and birds (Boydell, unpublished data). The transducer tip may be applied to the anterior lens capsule to remove the cells which can otherwise proliferate and lead to aftercataract formation (Nishi, 1989).

High-frequency ultrasound has also been used to produce controlled ocular tissue damage (Coleman *et al.*, 1978), to assist the clearing of vitreous opacities (Coleman *et al.*, 1980) and to reduce the intraocular pressure in glaucoma patients (Lizzi *et al.*, 1984).

References

Baum, G. and Greenwood, I. (1958) The application of ultrasonic locating techniques to ophthalmology. *American Journal of Ophthalmology*, 46, 319–329.

Boydell, P. (1990) Ultrasonographic ocular examination in the dog. *Abstracts of the 22nd Annual Meeting of the British Medical Ultrasound Society*, p. 54.

Boydell, P. (1991a) Fine needle aspiration biopsy in the diagnosis of exophthalmos. *Journal of Small Animal Practice*, 32, 542–546.

Boydell, P. (1991b) Ultrasonographic differentiation of vitreous membranes and retinal detachments in the dog. *Abstracts of the International Society of Veterinary Ophthalmology Congress*, p. 30.

Boydell, P. (1992) The significance of posterior vitreous detachment in dogs undergoing cataract surgery. *Paper synopses of the British Small Animal Veterinary Association Congress*, p. 165.

Boydell, P. (1993a) Ultrasonic findings in 1638 canine eyes with cataract. *Transactions of the 24th Annual Meeting of the American College of Veterinary Ophthalmologists*, p. 152.

Boydell, P. (1993b) Retinal detachment following lentectomy and posterior capsulectomy in eyes with posterior vitreous detatchment. *Transactions of the 24th Annual Meeting of the American College of Veterinary Ophthalmologists*, p. 185.

Boydell, P. (1994) Surgical treatment of cataract complicated by persistent hyperplastic primary vitreous. *Transactions of the 25th Annual Meeting of the American College of Veterinary Ophthalmologists*, p. 77.

Bronson, N.R. and Southampton, N.Y. (1969) Quantitative ultrasonography. *Archives of Ophthalmology*, 81, 460–472.

Cohen, J.S., Stone, R.D., Hetherington, J. and Bullock, J. (1976) Glaucomatous cupping of the optic disc by ultrasonography. *American Journal of Ophthalmology*, 82, 24–26.

Coleman, D.J. (1972) Reliability of ocular and orbital diagnosis with B-scan ultrasound. 1. Ocular diagnosis. *American Journal of Ophthalmology*, 73, 501–516.

Coleman, D.J. and Franzen, L.A. (1974) Vitreous surgery. Preoperative evaluation and prognostic value of ultrasonic display of vitreous haemorrhage. *Archives of Ophthalmology*, 92, 373–381.

Coleman, D.J. and Katz, L. (1974) Colour-coding of B-scan ultrasonograms. *Archives of Ophthalmology*, 91, 429–431.

Coleman, D.J. and Lizzi, F.L. (1983) Computerized ultrasonic tissue characterization of ocular tumours. *American Journal of Ophthalmology*, 96, 165–175.

Coleman, D.J. and Weininger, R. (1969) Ultrasonic M-mode technique in ophthalmology. *Archives of Ophthalmology*, 82, 475–479.

Coleman, D.J., Konig, W.F. and Katz, L. (1969) A hand operated ultrasound scan system for ophthalmic evaluation. *American Journal of Ophthalmology*, 68, 256–263.

Coleman, D.J., Katz, L., and Lizzi, F.L. (1975) Isometric, three-dimensional viewing of ultrasonograms. *Archives of Ophthalmology*, 93, 1362–1365.

Coleman, D.J., Lizzi, F.L. and Jakobiec, F.A. (1978) Therapeutic ultrasound in the production of ocular lesions. *American Journal of Ophthalmology*, 86, 185–192.

Coleman, D.J., Lizzi, F.L., El-Mofty, A.A.M., Driller, J and Franzen, L.A. (1980) Ultrasonically accelerated resorption of vitreous membranes. *American Journal of Ophthalmology*, 89, 490–499.

Dallow, R.L., Momose, K.J., Weber, A.L. and Wray, S.H. (1976) Comparison of ultrasonography, computerized tomography (EMI scan) and radiographic techniques in evaluation of exophthalmos. *Transcripts of the American Academy of Ophthalmology and Otolaryngology*, 81, 305–322.

Darnley-Fisch, D.A., Byrne, S.F., Hughes, J.R., Parrish, R.K. and Feuer, W.J. (1990) Contact B-scan echography in the assessment of optic nerve cupping. *American Journal of Ophthalmology*, 109, 55–61.

Dziezyc, J., Millichamp, N.J. and Keller, C.N. (1991) Use of phacofragmentation for cataract removal in horses: 12 cases (1985–1989). *Journal of the American Veterinary Medical Association*, 198, 1774–1778.

Erickson, S.J., Hendrix, L.E., Massaro, B.M., Harris, G.J., Lewandowski, M.F., Foley, W.D. and Lawson, T.L. (1989) Color doppler flow imaging of the normal and abnormal orbit. *Radiology*, 173, 511–516.

Fisher, Y.L. (1989) Advances in contact ophthalmic ultrasonography: ocular trauma and intraocular foreign body patients. *Developments in Ophthalmology*, 18, 69–74.

Gaiddon, G., Rosolen, S. and Steru, L. (1989) Study of biometry and keratometry and calculation of the power of an implant in the dog. *Pratique Medicale et Chirurgicale de l'Animale de Compagnie*, 24, 683–691.

Gelatt, K.N., Samuelson, D.A., Barrie, K.P., Das, N.D., Wolf, E.D., Bauer, J.E. and Andreson, T.L. (1983) Biometry and clinical characteristics of congenital cataracts and microphthalmia in the Miniature Schnauzer. *Journal of the American Veterinary Medical Association*, 183, 99–102.

Gilger, B.C., McLaughlin, S.A. and Whitley, R.D. (1990) Corneal pachymetry. *Proceedings of the 21st Annual Meeting of the American College of Veterinary Ophthalmologists*, pp. 8–16.

Hendrix, D.V.H., Nasisse, M.P. and Davidson, M.G. (1991) Clinical findings and risk factors associated with retinal detachment in dogs: a study of 1909 cases. *Proceedings of the 22nd Annual Meeting of the American College of Veterinary Ophthalmologists*, p. 63.

Jack, R.L., Hutton, W.L. and Machemer, R. (1974) Ultrasonography and vitrectomy. *American Journal of Ophthalmology*, 78, 265–274.

Kelman, C.D. (1967) Phaco-emulsification and aspiration. A new technique of cataract removal. A preliminary report. *American Journal of Ophthalmology*, 64, 23–35.

Kennerdell, J.S., Slamovits, T.L., Dekker, A. and Johnson, B.L. (1985) Orbital fine needle aspiration biopsy; the results of its use in fifty patients. *American Journal of Ophthalmology*, 99, 547–551.

Kerlen, C.H. (1981) B-scan ultrasonography in optic neuropathy. *Documenta Ophthalmologica Proceedings Series*, 29, 353–358.

Krohne, S.G. and Lindley, D.M. (1991) Aqueous humour flare and cells measured by laser flaremetry before and after cataract phacoemulsification in the dog. *International Society of Veterinary Ophthalmology Congress*, 1991, p. 25.

Lizzi, F.L., Driller, J. and Ostromogilsky, M. (1984) Thermal model for ultrasonic treatment of glaucoma. *Ultrasound in Medicine and Biology*, 10, 289–298.

Marmor, M.F., Wickramasinghe, H.K. and Lemons, R.A. (1977) Acoustic microscopy of the human retina and pigment epithelium. *Investigative Ophthalmology and Visual Science*, 16, 660–666.

Miller, T.R., Whitley, R.D., Meek, L.A., Garcia, G.A., Wilson, M.C. and Rawls, B.H. (1987) Phacofragmentation and aspiration for cataract extraction in dogs: 56 cases (1980–1984). *Journal of the American Veterinary Medical Association*, 190, 1577–1580.

Moore, P.A. and Fischer, C.A. (1990) Endocapsular phacofragmentation and aspiration. A retrospective study of the first 107 eyes. *Transcripts of the 21st Annual Meeting of the American College of Veterinary Ophthalmologists*, pp. 167–168.

Mundt, G.H. and Hughes, W.F. (1956) Ultrasonics in ocular diagnosis. *American Journal of Ophthalmology*, 41, 488–498.

Nishi, O. (1989) Lens epithelial removal by ultrasound: access to 12 o'clock. *Journal of Cataract and Refractive Surgery*, 15, 704–706.

Oksala, A. and Lehtinen, A. (1957) Diagnostic value of ultrasonics in ophthalmology. *Ophthalmologica*, 134, 387–395.

Ossoinig, K.C. (1974) Quantitative echography – the basis of tissue differentiation. *Journal of Clinical Ultrasound*, 2, 33–46.

Paunksnis, A.I., Daktaravichene, E.I. and Lukoshiavichius, A.I. (1989) Ways to increase the information value of ultrasonic studies in the diagnosis of intraocular tumours. *Oftalmologicheskii Zhurnal*, 6, 325–330.

Pavlin, C.J., Sherar, M.D., Haraswiewicz, K. and Foster, F.S. (1991) Clinical use of ultrasound biomicroscopy. *Ophthalmology*, 98, 287–295.

Restori, M. (1978) Ultrasonic holography in ophthalmic diagnosis. *British Journal of Clinical Equipment*, March, pp. 71–75.

Restori, M. and Wright, J.E. (1977) C-scan ultrasonography in orbital diagnosis. *British Journal of Ophthalmology*, 61, 735–740.

Rubin, L.F. and Koch, S.A. (1968) Ocular diagnostic ultrasonography. *Journal of the American Veterinary Medical Association*, 153, 1706–1716.

Schroeder, W. and Guthoff, R. (1981) Ultrasonography of the optic nerve. *Documenta Ophthalmologica Proceedings Series*, 29, 359–362.

Skalka, H.W. (1981) Ultrasonography and percutaneous orbital aspiration. *Documenta Ophthalmologica Proceedings Series*, 29, 375–383.

Skalka, H.W. and Kline, L.B. (1984) Comparative value of ultrasound and CT scanning in orbital optic nerve evaluation. *Proceedings of the 9th Societas Internationalis Prodiagnostica Ultrasonica Ophthalmologica Congress*, pp. 365–370.

Spoor, T.C., Kennerdell, J.S., Dekker, A., Johnson, B.L. and Rehkopf, P. (1980) Orbital fine needle aspiration biopsy with B-scan guidance. *American Journal of Ophthalmology*, 89, 274–277.

Torchia, R.T., Purnell, E.W. and Sokollu, A. (1967) Cataract production by ultrasound. *American Journal of Ophthalmology*, 64, 305–309.

Ziskin, M., Romayandanda, N. and Harris, K. (1974) Ophthalmological effect of ultrasound at diagnostic intensities. *Journal of Clinical Ultrasound*, 2, 119–122.

5 Large Animal Echocardiography

K.J. Long

Department of Veterinary Clinical Studies, Royal (Dick) School of Veterinary Studies, University of Edinburgh, Large Animal Hospital, Veterinary Field Station, Easter Bush, Roslin, Midlothian EH25 9RG, UK

Introduction

The investigation of heart disease in large animals is hindered by the limitations of conventional radiographic and electrocardiographic techniques. The ability to record dynamic images of the heart by two-dimensional (2-D) ultrasonography has greatly improved our diagnostic capabilities. 2-D echocardiography has proved invaluable in the diagnosis of congenital cardiac disorders, pericardial effusions and severe valvular dysfunction. It can also be used to monitor ventricular function and assess the response of the heart to abnormal blood flow. However, 2-D echocardiography is of limited value in cases of valvular dysfunction where the valve appears structurally normal. This is a major problem in equine cardiology where valvular regurgitation is commonly associated with minimal or no gross valvular lesions. Doppler echocardiography is a sensitive technique for the detection of abnormal blood flow and is the only noninvasive method of identifying valvular regurgitation. By combining information from 2-D, M-mode and Doppler techniques it is now possible accurately to diagnose cardiac disease, quantify ventricular function and determine the severity of valvular dysfunction in large animals.

Equipment

A sector scanner is more useful for echocardiography than a linear scanner, because the ultrasound beam of a sector scanner diverges from a relatively small footprint, which can be easily positioned between the ribs (see Chapter 1). This is especially important in foals and small ruminants where the intercostal spaces are narrow. With linear scanners, the number of image planes that can be produced is limited, as the transducer must be placed vertically between the ribs to maintain good contact with the skin surface.

Cardiac images are obtained from adult horses and cattle with low-frequency transducers (2.25 MHz–3 MHz). The resolution of these low-frequency transducers is poor, but higher frequency transducers do not penetrate to a sufficient depth to produce adequate images in large animals. Where maximum imaging depth is not required, e.g. in calves, sheep or foals, higher frequency transducers (3.5 MHz–5 MHz) may be used to obtain better quality images.

Rapidly moving structures are studied using M-mode echocardiography because of its high temporal resolution (Fig. 5.5a below). M-mode studies are used for measurement of cardiac dimensions, as the timing of measurements within the cardiac cycle is more precise. A simultaneously recorded electrocardiogram (ECG) allows accurate timing of these measurements.

With modern equipment, the 2-D image can be used to guide placement of the M-mode cursor into an area of interest. This is easily performed if the M-mode cursor can be moved within the 2-D sector. With many machines, however, the cursor is fixed and M-mode images are recorded by moving the 2-D image into the path of the cursor. This method is much more difficult.

Doppler echocardiography requires the use of equipment with additional features.

Basic Principles of Doppler Echocardiography

The Doppler principle was defined by Christian Andreas Doppler, who showed that an apparent shift in transmitted frequency occurs as a result of motion of either the source or the observer. In Doppler echocardiography, ultrasound is directed towards the area of interest in the heart, and is reflected by moving structures (e.g. red blood cells). The frequency of the reflected signal is altered in relation to the velocity of these reflectors. This change in frequency of the Doppler signal can be used to calculate the direction and speed of the moving target. Doppler ultrasound techniques differ in a number of ways from those used in 2-D and M-mode echocardiography. During 2-D and M-mode imaging, the best images are obtained when the ultrasound beam is directed at right angles to the reflective surfaces of the heart. With Doppler ultrasound the converse is true: the most accurate flow information is obtained when the ultrasound beam is directed parallel to the moving target, that is, parallel to blood flow (see Chapter 1). In 2-D and M-mode imaging the best images are obtained using high-frequency transducers which have high resolution. However, in Doppler ultrasonography lower frequency transducers are favoured as they are able to record higher velocities. Also, for a given velocity, a lower frequency transducer will be able to record that velocity at a greater depth. This becomes important when imaging larger animals, for example adult horses and cattle.

Doppler ultrasound can be used to record blood flow velocities from a specific location (pulsed Doppler), along a specific line (continuous wave Doppler; CWD), or from a given area comprising numerous sampling points (colour-coded Doppler). Each technique has its own advantages and disadvantages. By convention, the direction of flow is recorded as positive (above the baseline) or coded in red when flow is towards the transducer, and negative (below the baseline) or coded in blue when flow is in the opposite direction.

Pulsed Doppler echocardiography enables flow velocities to be recorded from a specific location within the heart. In this technique, one pulse of ultrasound is emitted and the frequency shifts caused by reflections at the specific sampling site (sample volume) are analysed (range gating). A further pulse of ultrasound is emitted after a time delay to allow echoes to return from the area of interest. This technique is called low pulse repetition frequency (LPRF) Doppler echocardiography. It allows flow velocities to be recorded at specific inflow and outflow points, and enables specific areas of the heart to be examined for the presence of abnormal flow. The disadvantage of pulsed Doppler echocardiography arises from the low pulse repetition frequencies available at greater depths: the maximum velocity that can be recorded by a transducer is equal to half the pulse repetition frequency (the Nyquist limit). The flow velocity cannot be accurately recorded if it exceeds this value.

It is often useful to record the maximum flow velocity, as this can be used to calculate the pressure gradient between the cardiac chambers and the great vessels. This calculated pressure gradient provides valuable information regarding the significance of any abnormal findings. The pressure gradient (e.g. between two chambers) is calculated from the formula:

$$\text{pressure gradient} = 4 \times (V_2{}^2 - V_1{}^2)$$

where V_1 is the peak velocity proximally and V_2 is the peak velocity distally. Underestimation of the maximum flow velocity would cause the severity of a given lesion to be incorrectly assessed.

Where blood flow velocity exceeds the Nyquist limit of the transducer, the calculated flow velocity will be displayed as though it were going in the opposite direction (aliasing), and the signal will 'wrap around' the baseline of the velocity display (Fig. 5.1). To overcome this problem, high pulse repetition frequency (HPRF) Doppler has been developed. With this technique, further ultrasound pulses are emitted before the initial pulse has returned to the transducer. This increases the pulse repetition frequency and therefore enables higher velocities to be recorded without aliasing. The disadvantage of this technique is the loss of specificity of the sampling site compared to conventional pulsed Doppler, and range ambiguity is a problem.

Continuous wave Doppler has the advantage of recording very high velocities accurately. Using this technique, one crystal continuously emits ultrasound and another crystal continuously receives it. However, as the velocity data are collected along the entire beam length, there is no way of knowing the exact location of the high velocity flow, and range ambiguity is again a problem.

Colour flow/colour coded Doppler is a form of pulsed Doppler and therefore has the same disadvantage of aliasing at velocities above the Nyquist limit. In colour-coded Doppler, velocities are recorded from numerous sampling points within a sector, which is positioned anywhere within the 2-D image, thus enabling large areas of the heart to be screened for abnormal flow at one time. This is useful in the diagnosis of equine heart murmurs where chamber dimensions are large although the area of abnormal flow is often small. The Doppler

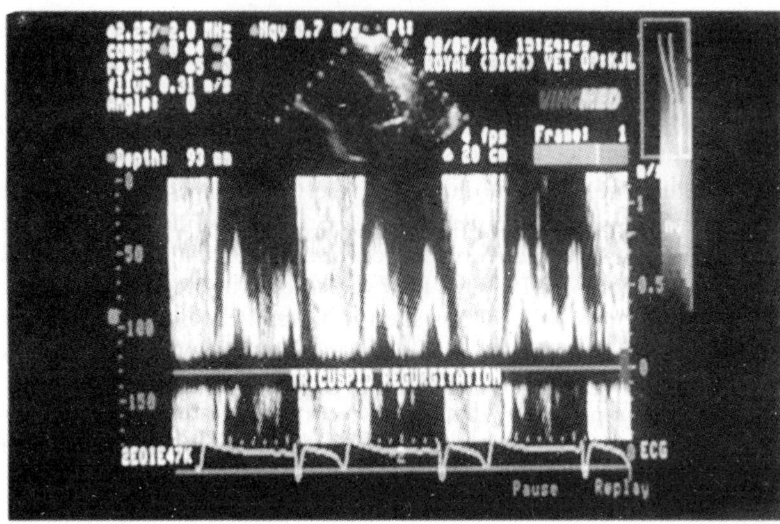

Fig. 5.1. Pulsed Doppler recording of blood flow through the tricuspid valve. During diastole the normal tricuspid inflow velocities are displayed above the baseline, and during systole tricuspid regurgitation is present. The regurgitant flow is in the opposite direction to the normal inflow, yet it is displayed above and below the baseline. This is termed aliasing. Aliasing occurs when the flow velocity exceeds the Nyquist limit of the transducer.

information is colour-coded for velocity and direction of flow (Plate 1, frontispiece), and in most instruments disturbed flow is also indicated. By convention, the flow towards the transducer is shown in red and that away is shown in blue, as mentioned earlier. Some indication of velocity is given by the brightness of the colours. Turbulent or disturbed flow is often shown in yellow or green (Plate 2, frontispiece). The actual velocity of flow is not quantified, and this must be measured by pulsed or continuous wave Doppler.

Colour-coded Doppler information can also be superimposed on an M-mode image (Plate 3, frontispiece). As M-mode images are constructed from a single imaging beam, blood flow information is updated rapidly. These images are therefore useful for accurate timing of the duration of abnormal flow.

Detection of normal and disturbed flow

Blood flow within the heart is normally laminar. A pulsed Doppler tracing from an area of laminar blood flow will show that all of the cells are travelling in the same direction with approximately the same velocity. When the operator has aligned the ultrasound beam accurately with the flow, the maximum flow velocity will be recorded and the Doppler waveform will show a minimal velocity spread. This is demonstrated by the tricuspid inflow signal in Fig. 5.1. The audible Doppler frequency shift at this point will be pure. Disturbed flow consists of cells moving in different directions and with different velocities as shown by the tricuspid regurgitant signal in Fig. 5.1. Disturbed flow occurs when blood flows over uneven surfaces or through a restrictive orifice. The audio signal obtained from areas of disturbed flow is coarse and contains a large number of frequencies.

Occasionally, abnormal flow appears laminar. This occurs when the sample volume is placed in the centre of a high velocity jet. In this case flow can be recognized as abnormal by its velocity, which is much higher than that found in normal hearts (Fig. 5.2).

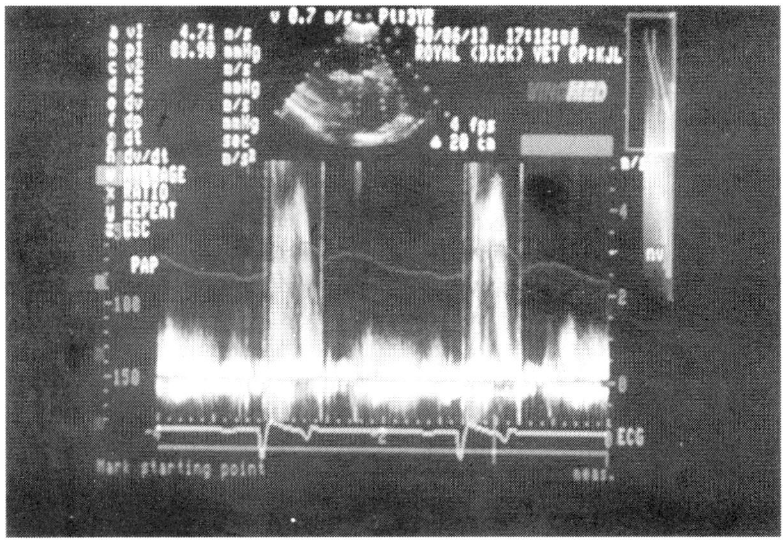

Fig. 5.2. High pulse repetition frequency Doppler study of blood flow through a ventricular septal defect in a three-year-old Thoroughbred mare. The blood flow is laminar, with most cells travelling at the same velocity. The maximum flow velocity is 4.71 m s^{-1}. Note the multiple sample volumes on the 2-D image. PAP = pulmonary artery pressure trace.

Normal Echocardiographic Examination

A systematic approach to the echocardiographic examination is advisable, to prevent oversight of important information when attention is focused by a positive finding in another chamber.

Cardiac images are usually obtained from the right side of the thorax first, as right-sided images are usually of better quality and most cardiac structures can be easily identified. The animal is stood squarely, and the hair coat is clipped in a vertical strip, immediately caudal to the triceps mass, commencing at the level of the olecranon process and extending 10 cm dorsally. A second strip of hair is clipped from the caudal edge of the triceps mass. In slim, fine-coated Thoroughbred horses, adequate images can often be obtained without clipping. The clipped area is wiped with surgical spirit prior to scanning to improve image quality.

The ultrasound transducer is held with the index mark, which indicates the edge of the imaging sector, under the thumb of the left hand when scanning from the right hemithorax, and under the thumb of the right hand when scanning from the left hemithorax.

2-D images from the right hemithorax

The transducer is held perpendicular to the thoracic wall, with the index mark in the 12 o'clock position (0°). The transducer is then placed in the fourth or fifth intercostal space just above the olecranon process. This produces a long-axis, four-chambered reference view of the ventricular inlets (Fig. 5.3a). The interventricular septum (IVS) will be orientated horizontally across the sector, with the axial or central beam crossing the image at the level of the chordae tendineae. In some animals it will be necessary to angle the transducer slightly caudally to obtain this view. In animals which require the more cranial transducer placement (usually heavy hunter horses and cobs) this is made easier by placing the right foreleg slightly forward, and by pushing the hindquarters away from the operator so that the olecranon process is clear of the body wall. Cattle are more difficult to scan, as the olecranon process is held close to the thoracic wall and they tend to stand with the forelegs positioned more caudally. More cranial placement of the transducer is required to produce the reference view. Care must be taken, when scanning cattle, not to damage the transducer, which is easily trapped beneath the olecranon process if the forelimb is suddenly moved caudally. Cattle are more easily scanned in a crush, with the appropriate foreleg held forward and either positioned cranially over a straw bale or elevated on a block. No advantage is gained by merely elevating the forelimb, as this results in flexion of the leg at the elbow with more caudal placement of the triceps muscle mass. Quiet halter-trained cattle can be stood freely and positioned as described for horses. Broad-chested animals and overweight animals tend to produce images of poorer quality. Calves and sheep may be scanned standing, or they may be positioned in lateral recumbency and scanned from underneath, as described for dogs and cats (see Chapter 6). Care must be taken to ensure that ruminants do not become bloated when held in lateral recumbency for long periods of time.

If the reference view is not obtained when the transducer is first placed on the animal, but the aorta can be seen in the centre of the screen, more caudal placement of the transducer or caudal angulation is required. If both the left ventricular outflow tract and the aorta are present in the image, clockwise rotation of the transducer or cranial angulation must have occurred. If the IVS is not perpendicular to the axial (central) beam, but the cardiac apex is tilted to the top of the sector, dorsal angulation of the transducer must have occurred (Fig. 5.3b).

It is important to appreciate that slight changes in angulation and rotation of the transducer will result in large changes in beam position at depths of 24–30 cm. For this reason, gradual movement of the transducer is recommended.

Once the reference view has been obtained, the whole heart can be examined systematically. As indicated above, the position of the axial beam in relation to intracardiac landmarks can be used to identify the location and angulation of the transducer. Therefore, it is possible to determine the transducer position required to obtain a subsequent view from any given image. From the reference view, if the transducer is slid ventrally on the body wall, more of the cardiac apex will appear in the image. If the transducer is moved dorsally, the tricuspid valve will move into the axial beam. More of the right atrium can be visualized from this image by rotating the transducer slightly clockwise and angling cranially (Fig. 5.3c). Slight cranial angulation and clockwise rotation (+30°) from the reference view, will produce a long-axis view of the aorta (Fig. 5.3d).

Short-axis images or cross-sectional views of the heart are obtained by rotating the transducer 90° in an anti-clockwise direction. A 90° rotation of the transducer from the reference position will give a cross-section of the left ventricle at the chordal level (Fig. 5.4a). If the transducer is angled ventrally from this position, images of the papillary muscles and left ventricular apex are obtained. Angling the transducer slightly dorsally from the chordal level with less anti-clockwise rotation (−80°) will give an image of the mitral valve (Fig. 5.4b). Further dorsal angulation, less anti-clockwise rotation (−30°) and slight cranial angulation, will produce a cross-sectional image of the aortic valve (Fig. 5.4c). If the transducer is angled still further cranially, with less anti-clockwise rotation (−20° to −30°) the right ventricular outflow tract, pulmonary artery and coronary artery will be visualized (Fig. 5.4d).

M-mode images from the right hemithorax

The left and right ventricular diameter and IVS and left ventricular wall thicknesses are measured from an M-mode study recorded from a short-axis view at the chordal level (Fig. 5.5b). By using short-axis images to guide placement of the M-mode cursor, the operator can ensure that the cursor is placed across the widest part of the chamber or vessel to be measured. The American Society of Echocardiography recommends that M-mode measurements are made using the 'leading edge' method. Measurements are made from the leading edge of the first endocardial surface to the leading edge of the second endocardial surface. End diastolic measurements are taken at the onset of the QRS complex of the ECG. Systolic measurements are taken during the maximum excursion of the ventricular septum, unless septal movement is abnormal, when they are timed from the maximum movement of the left ventricular free wall.

An assessment of the contractility of the left ventricle can be obtained by subtracting the left ventricular internal diameter at systole (LVIDs) from the diastolic dimension (LVIDd), and dividing this by the diastolic dimension. This is termed the fractional shortening (FS) of the ventricle and is usually expressed as a percentage:

$$FS = 100 \times (LVIDd - LVIDs)/LVIDd$$

If ultrasound images are limited to a depth of 24 cm or less, the far wall of the left ventricle may not be included in this image and therefore the measurement of left ventricular diameter cannot be made. In these cases, the left ventricle can be measured from short-axis images obtained from the left side of the thorax. Equipment with a maximum imaging depth of 30 cm enables all measurements to be made from this right parasternal image.

The aortic diameter is measured from an M-mode study taken at the aortic valve level (Fig. 5.5c). Measurements from guided M-mode studies recorded from 40 normal Thoroughbred and Thoroughbred cross horses are given in Table 5.1. Measurements from normal calves have also been reported (Amory *et al.*, 1991).

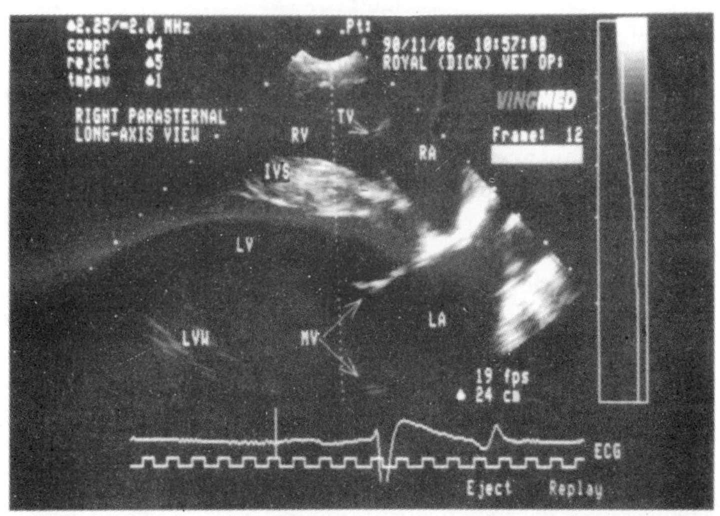
2.25/=2.0 MHz
compr   44
rejct   45
tmpav   41
RIGHT PARASTERNAL
LONG-AXIS VIEW
.Pt:
90/11/06   10:57:00
ROYAL (DICK) VET OP:
VINGMED
Frame: 12
RV
TV
IVS
RA
LV
LA
LVW
MV
19 fps
24 cm
ECG
Eject   Replay
a

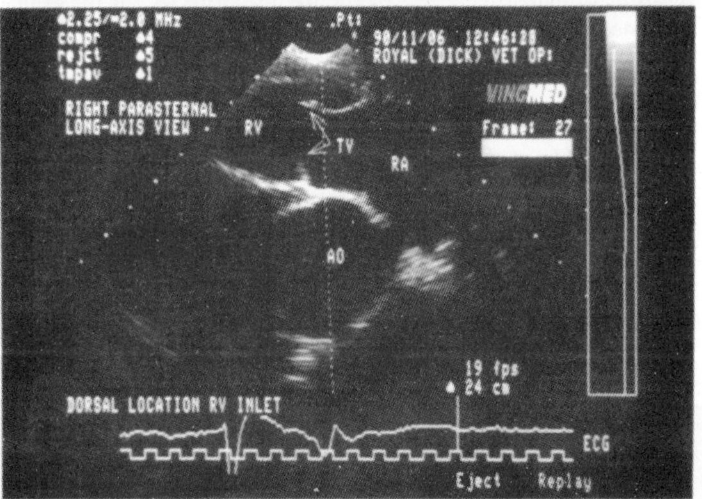
2.25/=2.0 MHz
compr   44
rejct   45
tmpav   41
RIGHT PARASTERNAL
LONG-AXIS VIEW
.Pt:
90/11/06   11:56:00
ROYAL (DICK) VET OP:
VINGMED
Frame: 33
RV
TV
LV
RA
MV
LA
19 fps
24 cm
ECG
Eject   Replay
b

2.25/=2.0 MHz
compr   44
rejct   45
tmpav   41
RIGHT PARASTERNAL
LONG-AXIS VIEW
.Pt:
90/11/06   12:46:20
ROYAL (DICK) VET OP:
VINGMED
Frame: 27
RV
TV
RA
AO
19 fps
24 cm
DORSAL LOCATION RV INLET
ECG
Eject   Replay
c

2-D and M-mode images from the left hemithorax

When imaging from the left hemithorax, the hair coat is clipped in a vertical strip behind the triceps mass. The reference image (Fig. 5.6a) is obtained by holding the transducer perpendicular to the chest wall with the index mark in the 12 o'clock position (0°). The transducer is then placed caudal to the olecranon process and dorsal to the apical impulse. This is a more caudal transducer placement than that used to obtain right-sided images. Sliding the transducer ventrally from this position results in a more apical image of the heart, whereas sliding the transducer dorsally results in the axial beam crossing the ventricle at the level of the mitral valve. If the transducer is placed ventrally and angled dorsally, the image will be tilted so that the IVS crosses the axial beam at an angle (Fig. 5.6b). The parasternal long-axis five-chambered view (Fig. 5.6c) is obtained from the reference position by pivoting the transducer on its caudal border and angling cranially. Short-axis images of the left ventricle are obtained by rotating the transducer 90° clockwise from the reference view. Left ventricular dimensions can be measured from an

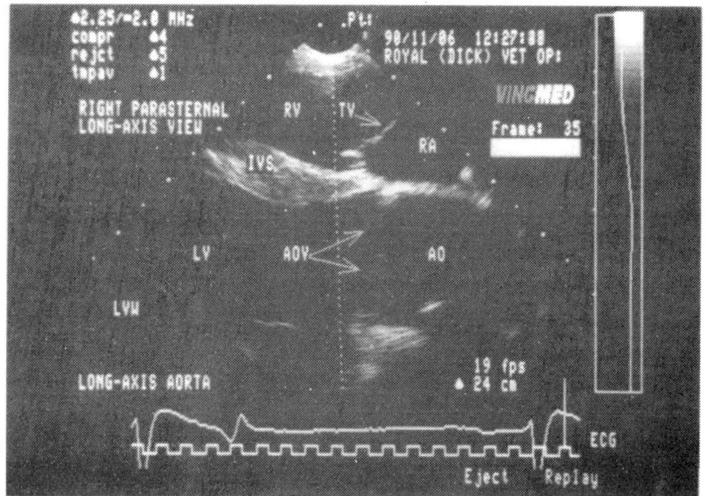

d

Fig. 5.3. Long-axis images from the right hemithorax. **(a)** Right parasternal long-axis view. Reference view, ventricular inlets. The transducer is placed at the fourth or fifth intercostal space with the index mark dorsal (0°). The axial beam should cross the left ventricle at the level of the chordae tendineae, with the interventricular septum orientated horizontally across the sector. **(b)** Right parasternal long-axis view. Apical view, ventricular inlets. The transducer is placed at the fourth or fifth intercostal space in a ventral location. The axial beam is angled dorsally and, in some horses, slightly cranially. **(c)** Right parasternal long-axis view. Dorsal location, right ventricular inlet. The transducer is placed at the fourth or fifth intercostal space in a dorsal location. The axial beam is angled cranially and rotated clockwise to image more of the right atrium. **(d)** Right parasternal long-axis view. Long-axis aorta. The transducer is rotated clockwise (+30°) and angled slightly cranially from the reference position. RA = right atrium; RV = right ventricle; TV = tricuspid valve; LA = left atrium; LV = left ventricle; MV = mitral valve; LVW = left ventricular wall; IVS = interventricular septum; AO = aorta; AOV = aortic valve; LVOT = left ventricular outflow tract.

2.25/~2.0 MHz
compr   4
rejct   5
tmpav   1
.Pt:
90/11/06 11:28:00
ROYAL (DICK) VET OP:
VINGMED
RIGHT PARASTERNAL
SHORT-AXIS VIEW
RV
Frame: 42
IVS
LV
CHORDAE
19 fps
24 cm
CHORDAL LEVEL
ECG
Eject   Replay

a

2.25/~2.0 MHz
compr   4
rejct   5
tmpav   1
.Pt:
90/11/06 11:48:00
ROYAL (DICK) VET OP:
VINGMED
RIGHT PARASTERNAL
SHORT-AXIS VIEW
RV
Frame: 41
IVS
MITRAL VALVE
19 fps
24 cm
MITRAL VALVE LEVEL
ECG
Eject   Replay

b

2.25/~2.0 MHz
compr   4
rejct   5
tmpav   1
.Pt:
90/11/02 14:10:28
ROYAL (DICK) VET OP:
VINGMED
RIGHT PARASTERNAL
SHORT-AXIS
RV
TV
RA
AORTIC VALVE
19 fps
24 cm
AORTIC VALVE LEVEL
ECG
Recall frame (4) :
Eject   Not Active

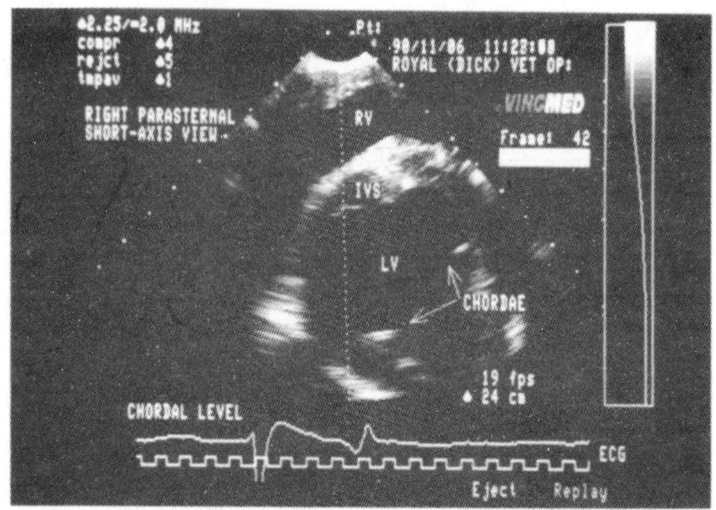

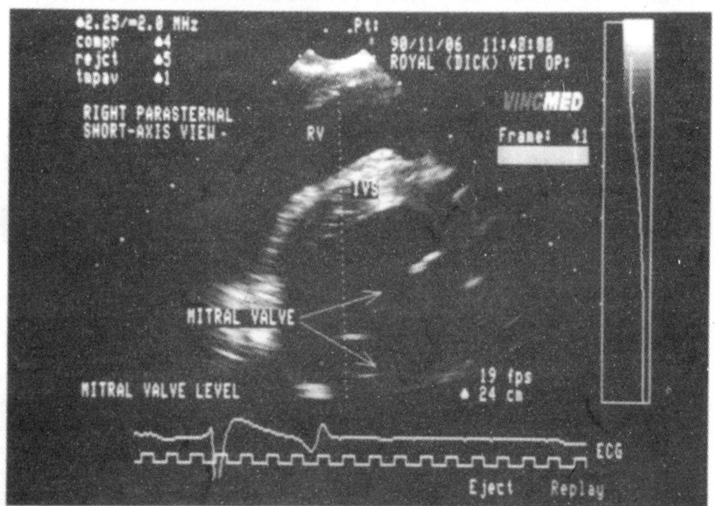

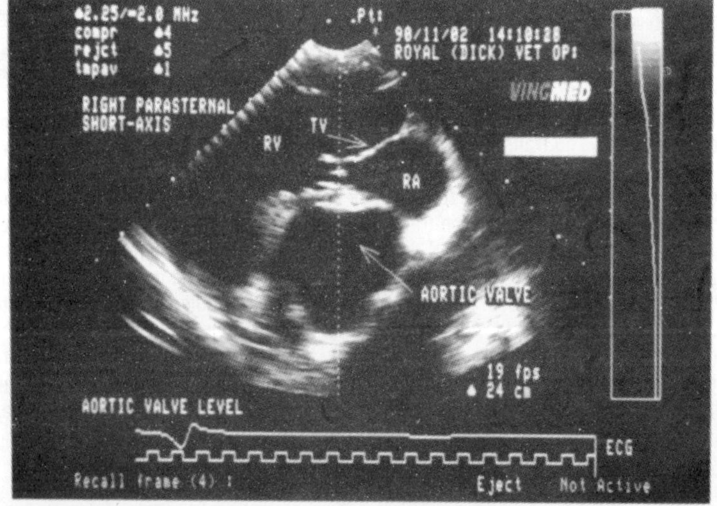

c

M-mode image taken at the chordal level. Care must be taken to ensure that the M-mode image is recorded from a true short-axis view without inclusion of the aorta or posterior papillary muscle (Fig. 5.6d). It is often helpful initially to align the axial beam in the long-axis view at the chordal level before rotating the transducer.

The normal Doppler examination

The Doppler examination is usually performed concurrently with the 2-D and M-mode studies, and again a systematic approach ensures that important information is not overlooked. The normal tricuspid inflow velocity is recorded from the right side of the animal from an apical view of the ventricular inlets (Fig. 5.3b above). The 2-D reference image is first obtained, then the transducer is slid ventrally on the thoracic wall and angled dorsally until the Doppler ultrasound beam can be aligned with the tricuspid inlet. The sampling site (sample volume) is placed on the ventricular side of the tricuspid valve at the valve tips. The operator must ensure that the sample volume does not move into the right atrium as the heart relaxes during diastole. Initial alignment with flow is determined from the 2-D image. This image is then frozen, and the transducer is adjusted until a pure audio signal and a clear visual signal are obtained. If colour flow technology is

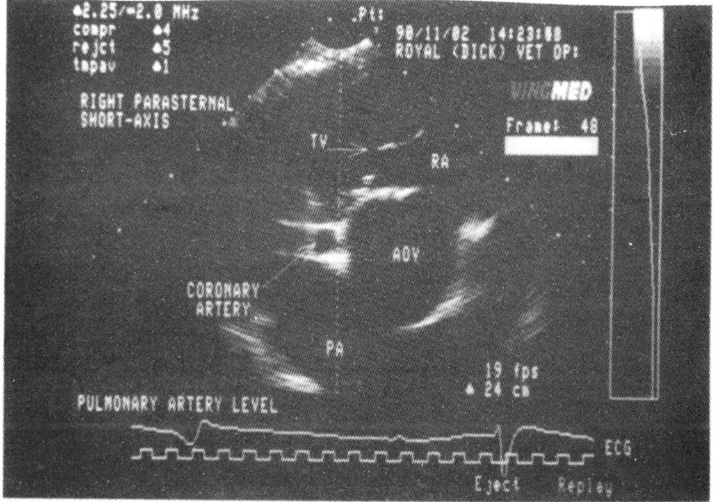

Fig. 5.4. Short-axis images from the right hemithorax. **(a)** Chordal level. The transducer is rotated anti-clockwise (–90°) from the reference position. The transducer is angled slightly caudal and dorsal. The degree of rotation should be adjusted to obtain a true short-axis. **(b)** Mitral valve level. The transducer is rotated anti-clockwise (–80°) from the reference position. The transducer is angled slightly caudal and dorsal. The degree of rotation should be adjusted to obtain a true short-axis. **(c)** Aortic valve level. The transducer is rotated anti-clockwise (–30°) from the reference position. Cranial and dorsal angulation is required. Rotation is then adjusted to obtain a true cross-section of the aorta. **(d)** Pulmonary artery (PA) level. The transducer is rotated anti-clockwise (–20° to –30°) from the reference position. Dorsal angulation and maximal cranial angulation are required. For abbreviations see Fig. 5.3.

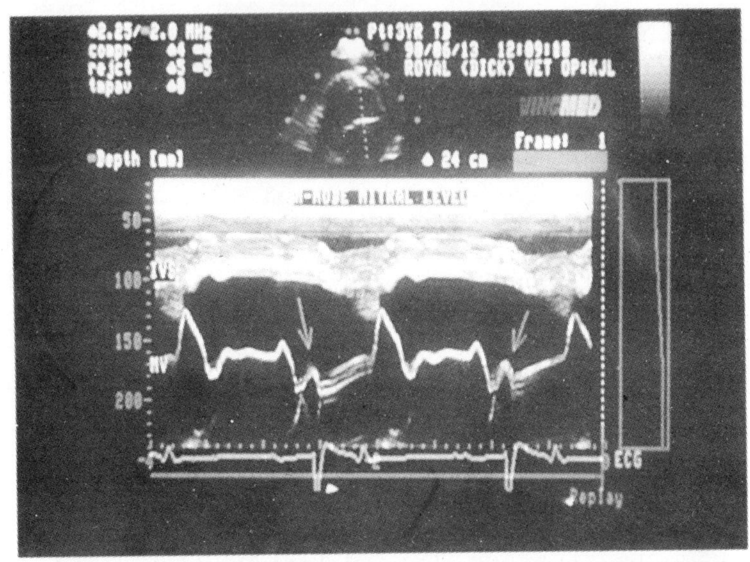

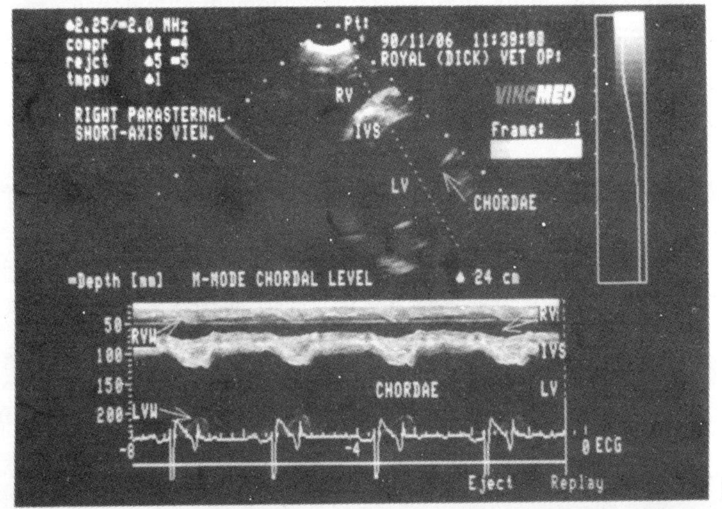

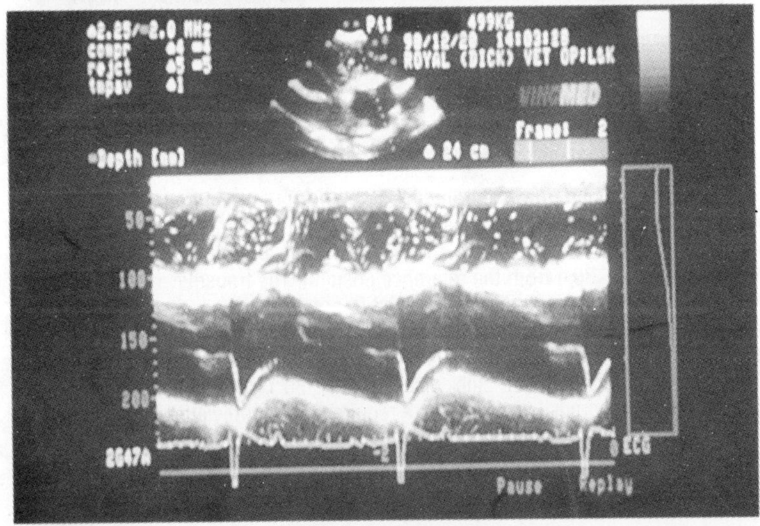

available, this can be used to guide the initial placement. Fig. 5.7a shows the typical inflow recording from the right ventricle. The E wave represents the initial rapid filling phase of the ventricle, and the A wave represents the atrial contraction. In humans, the E wave is normally larger than the A wave. A reversal of this pattern, with the A wave larger than the E wave, is seen in cases of diastolic dysfunction of the ventricle. This is also true for the left ventricular inflow. In horses, however, the A wave is very variable, and in some normal horses appears larger than the E wave. This may be due to differences in alignment with the two phases of the inflow. In some horses optimal alignment with the A wave is achieved from a different angle than with the E wave. If good alignment with the E wave cannot be achieved, the A wave will appear larger. In the normal horse, the E wave ranges from 0.43 to 1.01 m s^{-1}, and the A wave from 0.25 to 0.86 m s^{-1}. Normal Doppler values have not been reported for ruminants, although it is likely that they would show similar intracardiac flow velocities to other species.

The maximum velocity of the E and A waves increases with increasing heart rate, until at higher heart rates the E and A peaks combine to give a single inflow velocity.

Physiological back-flow is a common finding at the tricuspid valve in normal horses. This may be detected by pulsed and continuous wave Doppler as high velocity disturbed flow on the atrial side of the valve. It can be differentiated from significant tricuspid regurgitation by the short duration of the signal, which often occurs at the onset of the QRS complex of the ECG or after the T wave, and also is only detectable close to the tricuspid valve. Signals of short duration, indicative of physiological back-flow, can also be recorded at the mitral and aortic valves. Regurgitant signals of longer duration are detected close to the pulmonary valve in normal horses.

The pulmonary outflow velocity is recorded from the right parasternal short-axis view at the pulmonary artery level (Fig. 5.4d). The sample volume is placed on the arterial side of the valve, just beyond the valve tips. Alignment with flow is initially assessed from the 2-D image and then adjustments of the transducer are made, as described for the tricuspid inflow. Most equipment will allow the operator to assess the angle between the ultrasound beam and the blood flow as judged from the 2-D image. This angle can then be used to correct the flow

Fig. 5.5. M-mode images from the right hemithorax. **(a)** M-mode echocardiogram of the mitral valve (MV) taken from a short-axis view of the left ventricle. The anterior mitral valve leaflet can be seen in the lower half of the M-mode image. The valve leaflet moves towards the interventricular septum (IVS) during the rapid filling phase of the ventricle (E peak). The valve leaflets are then drawn towards each other, and then move apart (A peak) immediately following the P wave of atrial contraction. The valve leaflets are closed during systole. In this horse, the valve leaflets can be seen to open again immediately before the onset of systole (arrows). **(b)** M-mode taken from the right parasternal short-axis view, chordal level. The image of the left ventricle has been positioned at the far right of the sector display to enable the cursor to bisect the ventricle. The simultaneously recorded ECG allows accurate timing of measurements relative to the cardiac cycle. **(c)** M-mode taken from a right parasternal short-axis view, aortic valve level. The aorta is in the centre of the image. At least one valve leaflet should be present if aortic measurements are to be made. A contrast agent can be clearly seen in the top half of the image passing through the tricuspid valve. For abbreviations see Fig. 5.3.

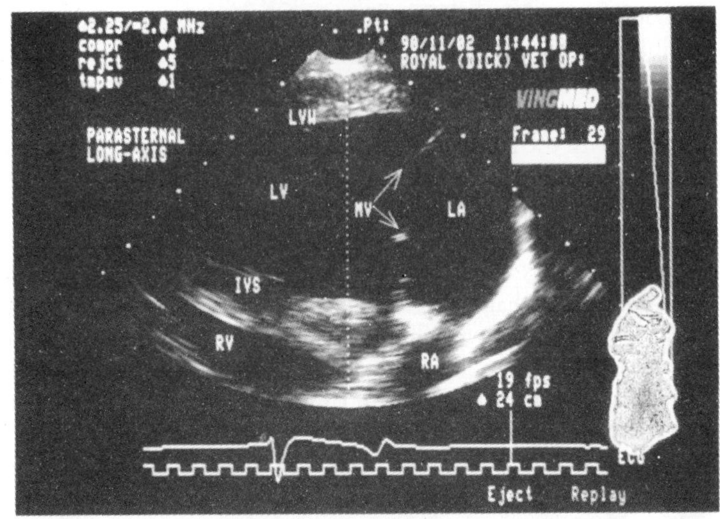

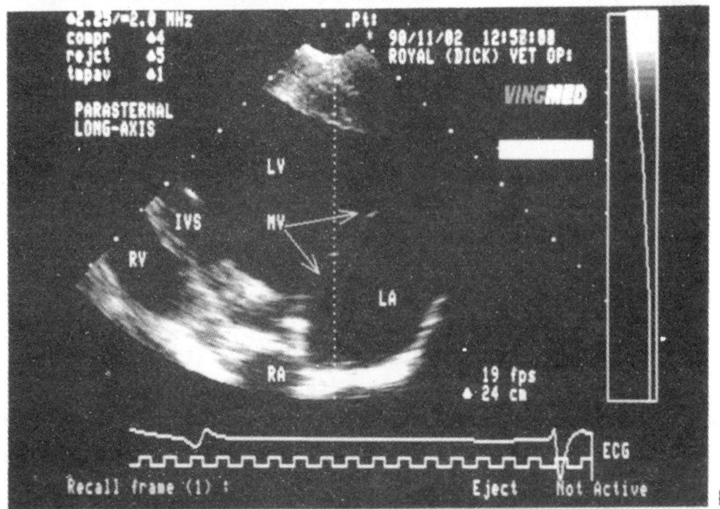

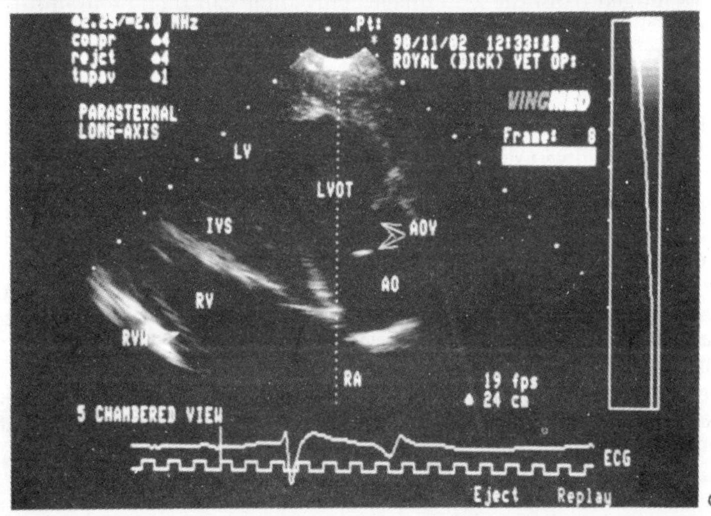

Table 5.1. Summary statistics of median measurements (cm) of five consecutive cardiac cycles, from a group of normal Thoroughbred and Thoroughbred cross horses, obtained by the methods described by Long *et al.* (1992).

Dimension	N	Mean	Max	Min	SD	CV(%)
LVIDs	40	7.577	9.15	6.18	0.733	9.67
LVIDd	34	11.870	13.50	10.02	0.706	5.95
LVWs	16	3.709	4.62	3.31	0.330	8.90
LVWd	5	2.162	2.53	1.92	0.226	10.45
IVSs	40	4.413	5.23	3.75	0.410	9.28
IVSd	40	3.042	3.66	2.35	0.366	12.02
RVIDs	38	2.985	4.88	1.05	0.943	31.59
RVIDd	39	3.937	5.92	2.09	0.851	21.61
FS (%)	34	36.4	44	28	4.04	11.10
Aod	39	8.305	9.41	6.71	0.625	7.53
LIVSd	29	2.968	3.36	2.49	0.207	6.97
LLVWd	29	2.355	2.91	1.68	0.248	10.55
LRVWd	29	1.337	1.83	1.13	0.184	13.74
LRVWs	29	2.361	3.31	1.74	0.355	15.05
LLVIDs	40	7.753	9.49	6.10	0.730	9.42
LLVIDd	40	12.455	14.20	10.54	0.782	6.28

N = number of horses, SD = standard deviation, CV = coefficient of variation.
s = in systole, d = in diastole.
LVID = left ventricular internal diameter, LVW = left ventricular wall, IVS = interventricular septum, RVID = right ventricular internal diameter, FS = fractional shortening calculated from measurements obtained from the right hemithorax, Ao = aortic diameter, LIVS = interventricular septum measured from the left hemithorax, LLVW = left ventricular wall measured from the left hemithorax, LRVW = right ventricular wall measured from the left hemithorax, LLVID = left ventricular internal diameter measured from the left hemithorax.

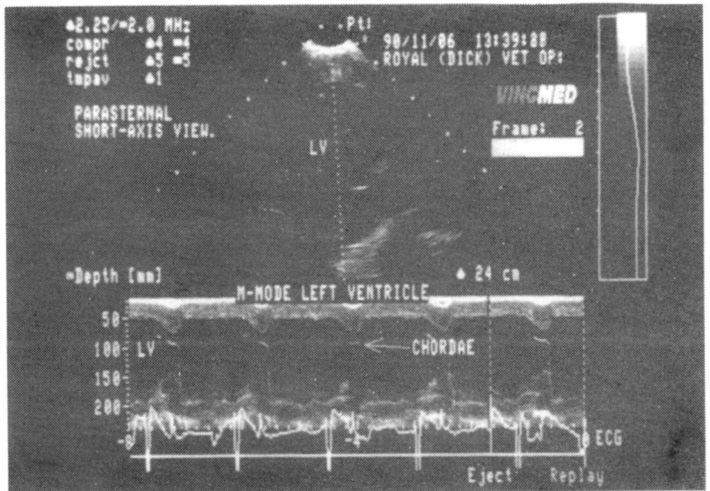

Fig. 5.6. Images from the left hemithorax. **(a)** Left parasternal long-axis view. Reference view. Left ventricular inlet. The transducer is placed caudal to the olecranon process and dorsal to the left apical impulse. The index mark indicating the sector edge is held dorsal. **(b)** Left parasternal long-axis view. Apical view, left ventricular inlet. The transducer is placed ventrally from the reference position and is angled steeply dorsally. **(c)** Left parasternal long-axis view. Five-chambered view. The transducer is slid to the caudal edge of the intercostal space used for the reference image, and is angled cranially. **(d)** M-mode recorded from the left parasternal short-axis view, chordal level. Care should be taken not to include the left ventricular outflow tract or the posterior papillary muscle in the image when measuring the internal dimension of the ventricle. For abbreviations see Fig. 5.3.

RIGHT VENTRICULAR INFLOW

PULMONARY OUTFLOW

LEFT VENTRICULAR INFLOW

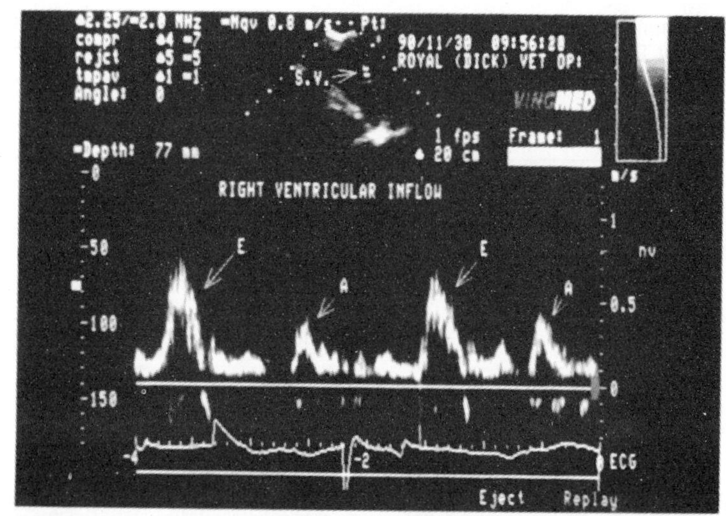

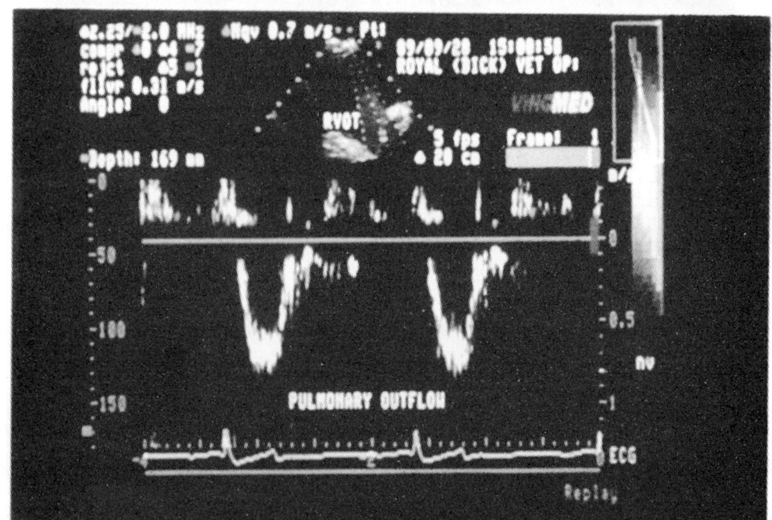

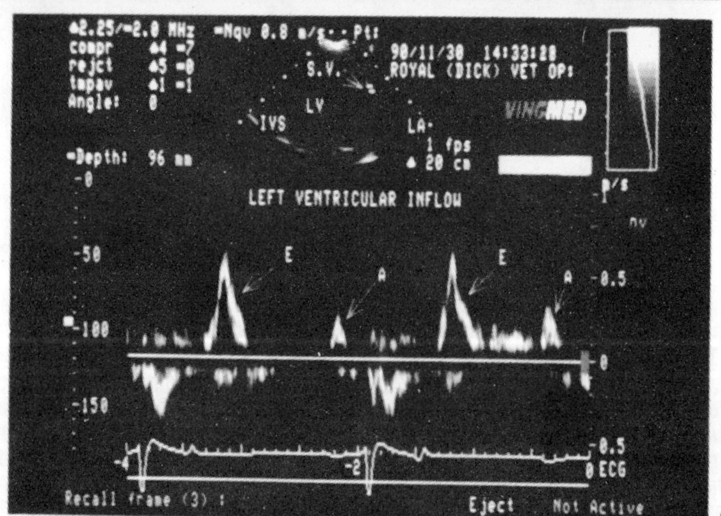

a

b

c

velocity that has been calculated from the Doppler frequency shift. This procedure should be avoided, however, as the 2-D image only indicates alignment in two dimensions, not in three dimensions. Also, the 2-D image is frozen during the final alignment of the transducer and therefore the 2-D image will not give an accurate indication of the final alignment. Correction of the Doppler calculation based on the 2-D image can result in overestimation of the maximum velocity and misinterpretation of the severity of any abnormal flow.

Care should be taken to ensure that the sample volume stays in the centre of the pulmonary artery during systole, to avoid shortening or pointing of the velocity profile. The pulmonary outflow velocity in normal horses varies between 0.73 and 1.11 m s^{-1} at resting heart rates (Fig. 5.7b). At elevated heart rates the maximum velocity will increase. Trivial pulmonary back-flow is a common finding in normal horses.

The left ventricular inflow and outflow velocities are recorded from the left side of the thorax. The mitral inflow velocity is recorded from an apical view of the ventricular inlet (Fig. 5.6b), which is obtained by sliding the transducer ventrally from the reference position and angling dorsally. The sample volume is positioned as described for the tricuspid valve. The E and A velocities of the mitral inflow are often lower than those recorded at the tricuspid inflow: E = 0.33–1.12 m s^{-1}; A = 0.20–0.71 m s^{-1} (Fig. 5.7c). Again inflow velocities will

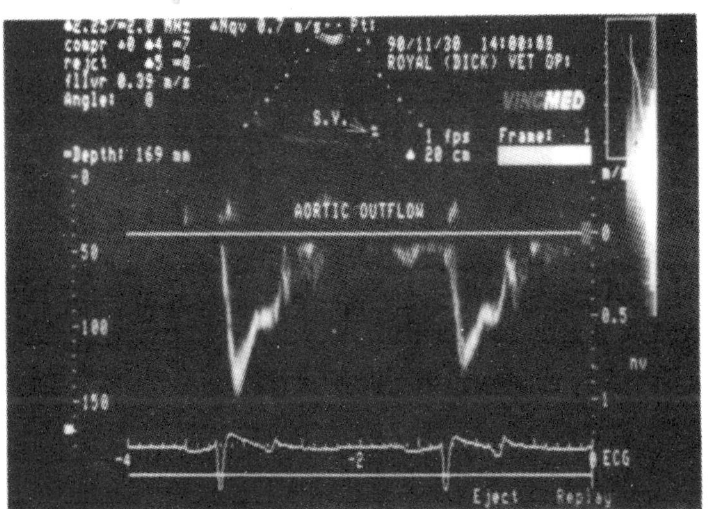

Fig. 5.7. Normal Doppler flow profiles. **(a)** Pulsed wave Doppler study, showing normal tricuspid inflow. The sampling site (S.V.) is shown on the 2-D image. The E wave represents rapid filling of the ventricle. The A wave corresponds to filling associated with atrial contraction. The velocity scale is on the right of the Doppler display. **(b)** Pulsed wave Doppler study of the pulmonary outflow. The sampling site is shown on the 2-D image. **(c)** Pulsed wave Doppler study of the mitral inflow recorded from a left parasternal apical view. E = rapid filling, A = atrial contraction. **(d)** Pulsed wave Doppler study of the aortic outflow. The pulsed Doppler sampling site is positioned just beyond the aortic valve using a left parasternal five-chambered view. For abbreviations see Fig. 5.3.

be increased at elevated heart rates, and will also increase in cases of mitral valve insufficiency due to increased flow through the mitral valve in diastole.

Aortic outflow velocities are recorded from the left parasternal long-axis five-chambered view (Fig. 5.6c). The sample volume is positioned as described for the pulmonary outflow. The velocity waveform differs from that obtained from the pulmonary artery. The waveform is more pointed, the peak velocity occurring earlier (range 0.72–1.16 m s^{-1}), with the acceleration or upstroke being faster (Fig. 5.7d).

Clinical Applications

Identification of congenital cardiac abnormalities

Ventricular septal defect (VSD) is the commonest congenital cardiac abnormality in large animals. It is most often located in the membranous portion of the septum, immediately below the tricuspid valve, and can be readily demonstrated from a 2-D right parasternal long-axis image of the aorta (Fig. 5.8a) and a short-axis view immediately below the aortic valve level. More rarely, septal defects occur in the muscular part of the septum (Fig. 5.8b) or beneath the pulmonary valve. Measurement of the VSD in two planes gives an indication of the size of the defect and its likely significance to future performance or production. Doppler recordings of blood flow velocity through the defect can be used to calculate the pressure gradient across the septum. This gives a more accurate indication of the likely significance of the defect. The maximum flow velocity recorded through the VSD in Fig. 5.8b was 1.9 m s^{-1}. This represents a pressure gradient between the left and right ventricle of 14.5 mmHg ($\Delta P = 4V^2$) and indicates that the right and left ventricular pressures have started to equalize due to significant blood flow across the VSD.

Congenital abnormalities of the cardiac valves can also be visualized by 2-D echocardiography. It is again helpful to obtain images in two planes so that the extent of valve dysfunction can be assessed fully. Fig. 5.9a shows a right parasternal long-axis view from a four-month-old Clydesdale foal. The tricuspid valve appears thickened but the valve appears to close normally during systole. A short-axis view of the same valve (Fig. 5.9b) shows the full extent of valve dysfunction, revealing incomplete valve closure during systole.

Atrial septal defects can easily be missed in large animals, due to the difficulty in visualizing the entire atrial septum. In calves and small foals a four-chambered image plane can be obtained (see Chapter 6) which allows an atrial septal defect to be seen more clearly. The injection of contrast agents into the jugular vein, or the use of Doppler colour flow technology, may assist in the diagnosis of a right-to-left shunt. The foramen ovale can be easily visualized in neonates from the right parasternal long-axis reference view. Care should be taken not to over diagnose atrial septal defects, as echo dropout is a common finding in the normal septum, whereas atrial septal defects are rare.

The patent ductus arteriosus is also difficult to visualize by 2-D echocardiography. Colour flow Doppler techniques can be used to record abnormal ductal

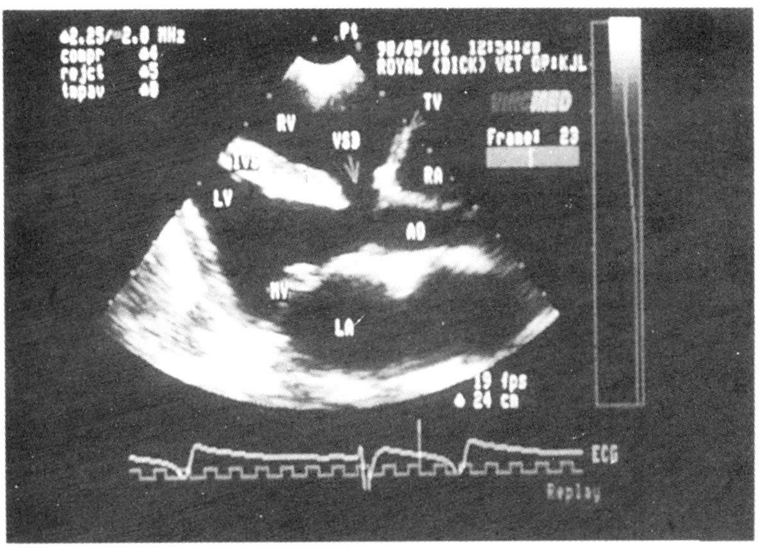

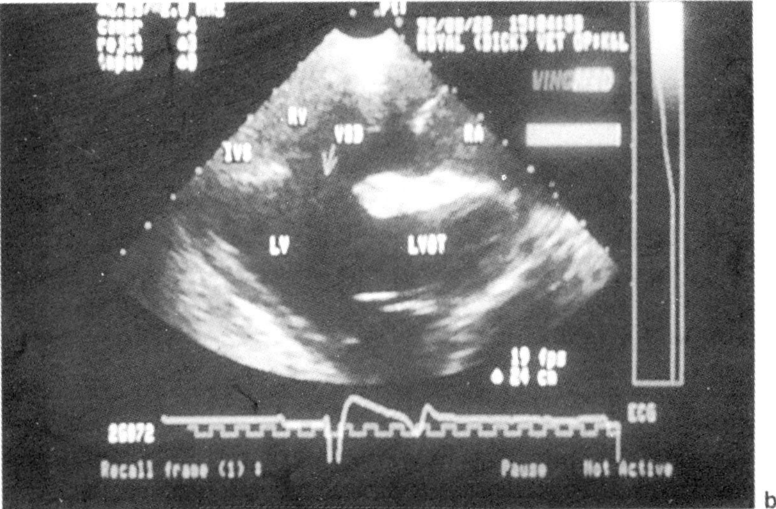

Fig. 5.8. (a) Right parasternal long-axis view. A ventricular septal defect (VSD) can be seen in the membranous portion of the septum immediately below the tricuspid valve. **(b)** Right parasternal long-axis view. A large VSD can be seen in the muscular portion of the septum. For abbreviations see Fig. 5.3.

flow, but lack of imaging depth makes this difficult in larger animals. In small calves and foals the patent ductus is observed from the image planes described for dogs in Chapter 6.

Complex congenital abnormalities can also be detected by 2-D echocardiography. A thorough appreciation of the normal anatomy is required and a systematic examination of cardiac structures is essential.

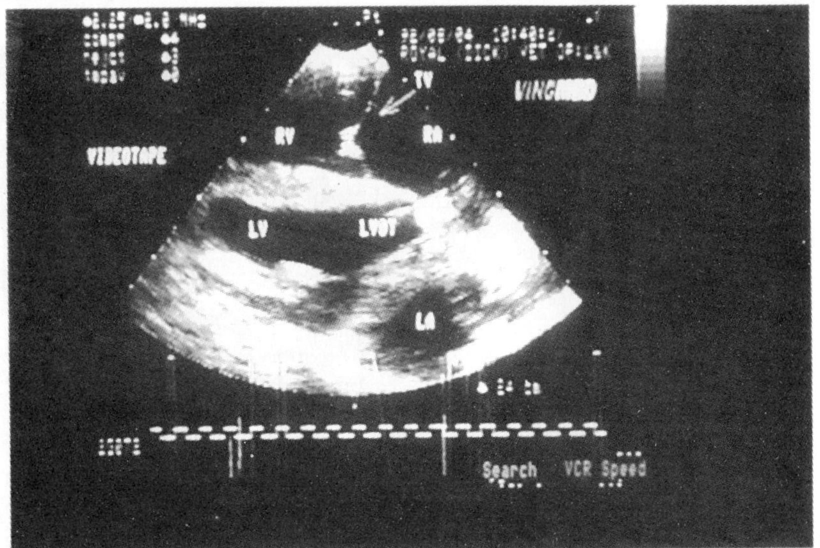

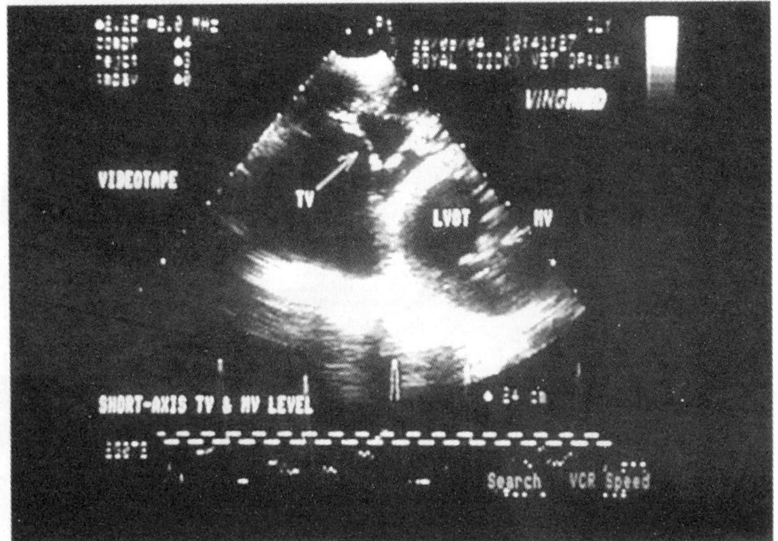

Fig. 5.9. (a) Right parasternal long-axis view from a four-month-old Clydesdale foal. The tricuspid valve (TV) is thickened but the valve appears to close normally. **(b)** Right parasternal short-axis view of the tricuspid valve (TV) shown in Fig. 5.9a. The short-axis view reveals incomplete closure of the valve during systole. For abbreviations see Fig. 5.3.

Investigation of valvular disease

Valve lesions caused by endocarditis are a common finding in cattle and are readily detected by 2-D echocardiography (Fig. 5.10a). Fig. 5.10b shows a mass on the tricuspid valve which produced reverberation artifacts obliterating the far field image. It must be remembered, however, that masses may be present on cardiac valves which are unassociated with endocarditis. Excessive amplification (gain) of returning echoes decreases lateral resolution, and this can make valve leaflets appear thicker than they really are.

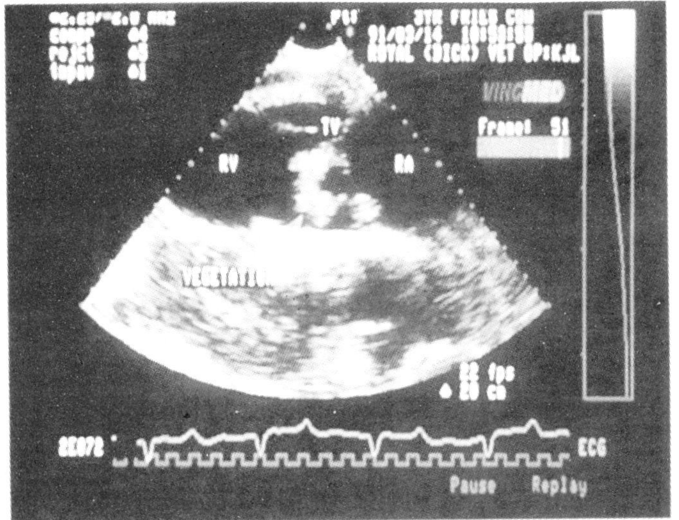

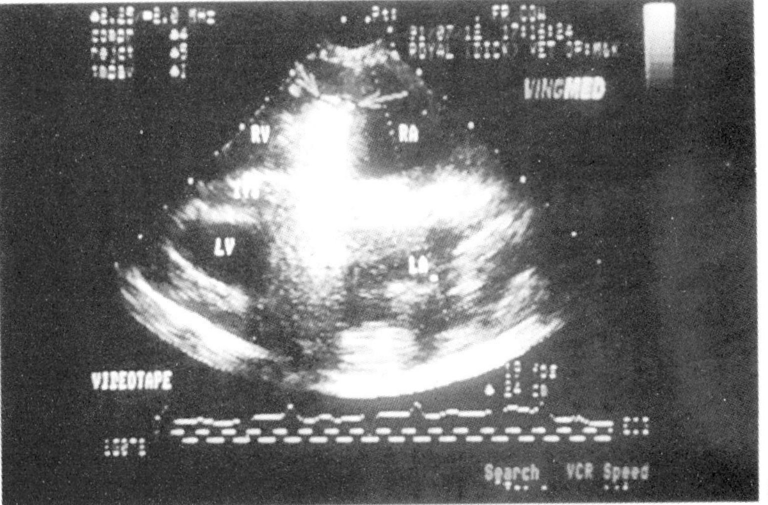

Fig. 5.10. (a) Three-year-old Friesian cow with endocarditis. Right parasternal long-axis view. A vegetative lesion is evident on the tricuspid valve (TV). **(b)** Right parasternal long-axis view from a Friesian cow with endocarditis. Reverberation artifacts from the mass on the tricuspid valve have obliterated the far field image. For abbreviations see Fig. 5.3.

Reverberation artifacts can also produce images which appear to show 'masses' in cardiac chambers and on cardiac valves. An artifact caused by reverberations from the coronary artery in the near field often gives the appearance of a mass in the left or right atrium. When an abnormality appears to be present, it is advisable to try to reproduce it in another image plane to avoid misinterpretation. Apparent masses on cardiac valves can be created by unusual angulation of the transducer through the valve annulus, and by reflections from underlying structures.

Endocarditis is less common in horses, although valvular regurgitation is a very common finding. Most adult horses with cardiac murmurs caused by valvular regurgitation show little or no obvious ultrasonic findings on the valve leaflets, even in cases with severe valvular regurgitation. As the ultrasonic appearance of the valve leaflets is often unremarkable, in the absence of more sophisticated Doppler techniques, the ultrasonographer has to carefully assess valve movement and look for other signs suggestive of valvular regurgitation.

In cases of tricuspid regurgitation, the tricuspid valve tends to have a 'floppy' motion and may be seen to buckle back into the right atrium during systole. This is also seen in some cases with mitral regurgitation. Care must be taken not to misdiagnose this abnormality by taking a skewed view through the valve annulus.

Aortic regurgitation can often be detected by M-mode studies of the mitral valve, as the regurgitant flow causes vibration of the anterior mitral valve leaflet in diastole (Fig. 5.11).

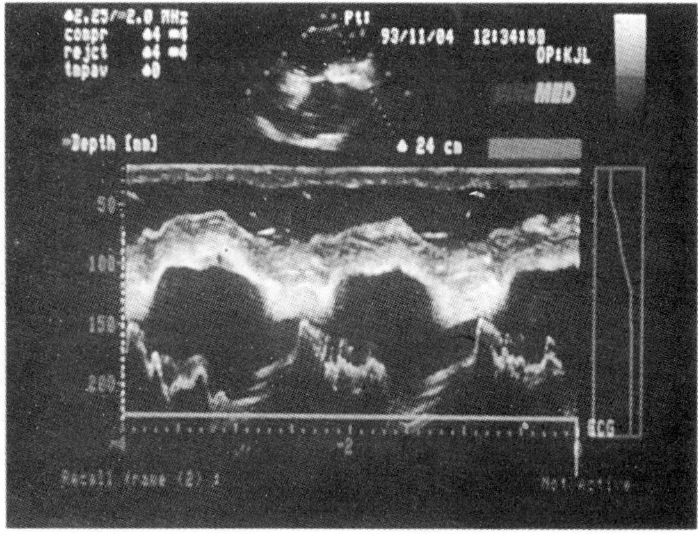

Fig. 5.11. M-mode study of mitral valve from a horse with aortic regurgitation. The anterior leaflet of the mitral valve can be seen to vibrate during diastole. Compare with Fig. 5.5a.

Where valve regurgitation is due to rupture of the chordae tendineae, the valve may be seen to have a 'flail leaflet' which moves into the atrium during systole. In some cases the free chorda may be visualized. However, many cases of mitral chordal rupture involve a minor chorda of the right commissural cusp of the valve. In these cases the affected valve may not prolapse into the atrium and the ruptured chorda may not flail freely. Therefore, failure to identify a flail leaflet or chorda does not rule out this condition, although abnormal movement will be seen either in the M-mode or the 2-D short-axis view of the mitral valve.

Valvular regurgitation can be diagnosed using Doppler echocardiography, by recording high velocity disturbed flow on the atrial side of the atrioventricular valves during systole or on the ventricular side of the semilunar valves in diastole. As the regurgitant jet may pass through the valve at any angle, and from any point, the sample volume must be placed at multiple sites along the valve, and in multiple image planes, to search for abnormal flow. The jet of tricuspid regurgitation is rarely found in the apical long-axis view used to record inflow velocities. In most cases it is detected in a dorsal location view of the right ventricular inlet (see Fig. 5.3c), or a long-axis view of the aorta (see Fig. 5.3d).

The jets of mitral regurgitation are more difficult to detect as they are often small, tend to enter the atria at various angles (Plate 2, frontispiece), and are detected in different image planes in different horses.

The volume of regurgitant flow can be semi-quantified by mapping the area of the disturbed flow (Plate 4, frontispiece) and by the intensity and duration of the regurgitant signal. Severity can be assessed by calculating the pressure gradient across the valve. The area of the regurgitant signal is more easily determined using colour flow Doppler echocardiography. It must be remembered that this represents the area of abnormal flow velocities, not the volume of the regurgitant flow. Therefore again the severity can only be semi-quantified by this technique. Further indications of severity are gained by measuring the width of origin and the timing of the abnormal flow, and also by calculating the volume of the convergence flow as it goes through the abnormal orifice.

Identification of pericardial disease

Echocardiography is the method of choice for the diagnosis of pericardial effusion. The ultrasonic appearance of this condition depends on the nature of the effusion. In some cases the heart will be separated from the pericardium by an anechoic (black) space. In other cases hyperechoic strands of fibrin will be seen, floating in the effusion and attached to the myocardium. This will give the heart a shaggy appearance.

Assessment of cardiac function

Echocardiography can also be used to monitor the response of the heart to abnormal blood flow. Chamber enlargement (volume overload) of the heart, secondary to valvular regurgitation and pressure overload, can be detected (Fig. 5.12). In cases of volume overload secondary to valvular regurgitation, changes may be noted in the calculation of FS. In cases of mitral regurgitation, depending on the severity, the FS may be increased, as part of the stroke volume is ejected into the low pressure left atrium. The FS may also be increased in cases of aortic insufficiency due to an augmented preload by the regurgitant fraction. The use of $\alpha 2$ agonist drugs (xylazine, romifidine, or detomidine) for sedation decreases ventricular contractility and decreases the FS.

Doppler techniques allow more accurate assessment of global ventricular function. The peak acceleration and peak velocity of blood ejected from the ventricle have been shown to be sensitive indicators of ventricular contractility, and

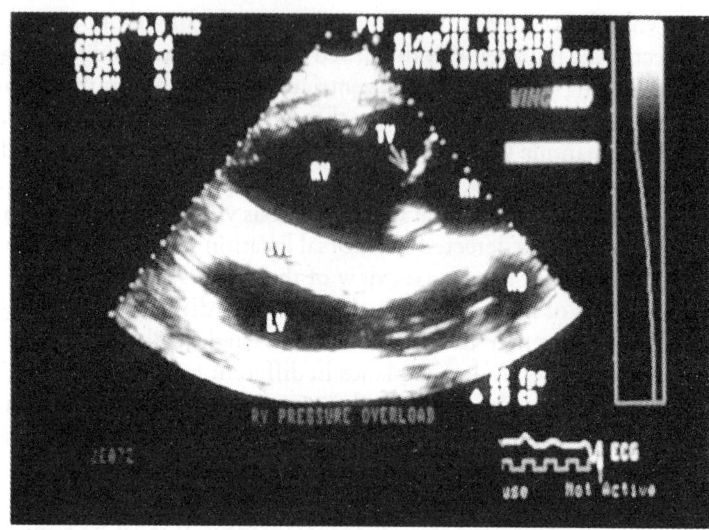

Fig. 5.12. Right parasternal long-axis view of a cow with endocarditis causing tricuspid regurgitation and pulmonary stenosis. The elevated right ventricular pressure has pushed the interventricular septum towards the left ventricle. The septum has a concave appearance. Compare with a normal septum in Fig. 5.3a. For abbreviations see Fig. 5.3.

are easily measured from the Doppler traces of the pulmonary and aortic outflow. The peak acceleration and peak velocity of blood flow are decreased in cases of dilated cardiomyopathy and following sedation.

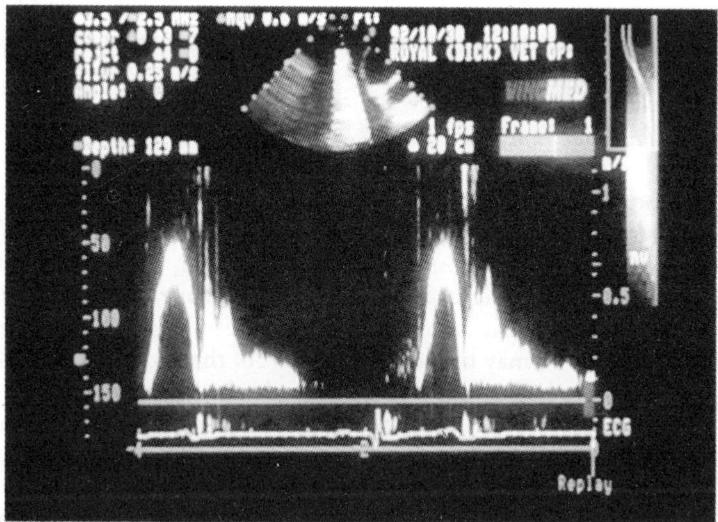

Fig. 5.13. Transoesophageal pulsed wave Doppler study of the aortic outflow. The use of transoesophageal transducers allows cardiac output to be monitored during anaesthesia.

Cardiac output can be calculated from the pulmonary and aortic Doppler flow profiles by measuring the area under the waveform and multiplying by the cross-sectional area of the vessel. The area of the vessel is calculated from the vessel diameter measured from the 2-D image. This method of calculating cardiac output correlates well with the invasive thermodilution technique in horses. Doppler transducers have now been located on endoscopes for transoesophageal use. These transducers enable cardiac function to be monitored during anaesthesia (Fig. 5.13).

References and Suggested Reading

Amory, H., Jakovljevic, S. and Lekeux, P. (1991) Quantitative M-mode and two-dimensional echocardiography in calves. *Veterinary Record*, 128, 25–31.

Bonagura, J.D., Herring, D.S. and Welker, F. (1985) Echocardiography. *Veterinary Clinics of North America, Equine Practice*, 1, 311–333.

Goldberg, S.J., Allen, H.D., Marx, G.R. and Donnerstein, R.L. (1988) *Doppler Echocardiography*, 2nd edn, Lea and Febiger, Philadelphia.

Long, K.J., Bonagura, J.D and Darke, P.G.G. (1992) Standardised imaging technique for guided M-mode and Doppler echocardiography in the horse. *Equine Veterinary Journal*, 24, 226–235.

Weyman, A.E. (1994) *Principles and Practice of Echocardiography*. Lea and Febiger, Philadelphia.

6 Small Animal Echocardiography

M.W.S. Martin
*Godiva Referrals, 207 Daventry Road,
Cheylesmore, Coventry CV3 5HH, UK*

Equipment

To perform a full cardiac ultrasound examination, real-time two-dimensional (2-D), M-mode and Doppler ultrasound are essential. The absence of a Doppler facility greatly reduces the information that can be obtained and leaves uncertainties about the source of abnormal blood flow, but there are many cardiac diseases which do not require Doppler ultrasound to reach a diagnosis, e.g. pericardial and myocardial diseases.

A sector scanner with a small transducer footprint is required to image between the rib spaces and allow good flexibility to obtain the various imaging planes. Ideally a choice of transducers, from 3.5 MHz to 7.5 MHz, is necessary to image the range of sizes of dogs and cats. The choice of only one probe (e.g. 5 MHz) is limiting, but two probes (e.g. 3.5 MHz and 7.5 MHz; or 5 MHz and 7.5 MHz) usually allow satisfactory examination. Some transducers contain crystals which allow frequency switching, with only a small reduction in image resolution.

A suitable table to lay the animal on and a comfortable position from which to perform an echocardiographic examination, which may take up to an hour, is essential. To obtain good images of the heart, the animal is placed in lateral recumbency and scanned from the dependent side. This brings the heart closer to the transducer. The weight of the heart presses the lungs to the side, reducing interference due to lung artifact. To achieve this position, it is necessary to lay the animal on a table with an appropriate U-shaped cut-out.

A record of the echocardiographic examination can be made using a video recording and/or a thermal printer or photography. A suitable video recorder should be able to scroll slowly and freeze on an image for closer study.

Animal Preparation

Clipping the animal over the transducer positions is usually necessary to prevent attenuation by air trapped in the animal's coat. Soaking the transducer positions with spirit or alcohol helps in reducing air artifact, and also reduces the amount of ultrasound gel required. Sparsely-coated animals may only require soaking with spirit, without clipping. A liberal application of acoustic coupling gel should then be placed on the transducer and/or the animal.

The animal is preferably placed, on a suitable table, as described above, in lateral recumbency with its legs towards the echocardiographer. Manual restraint is necessary, not only to keep the animal still while it is scanned, but also to prevent it damaging the ultrasound system or transducers. The underside foreleg should also be pulled forward, thus taking the animal's elbow away from the cardiac apex. In some cases it may be detrimental, or simply difficult, to restrain an animal in lateral recumbency. In these cases a different position of the animal is necessary. In many instances good images can be obtained with the animal standing, sitting or in sternal recumbency.

Sedation is not usually required in dogs, but is often necessary in cats to facilitate positioning. Sedation will not usually interfere with diagnosis, but it may alter the assessment of severity and therefore prognosis of a cardiac disease. However, one could equally argue that the stress of manual restraint in some animals might also alter this assessment.

Cardiac ultrasound systems have a single lead ECG monitor, for the purposes of a timing reference. The clips should be attached and a good ECG trace noted prior to commencement.

Normal Echocardiographic Examination

It is important that a regular and consistent routine is established, so that the heart is fully imaged and nothing is overlooked. The operator and animal must be comfortably positioned, and sufficient time must be allowed. The normal examination is described under the following sections: two-dimensional, M-mode, Doppler and contrast echocardiography. The basic principles of ultrasound have been described in Chapter 1. Doppler techniques are described in more detail in Chapter 5. (See also Feigenbaum, 1986; Goldberg *et al.*, 1988.)

Two-dimensional echocardiography

There are standardized views (Henry *et al.*, 1980) from which the heart is imaged. These can be explained as follows.

Transducer locations

Right parasternal position – right thorax over the palpable cardiac impulse, at the fourth to sixth intercostal spaces and between the sternum and costo-chondral junctions.
Left caudal parasternal position (or left apical position) – left thorax over the palpable cardiac impulse, at the fifth to seventh intercostal spaces and between the sternum and costo-chondral junctions.

Left cranial parasternal position – left thorax over the palpable cardiac impulse, at the third to fourth intercostal spaces and between the sternum and costo-chondral junctions.

Subcostal position – caudal to the xiphisternum and ribs.

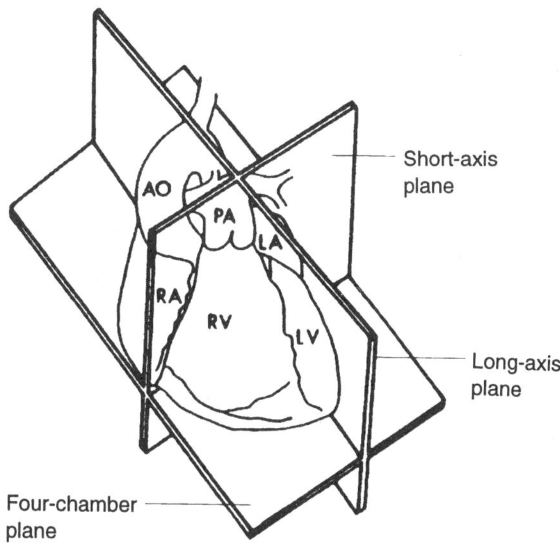

Fig. 6.1. Diagram showing the three orthogonal planes for two-dimensional echocardiographic imaging. AO = aorta; PA = pulmonary artery; LA = left atrium; RA = right atrium; LV = left ventricle; RV = right ventricle. Reproduced with kind permission from Henry *et al.* (1980). Copyright (1980) American Heart Association.

Imaging planes

There are three orthogonal planes (Fig. 6.1) for 2-D imaging:

Long-axis – imaging plane that transects the heart perpendicular to the ventral and dorsal surfaces of the body, and parallel to the long axis of the heart, i.e. from base to apex.

Short-axis – imaging plane that transects the heart perpendicular to its long axis, and also perpendicular to the ventral and dorsal surfaces of the body.

Four-chamber view – imaging plane that transects the heart parallel to the ventral and dorsal surfaces of the body.

Image orientation on the monitor

The transducer should have an index mark to indicate one edge of the imaging plane and should display that side of the imaging plane to the right on the monitor. Thus correct orientation will be maintained by holding the transducer such that the index mark is always to the animal's head or to its left. An image inversion switch will facilitate such positioning. As a general rule, right heart structures are viewed on the monitor to the right.

Standard echocardiographic views

Although it is possible to obtain an infinite number of 'slices' through the heart, there are a series of standard views. These have been documented by a number of authors and the reader is referred to these for a more detailed description (Thomas, 1984; O'Grady *et al.*, 1986; Yuill & O'Grady, 1991).

Right parasternal position

Long-axis views

Begin by placing the transducer over the palpable apex beat on the right side (fourth–sixth intercostal space, midway between the sternum and the costochondral junctions), with no angulation, i.e. vertically, and in a plane at right angles to the sternum. At this position the left side of the heart, ventricle and atrium should be well visualized, with part of the right side (Figs 6.2a and 6.3a). If the heart does not appear in a horizontal position on the monitor, but tilted (from base to apex), the transducer should be moved slightly dorsally or even a rib space cranially.

From the above position slightly rotate the transducer anticlockwise (supinate the wrist), while tilting it dorsally. This causes the sector plane to transect the aorta (Fig. 6.3b).

From the position in which Fig. 6.3b is obtained, tilt the transducer in a cranial and slightly ventral direction. The aorta will appear to close off, and the pulmonary artery will appear, crossing the aorta (Fig. 6.3c). The pulmonic valve will be evident at the 3 o'clock position on the monitor, and the right ventricular outflow tract above this, with the pulmonary artery below and an angled section of the left ventricle to the left. (Rotating the transducer anticlockwise 90° about its axis will produce Fig. 6.4g.)

To obtain a better view of the left atrium and atrial septum, tilt the transducer dorsally from the position in which Fig. 6.3a is obtained. The heart appears to rotate on the monitor and the left atrium comes more fully into view.

Short-axis views

From the position described as Fig. 6.3a, rotate the transducer anticlockwise 90° about its axis. This will result in a view which transects the left ventricle in its short axis, with the slim right ventricle around the left, from 11 o'clock to 4 o'clock. The transducer should be rotated or tilted to ensure that the left ventricle appears in true circular sections. The sector beam can now be tilted from the apex to the base of the heart by tilting the transducer ventrally or dorsally, retrospectively, at right angles to the plane of the sector beam (Fig. 6.4a).

At the apical level (Fig. 6.4b) the left ventricle appears circular, with a small portion of the right ventricle visible. Tilting the transducer dorsally from this, the papillary muscles are seen protruding into the ventricular chamber (Fig. 6.4c), at the 4–5 o'clock and the 8–9 o'clock positions. Tilting the transducer further dorsally, the chordae tendineae are seen arising from the papillary muscles (Figs 6.4d and 6.5a). The right ventricle is seen maximally at this level. Tilting the transducer further dorsally, the mitral valve begins to appear entering the section,

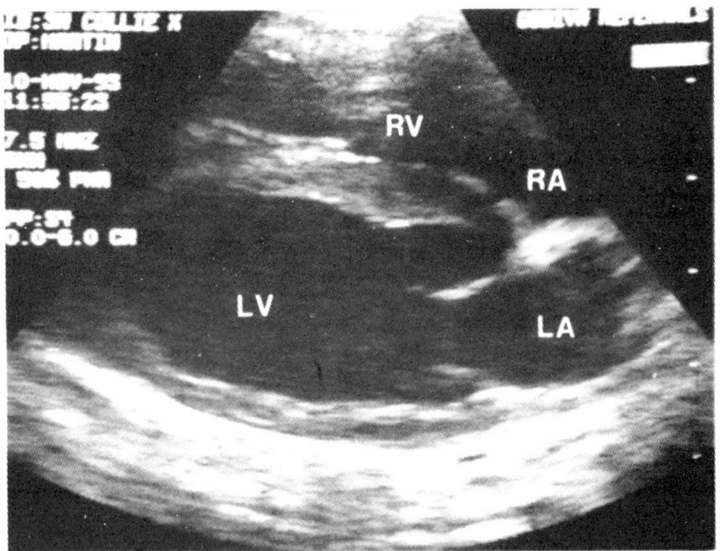

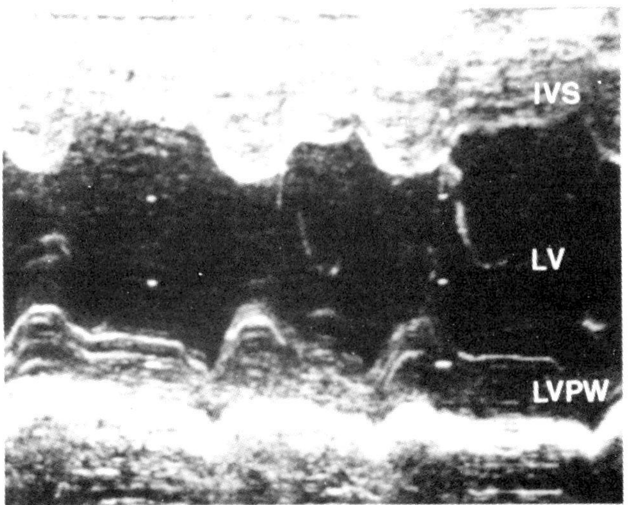

Fig. 6.2. (a) Two-dimensional echocardiogram obtained from the right parasternal position showing the long-axis (four-chamber) view of the left ventricle and atrium, and part of the right ventricle and atrium. (See Fig. 6.3a for a diagrammatic representation.) **(b)** M-mode echocardiogram obtained from the right parasternal position at the level of the chordae tendineae. (See Figs 6.10 and 6.13 for a diagrammatic representation.) The mitral valve cusps are just coming into view during the second and third beats. Left ventricular measurements are usually obtained from an M-mode echocardiogram at the level of the chordae tendineae (just below the mitral valve). The fractional shortening in this dog is 36%. LA = left atrium; RA = right atrium; LV = left ventricle; RV = right ventricle; IVS = interventricular septum; LVPW = left ventricular posterior wall; P = pericardium.

within the left ventricle. During diastole (when the valves are open) an image is created that has been described as a 'fish-mouth' (Fig. 6.4e). In systole, when the

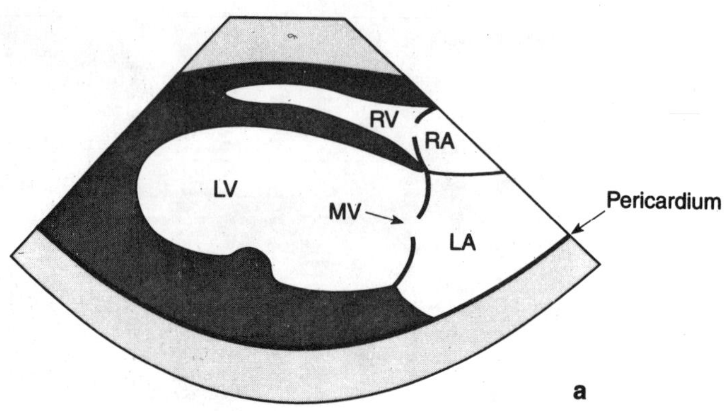
RV
RA
LV
MV
LA
Pericardium
a

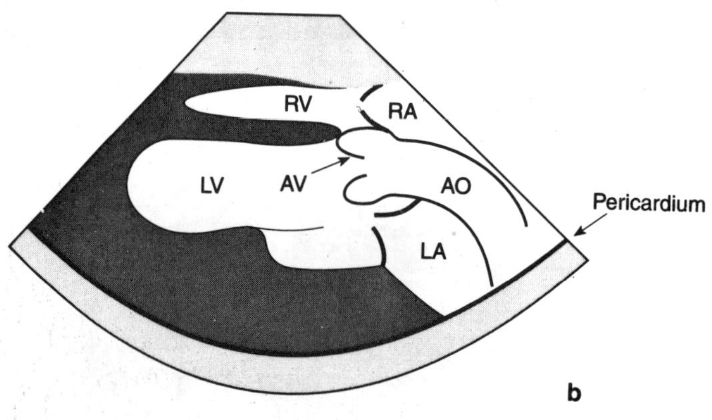
RV
RA
LV
AV
AO
LA
Pericardium
b

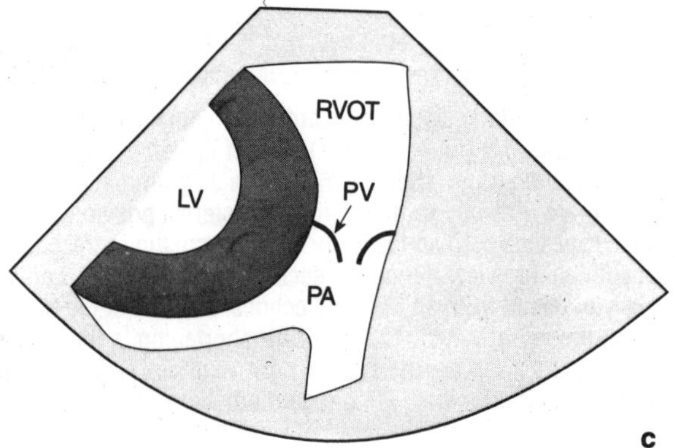
RVOT
LV
PV
PA
c

valves close, the two cusps coapt to form an irregular line. Further dorsal tilting of the transducer will image a cross-section of the aorta at valve level (Figs 6.4f and 6.5b). The image created by the three cusps is sometimes described as a 'Mercedes Benz symbol' or an inverted Y. To the lower left of the aorta is the left atrium, and the right side of the heart encircles the remaining portion of the aorta; the right atria and tricuspid valve are to the upper left, the right ventricle and its outflow tract to the upper right and the pulmonary artery and its valve to the right. Slight angulation of the transducer from this position can improve the image on the different parts of the right heart. The pulmonary artery and its two branches can be visualized by moving the position of the transducer slightly ventrally and/or cranially (Fig. 6.4g) (Rotating the transducer clockwise 90° about its axis will produce Fig. 6.3c.)

Left caudal parasternal position

Begin by placing the transducer as far caudally as is possible, while still visualizing the heart (at approximately the fifth to seventh intercostal space). Rotate the transducer slightly anticlockwise and tilt it steeply towards the base of the heart, i.e. cranially. This produces an image that transects all four chambers of the heart (Figs 6.6a and 6.7a): an apical, four-chambered view. The aorta can be viewed by rotating the transducer anticlockwise and tilting the transducer cranio-dorsally (Figs 6.6b and 6.7b). This view is optimized for the left ventricle, its outflow tract and the aorta.

Left cranial parasternal position

Place the transducer at the third to fourth intercostal space and rotate clockwise by 90° so that the sector beam runs cranio-caudally. With slight tilting, and some-times caudal angulation, a view of the aorta and left ventricle is obtained (Figs 6.8a and 6.9a). The aorta appears to lie horizontally on the monitor and the walls of the ascending aorta should be parallel to each other, indicating that the sector beam accurately transects the aorta. By tilting the beam dorsally, the aorta appears to close off and the pulmonary artery emerges at right angles to the aorta. The pulmonary valve is seen at the 12–1 o'clock position and the artery is seen dividing into its two branches at the 4–5 o'clock position (Figs 6.8b and 6.9b).

Fig. 6.3. Right parasternal long-axis views. **(a)** Optimized for the left atrium and mitral valve. **(b)** Optimized for the left ventricle, aortic valve and aorta. **(c)** Optimized for the right ventricular outflow tract, pulmonary valve and artery. AO = aorta; AV = aortic valve; PA = pulmonary artery; PV = pulmonic valve; LA = left atrium; RA = right atrium; LV = left ventricle; RV = right ventricle; MV = mitral valve; RVOT = right ventricular outflow tract.

With careful tilting and angulation, the right side of the heart can be followed back to the right atrium. Returning to the view maximized for the aorta, and then tilting ventrally, an image of the right atrium, tricuspid valve and right ventricle can be seen (Fig. 6.9c); the left ventricle appears closed off to the left.

Subcostal view

By placing the transducer caudal to the xiphoid, and then pushing the transducer slightly dorsal to it with rotation such that the sector beam runs from ventral to dorsal, an image of the heart is obtained that views the aorta parallel to the direction of the transducer beam. This view is good for obtaining Doppler velocity measurements in line with blood flow. The left ventricle appears above the aorta and the left atrium to the left.

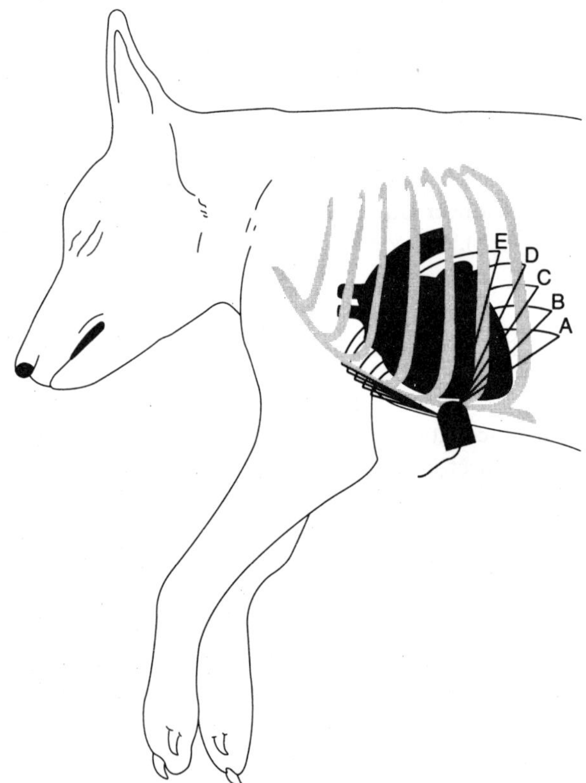

Fig. 6.4. Right parasternal short-axis views. **(a)** Diagram showing how the sector beam transects the heart from this position at different levels, from apex to base. **(b)** At the apical level. **(c)** At the papillary muscle level. **(d)** At the chordae tendineae level. **(e)** At the mitral valve level. **(f)** At the aortic valve level. **(g)** Optimized for the right ventricular outflow tract, pulmonary valve and artery. AO = aorta; PA = pulmonary artery; PV = pulmonic valve; LA = left atrium; RA = right atrium; LV = left ventricle; RV = right ventricle; TV = tricuspid valve; PM = papillary muscle; RVOT = right ventricular outflow tract; CT = chordae tendineae.

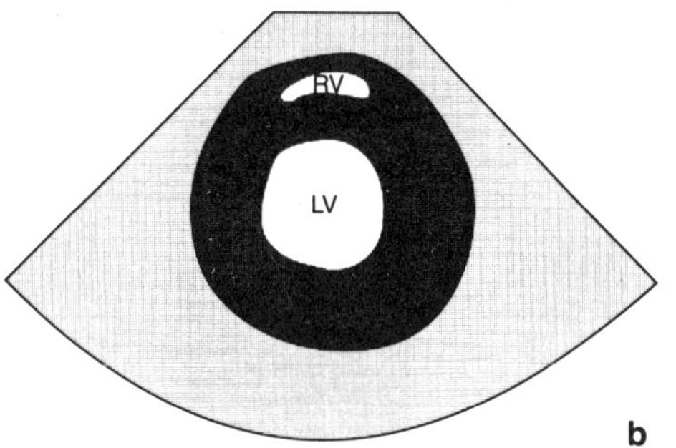
RV
LV
b

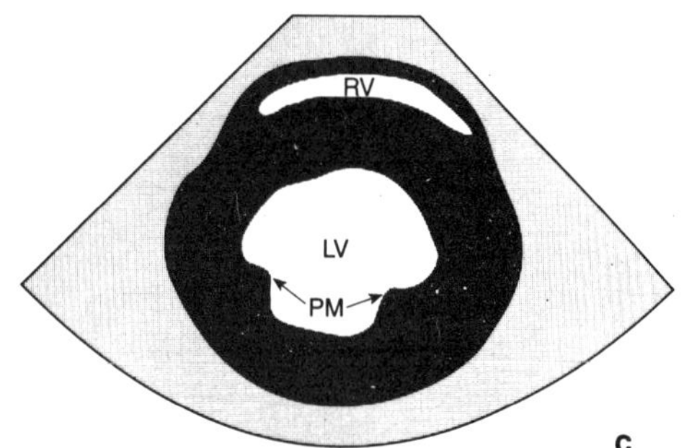
RV
LV
PM
c

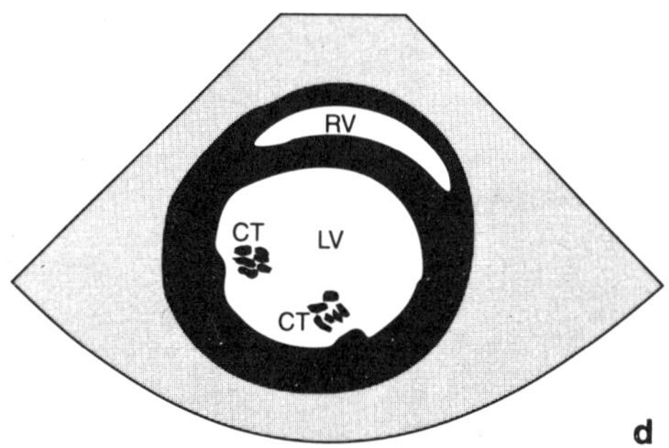
RV
CT
LV
CT
d

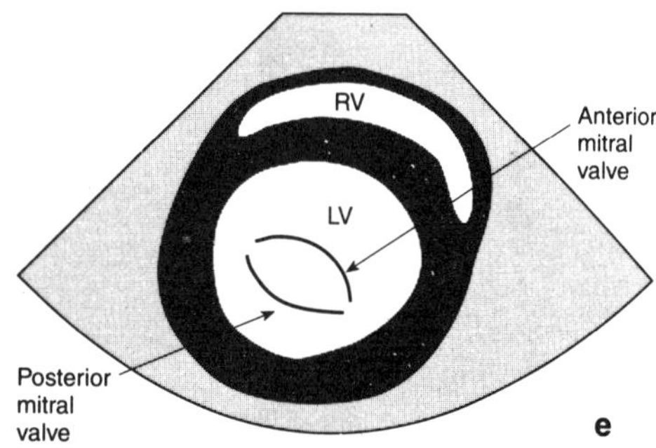
RV
LV
Anterior
mitral
valve
Posterior
mitral
valve
e

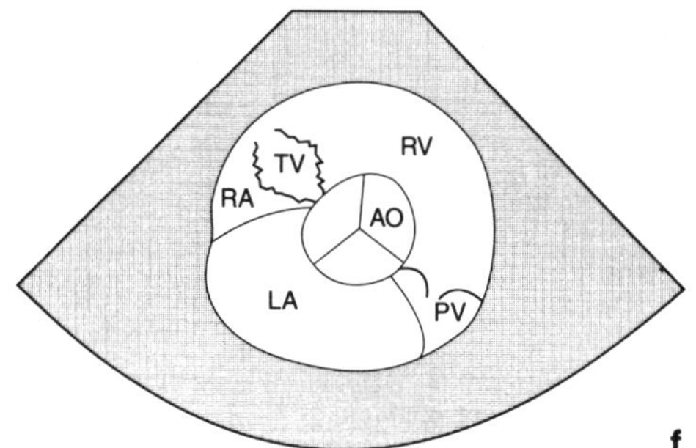
TV
RV
RA
AO
LA
PV
f

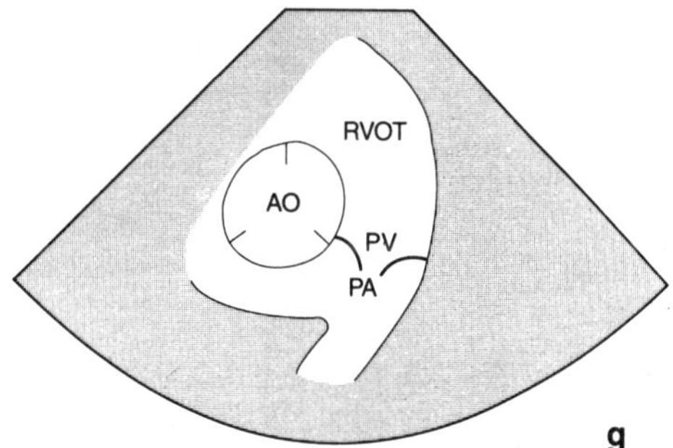
RVOT
AO
PV
PA
g

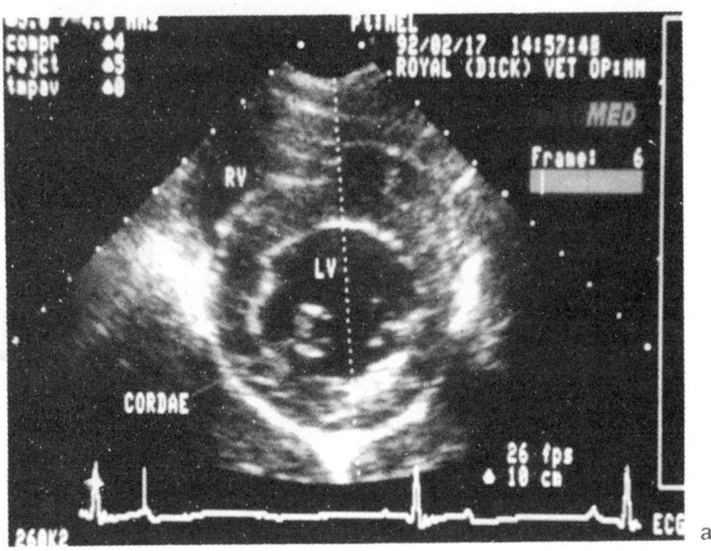

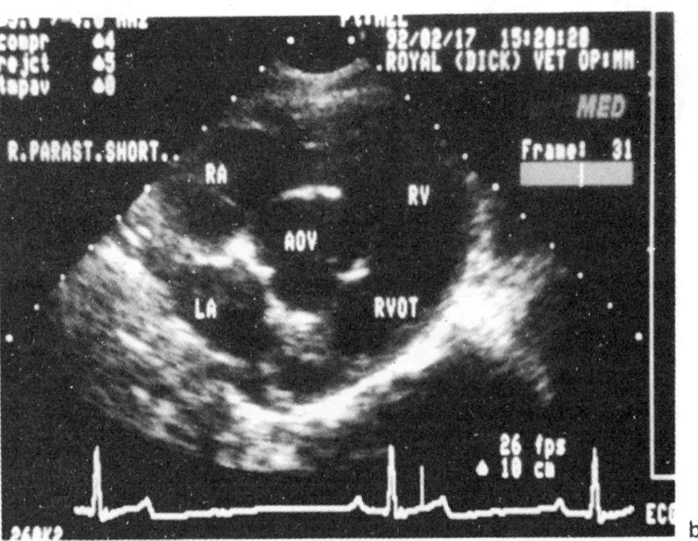

Fig. 6.5. (a) Two-dimensional echocardiogram obtained from the right parasternal position showing a short-axis view at the level of the chordae tendineae. (See Fig. 6.4d for a diagrammatic representation.) The orientation is not standard and should be reversed from left to right. The dotted line is the cursor in position for recording an M-mode echocardiogram. **(b)** Two-dimensional echocardiogram obtained from the right parasternal position showing a short-axis view at the level of the aortic valve. (See Fig. 6.4f for a diagrammatic representation.) The pulmonary valve is not visible on this echocardiogram, but would usually be seen where the RVOT label has been placed. AOV = aorta/aortic valve; CORDAE = chordae tendineae; RA = right atrium; RV = right ventricle; LA = left atrium; LV = left ventricle; RVOT = right ventricular outflow tract.

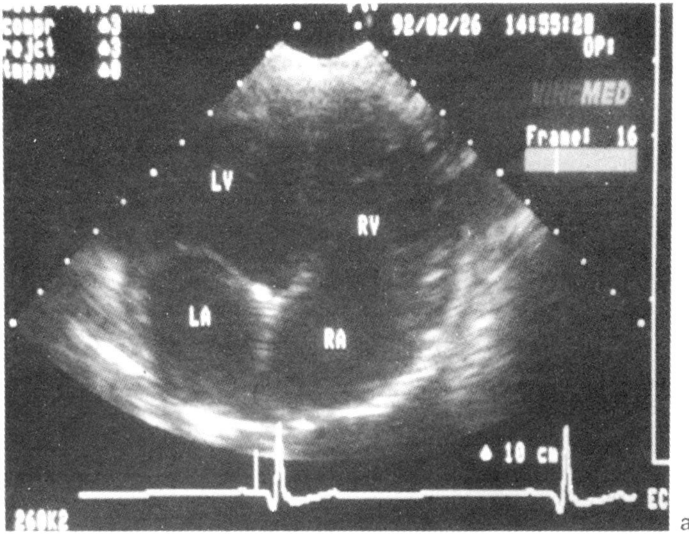

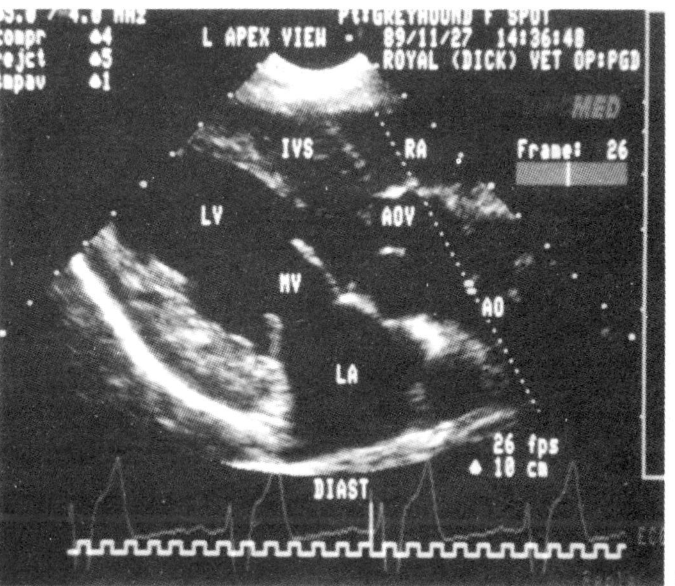

Fig. 6.6. (a) Two-dimensional echocardiogram obtained from the left caudal parasternal position showing a four-chambered (apical) view. (See Fig. 6.7a for a diagrammatic representation.) **(b)** Two-dimensional echocardiogram obtained from the left caudal parasternal position showing a long-axis view optimized for the left ventricle, its outflow tract and the aorta. (See Fig. 6.7b for a diagrammatic representation.) NB: The ECG shows a right bundle branch block pattern. LA = left atrium; RA = right atrium; LV = left ventricle; RV = right ventricle; MV = mitral valve; IVS = interventricular septum; AOV = aortic valve; AO = aorta. Reproduced by kind permission of Dr Peter Darke.

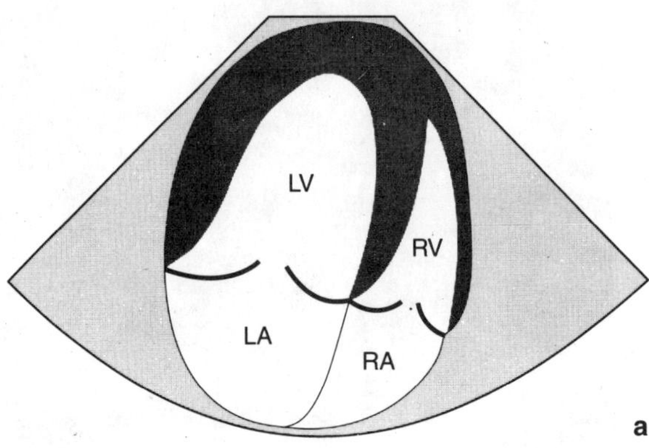

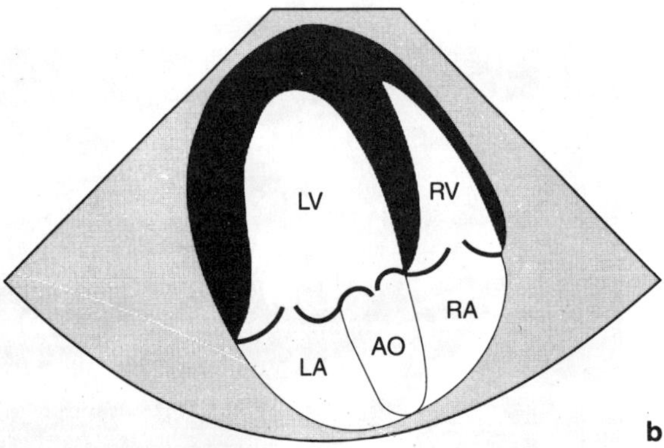

Fig. 6.7. Left caudal (apical) parasternal views. **(a)** Four-chambered view, showing the left and right atria and ventricles. **(b)** Long-axis view, optimized for the left ventricle, aortic valve and aorta. LA = left atrium; RA = right atrium; LV = left ventricle; RV = right ventricle; AO = aorta.

M-mode echocardiography

M-mode (motion mode) echocardiography is obtained by placing the cursor line through the heart, in an area of interest, and displaying the movement of the heart through that line against time (time-motion graph or display), where time is on the x-axis and motion on the y-axis. The ECG provides a timing reference. M-mode echocardiography is generally used when performing measurements or observing the motion of structures over time. Standardization of cardiac

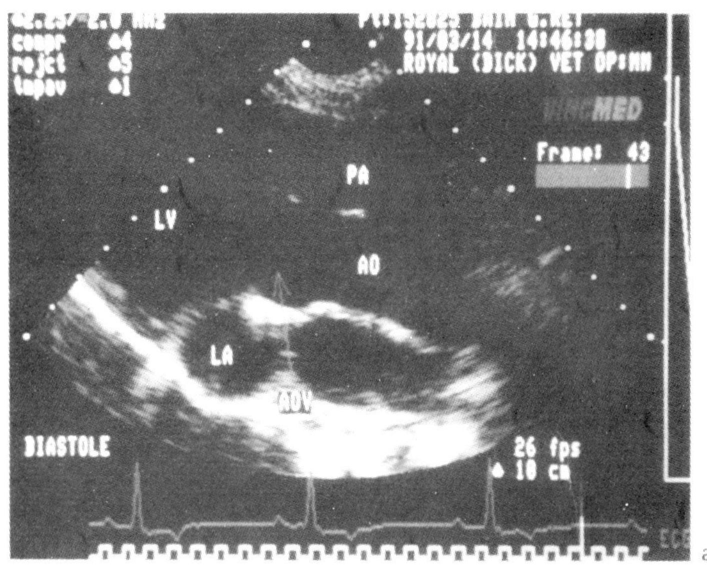

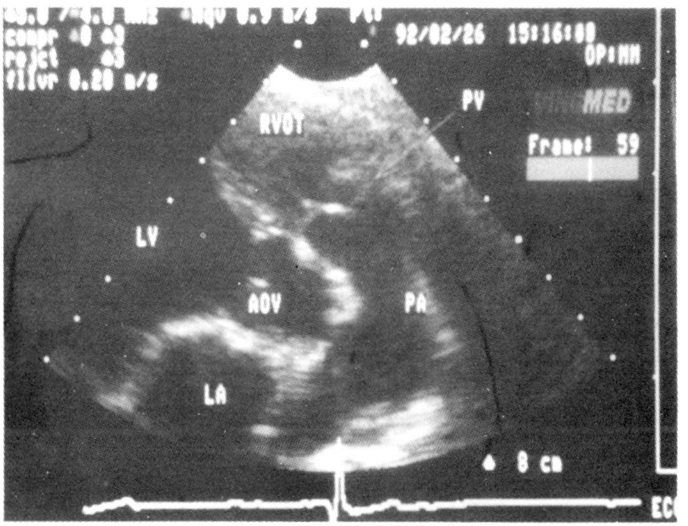

Fig. 6.8. (a) Two-dimensional echocardiogram obtained from the left cranial parasternal position, showing a long-axis view of the left ventricular outflow tract and aorta. The aortic valve (AOV) cannot be seen clearly in the photographic reproduction. (See Fig. 6.9a for a diagrammatic representation.) **(b)** Two-dimensional echocardiogram obtained from the left cranial parasternal position, showing a long-axis view of the right ventricular outflow tract and pulmonary artery. LA = left atrium; LV = left ventricle; AO = aorta; AOV = aortic valve; PA = pulmonary artery; PV = pulmonic valve; RVOT = right ventricular outflow tract.

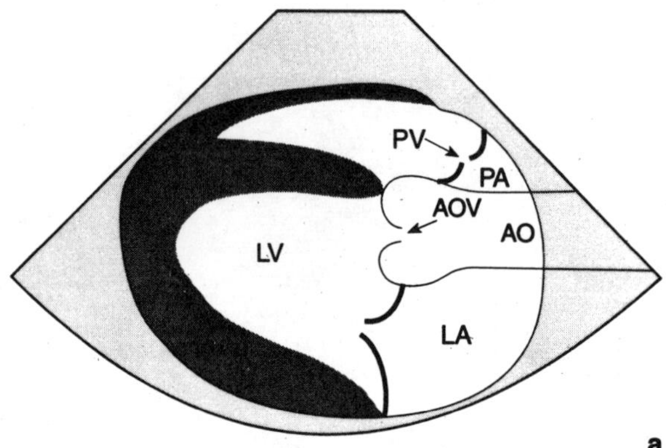
PV
PA
AOV
AO
LV
LA
a

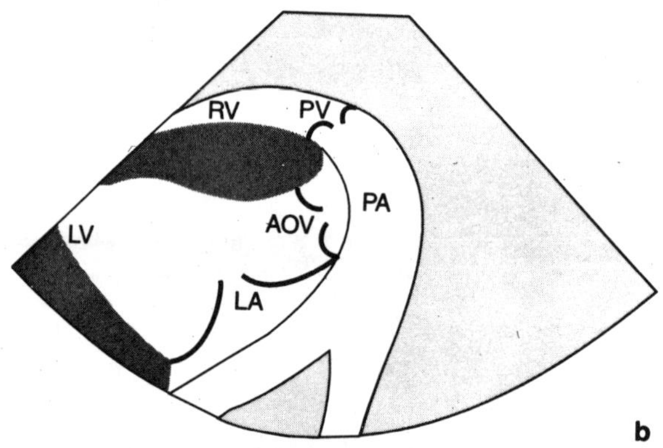
RV
PV
PA
AOV
LV
LA
b

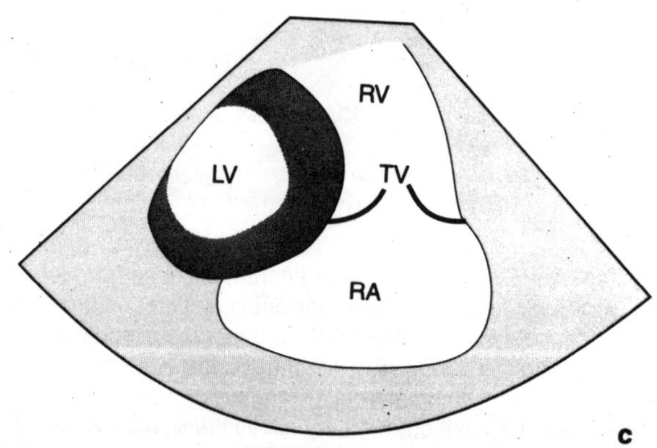
RV
LV
TV
RA
c

measurements from M-mode has been described by the American Society of Echocardiography (Sahn *et al.*, 1978; O'Rourke *et al.*, 1984).

Left ventricle

Place the cursor line through the centre of the left ventricle in the right parasternal short-axis view of the heart at the level of the chordae tendineae (Figs 6.4d and 6.5a). When the ultrasound unit is switched to M-mode, a typical tracing should be obtained (Figs 6.2b and 6.10).

When making the M-mode measurements, diastole should be taken at the onset of the QRS complex, and systole should be taken at the nadir of septal wall motion. If the wall motion is abnormal it should be taken at the peak of the posterior wall motion. The points at which the wall thicknesses and cavity dimension are measured should follow the leading edge methodology (Fig. 6.13), so that variations in epicardial and endocardial thickness due to the ultrasound system gain setting and signal processing are minimized.

Measurements of the ventricular septum and left ventricular posterior wall thicknesses and the left ventricular chamber diameter, in diastole and systole, can be obtained. Calculation of the fractional shortening percentage (FS, the percentage linear reduction in the left ventricular internal dimensions from diastole to systole) and the ejection fraction (the percentage volume reduction in the left ventricular internal dimension from diastole to systole) is usually performed by the computer. For the left ventricle:

$$FS = 100 \times (LVIDd - LVIDs)/LVIDd$$

where LVIDd is left ventricular internal diameter in diastole, and LVDIs is left ventricular internal diameter in systole. Normal echocardiographic values for small animals (Fig. 6.11 and Table 6.1) have been published (Boon *et al.*, 1983; Lombard 1984; Bonagura *et al.*, 1985; Jacobs and Knight, 1985; Morrison *et al.*, 1992). The normal FS in the dog ranges from 28 to 50%, and in the cat from 29 to 55%. This measurement is considered an estimate of contractility, but it varies with the preload and afterload on the heart.

The mean velocity of circumferential fibre shortening (VCF) (i.e. the rate at which the fractional shortening is performed) is calculated in circumferences per second (cir. s^{-1}) from the following formula:

$$VCF = FS/ET$$

where FS is fractional shortening percentage and ET is ejection time (from opening of aortic valve to closure). The normal VCF in dogs ranges from 1.6 to 2.8 cir. s^{-1}, and in cats from 1.3 to 4.5 cir. s^{-1}. A decrease in FS or VCF is considered

Fig. 6.9. Left cranial parasternal views. **(a)** Optimized for the left ventricle, aortic valve and aorta. **(b)** Optimized for the pulmonary valve and artery. **(c)** Optimized for the tricuspid valve and right atrium. LA = left atrium; RA = right atrium; LV = left ventricle; RV = right ventricle; TV = tricuspid valve; AO = aorta; AOV = aortic valve; PV = pulmonic valve; PA = pulmonary artery.

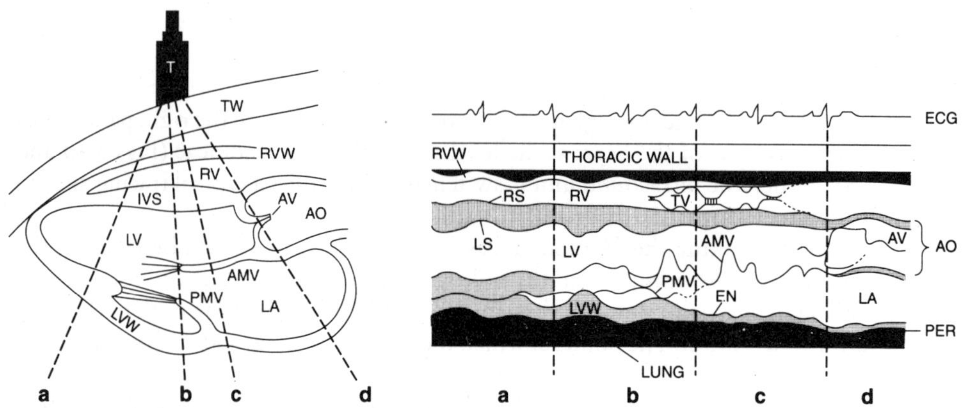

Fig. 6.10. Schematic illustrations of the standard M-mode echocardiographic positions and their approximate location on a 2–D image. **(a)** At the papillary muscle level. **(b)** and **(c)** At the mitral valve level. **(d)** At the aortic valve level. For abbreviations see Fig. 6.13. Reproduced with kind permission from Bonagura *et al.* (1985). Copyright (1985) W.B. Saunders Company.

Table 6.1. Normal M-mode values for cats. Reproduced with kind permission from Bonagura *et al.*, 1985. Copyright (1985) W.B. Saunders Company.

Dimension	Value
Left ventricle in diastole	11.0–16.0 mm
Left ventricle in systole	6.0–10.0 mm
Interventricular septum in diastole	2.5–5.0 mm
Interventricular septum in systole	5.0–9.0 mm
Left ventricle posterior wall in diastole	2.5–5.0 mm
Left ventricle posterior wall in systole	4.0–9.0 mm
Left atrium	8.5–12.5 mm
Aortic diameter	6.5–11.0 mm
Fractional shortening	25–55%

indicative of a reduction in ventricular contractility. FS and VCF are termed non-volume dependent indices, whereas ejection fraction is volume dependent. The ejection fraction (%) is a ratio of the stroke volume to the end-diastolic volume of the left ventricle. However, it is calculated from the same figures as fractional shortening percentage, but uses geometric assumptions to estimate the volume. Most echocardiographers tend not to use this latter measurement. More accurate measurements of volume are obtained from the 2-D echocardiogram. Other measurements sometimes used include ratio of septal to left ventricular posterior wall thickness (normally 1.0), percentage increase in wall thickening (septum and left ventricular posterior wall), or rate of thickening.

Normal and paradoxical ventricular septal wall motion has been well described by DeMadron *et al.* (1985). Flat or paradoxical septal wall motion indicates the presence of right ventricular volume or pressure overload.

Right ventricle

The epicardial and endocardial surfaces of the right ventricular anterior wall are rarely visualized. These can occasionally be measured while measuring the left ventricular dimensions from the same M-mode echocardiogram. Measurements are best obtained from 2-D echocardiograms (Schnittger *et al.*, 1983; O'Grady *et al.*, 1986).

Mitral valve

An M-mode sweep to the mitral valve, in the right parasternal short-axis view, will reveal a characteristic display traced by the movement of the anterior and posterior mitral valve cusps (Figs 6.10c and 6.12a). The anterior cusp inscribes a M shape, and the posterior cusp a W shape. Normal mitral valve motion has been described as follows (Fig. 6.13): C = point of mitral valve closure; D = end of systolic mitral valve closure; E = maximum early diastolic valve opening (passive filling phase); F = point of partial closure of mitral valve in mid-diastole; A = maximum late diastolic valve opening (atrial contraction phase). The E point to septal separation (EPSS), is commonly measured as an indication of left ventricular dilation (volume overload). A distance greater than 6 mm is considered significant. Premature closure of the mitral valve with anterior movement ('B' shoulder) between the A and C points on the M-mode, is considered indicative of a non-compliant (stiff) ventricle with a high end-diastolic ventricular pressure. Fluttering of the mitral valve can often result from moderate to severe aortic regurgitation (see Chapter 5, Fig. 5.11).

Aortic root and left atrium

The M-mode cursor is placed through the aortic valve and left atrium from right parasternal short- or long-axis views at aortic valve level. When the ultrasound unit is switched to M-mode, a characteristic display is obtained (Figs 6.10d and 6.12b). Measurements should be obtained from a point where at least two aortic valve cusps are seen (although frequently difficult to achieve in the dog), at end-diastole (start of QRS) (Fig. 6.13). The leading edge method should be employed, from the anterior to the posterior walls of the aorta. Reduced systolic movement of the aorta is considered indicative of a poor stroke volume. The left atrium should be measured at end-systole, including the thickness of the posterior wall of the aorta. The ratio of the left atrial length to the aortic diameter (LA:Ao) is approximately 0.8–1.2:1.0. When there is left atrial dilation, this ratio increases.

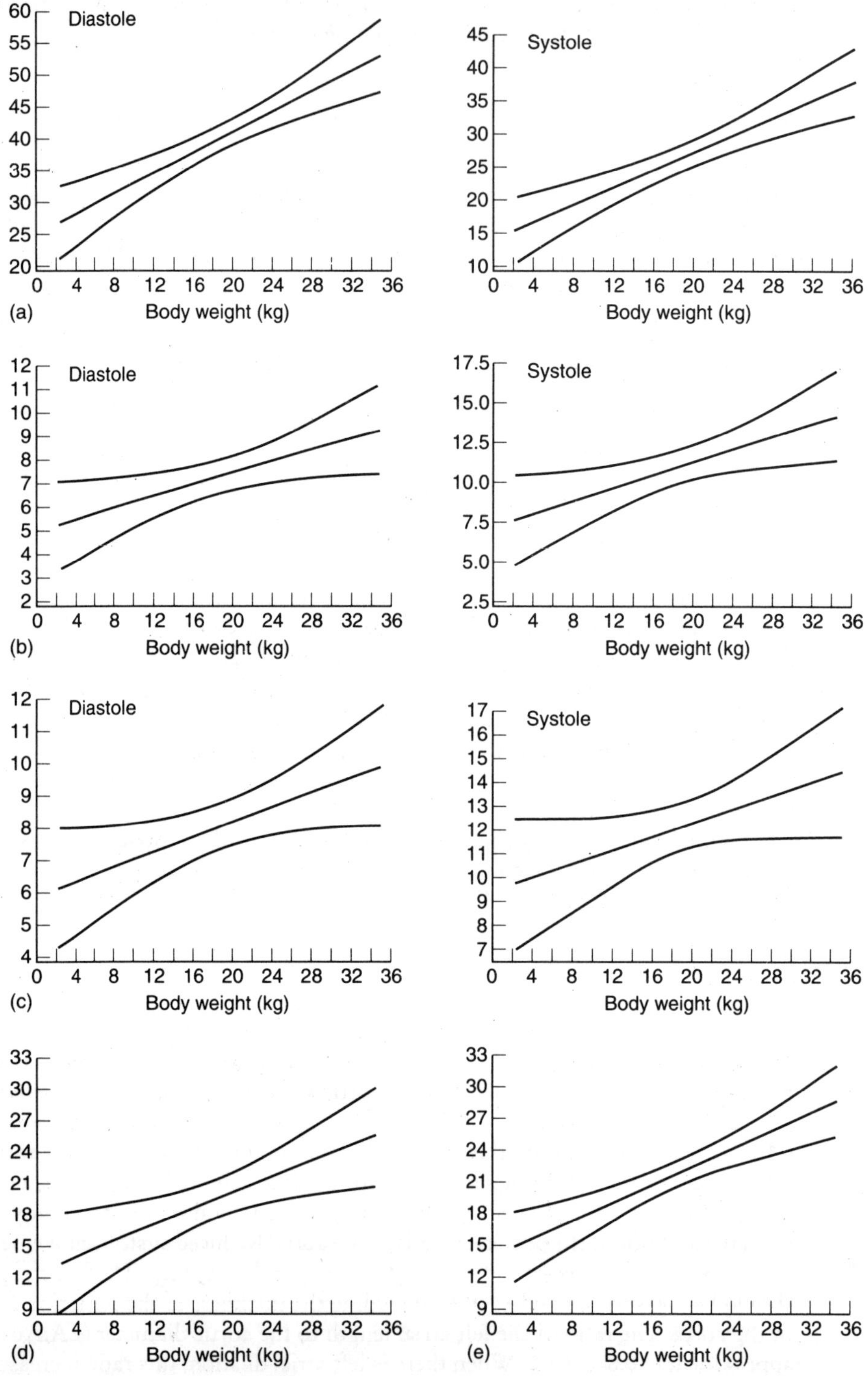
Diastole
Systole
Body weight (kg)
(a)
(b)
(c)
(d)
(e)

Table 6.2. Summary of the normal Doppler velocities (approximated) and optimal views for dogs and cats (Brown *et al.*, 1991; Yuill and O'Grady, 1991; Darke *et al.*, 1993).

Valve	Velocities (m s^{-1})		Views for optimal Doppler alignment
	Dogs	Cats	
Aortic valve	0.9–1.5	0.6–1.0	Subcostal view
			Left caudal parasternal (five-chamber) view
Pulmonic valve	0.7–1.2	0.5–1.0	Right parasternal long-axis view
			Right parasternal short-axis view
			Left cranial parasternal long-axis view
Mitral valve	E: 0.6–1.0	E: 0.5–0.9	Left caudal (four-chamber) parasternal view
	A: 0.3–0.7	A: no data	
Tricuspid valve	E: 0.4–0.8	E: 0.4–0.8	Left caudal long-axis view
	A: 0.3–0.6	A: no data	Left cranial short-axis view

Aortic valve

Early closure, and/or fluttering, of the aortic valve may sometimes be seen on M-mode, in animals with obstructive hypertrophic cardiomyopathy or subaortic stenosis. Gradual premature closure of the aortic valve is sometimes seen with mitral regurgitation or in low cardiac output situations.

Doppler echocardiography

The basic principles of Doppler echocardiography have been outlined in Chapter 5. Pulsed wave Doppler, continuous wave Doppler and colour coded Doppler can all be used in small animals as in large animals. Again, there are certain compromises which may mislead the echocardiographer if the principles of the technique are not understood.

The optimal echocardiographic views from which to record Doppler velocities and normal values have been described (Table 6.2) (Brown *et al.*, 1991; Yuill and O'Grady, 1991; Darke *et al.*, 1993). To record blood flow velocities, the Doppler beam or sample volume must be in-line with the direction of flow, and not exceed 20° out of line.

Regurgitation from the pulmonic valve has been found to occur in up to 70% of normal dogs and from the tricuspid valve in 50% of normal dogs (Yuill and

Fig. 6.11. Graphs showing normal M-mode values versus body weight for dogs. (Predicted values ± 95% confidence intervals). **(a)** Left ventricular internal dimensions (mm), in diastole and systole. **(b)** Left ventricular posterior wall thickness (mm), in diastole and systole. **(c)** Ventricular septal wall thickness (mm), in diastole and systole. **(d)** Left atrial dimensions (mm). **(e)** Aortic root dimensions (mm). Reproduced with kind permission from Bonagura *et al.* (1985). Copyright (1985) W.B. Saunders Company.

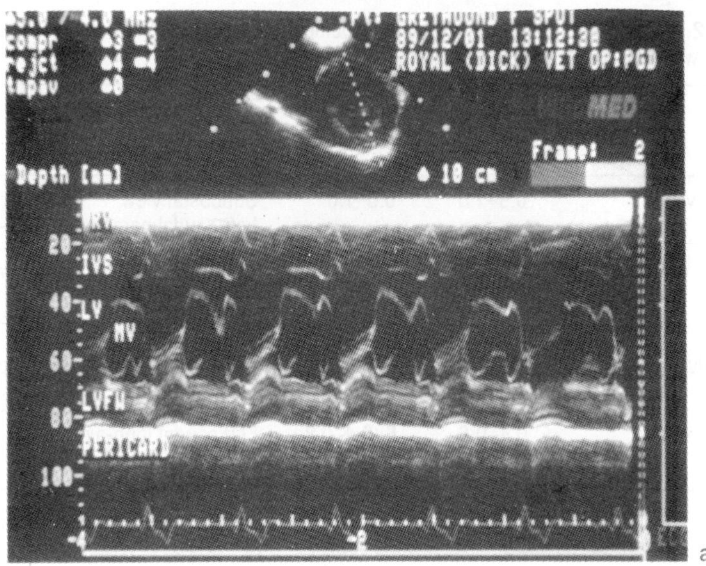

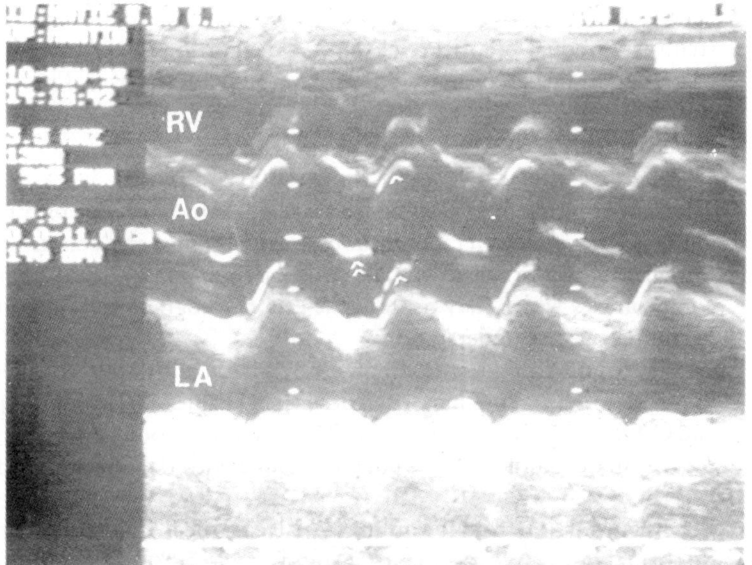

Fig. 6.12. (a) M-mode echocardiogram obtained from the right parasternal position at the level of the mitral valve. (See Figs 6.10b, 6.10c and 6.13 for a diagrammatic representation.) Note the M-shaped movement of the anterior cusp and the W-shaped movement of the posterior cusp. **(b)** M-mode echocardiogram obtained from the right parasternal position at the level of the aortic valve. (See Fig. 6.10d for a diagrammatic representation.) Double arrows point to the aortic valve cusps during diastole and single arrows point to the aortic valve cusps during systole. LA = left atrium; LV = left ventricle; RV = right ventricle; IVS = interventricular septum; MV = mitral valve; LVFW = left ventricular free wall; PERICARD = pericardium; Ao = aorta. Reproduced by kind permission of Dr Peter Darke.

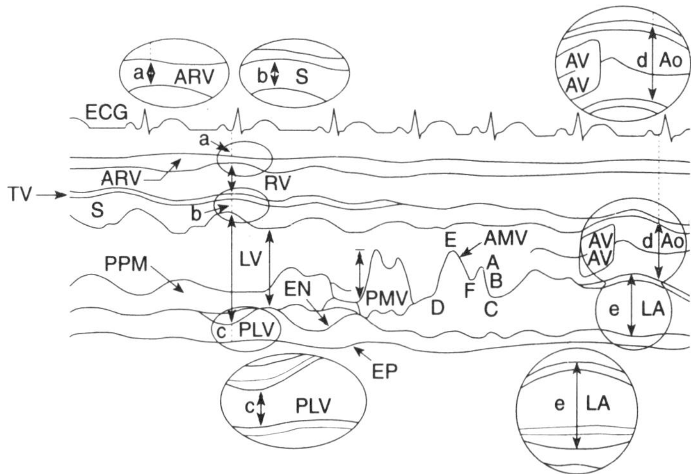

Fig. 6.13. Diagrammatic M-mode sweep, similar to Fig. 6.10, showing the recommended criteria for measurement. Diastolic measurements are made at the onset of the QRS complex on the ECG. Cavities and walls are measured at the level of the chordae, just below the mitral valve. The illustration and the elliptical inserts, a–e, show the leading edge method, together with measurements using the thinnest continuous echo lines. ARV = right ventricular anterior wall; RV = right ventricle; LV = left ventricle; PLV = left ventricular posterior wall; S = septum; PPM = papillary muscle; AMV and PMV = anterior and posterior mitral valve leaflets; A–F = points of mitral valve motion; EN = endocardium; EP = epicardium; TV = tricuspid valve; Ao = aorta; AV = aortic valve; LA = left atrium. Reproduced with kind permission from Sahn *et al.* (1978). Copyright (1978) American Heart Association.

O'Grady, 1991). Small and brief regurgitation found in the normal animal is often referred to as backflow. Regurgitation from the aortic or mitral valve has not been found in normal dogs, and therefore should be considered pathological.

Blood flow within the heart is usually laminar and the Doppler velocity display (termed the spectral velocity display) will show that the majority of red cells accelerate together to a similar peak velocity and decelerate at a similar rate. This is referred to as a 'clean envelope' or described as having minimal 'spectral dispersion' (Fig. 6.14a). Abnormal or turbulent flow, such as occurs distal to an obstruction, will produce a spectral velocity display with widespread spectral dispersion.

Abnormalities in blood flow (disturbed flow) may be due to valvular regurgitation, stenosis, or cardiac shunts. Thus, in the normal examination, the velocities should be recorded proximal and distal to every valve, and in areas where shunts are likely to be found, e.g. ventricular septal defect.

The pressure gradient between any two chambers, or the ventricles and great vessels, can be estimated from the peak velocity of blood flow between the two. For example, if the velocity is within the normal range proximal to a stenosis, and grossly elevated distal to it (Fig. 6.14b), the pressure gradient that is required to

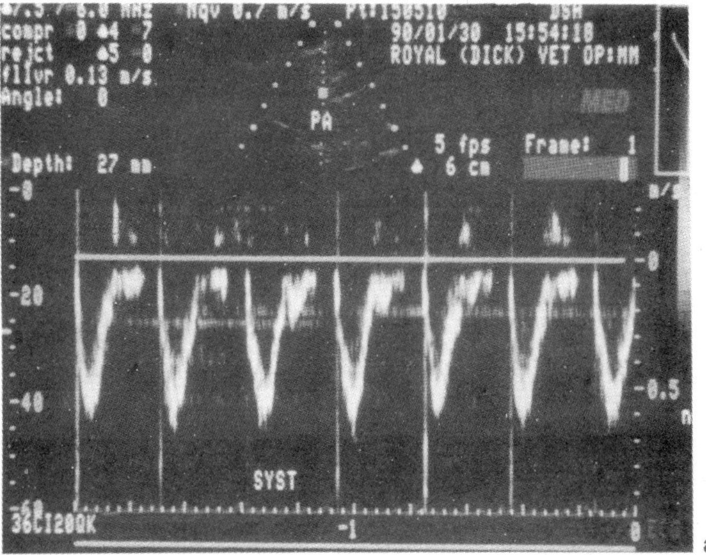

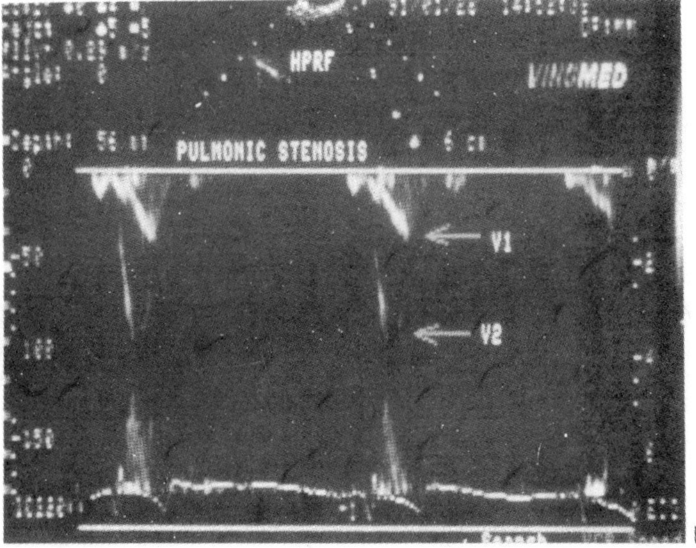

Fig. 6.14. (a) Doppler spectral velocity display obtained from the pulmonary artery of a cat. Note that the peak velocity is 0.6 m s⁻¹ (from the scale on the right). There is minimal spectral dispersion indicating that the blood flow is laminar. The narrow vertical lines seen at the start of systole are created by the opening of the pulmonic valve crossing the sample volume. SYST = systole. **(b)** Doppler spectral velocity display obtained from a dog with valvular pulmonic stenosis. V1 = velocity proximal to the stenosis. V2 = velocity distal to the stenosis. V2 is approximately 4 m s⁻¹ (from the scale on the right), which equates to a transvalvular pressure gradient of 64 mmHg using the modified Bernoulli equation (see text). In this dog, the pulmonic stenosis would therefore be classified as moderately severe. Reproduced with kind permission from Martin *et al.* (1992). Copyright (1992) British Small Animal Veterinary Association.

produce the peak velocity, can be estimated from the modified Bernoulli equation (Goldberg *et al.*, 1988):

$$\text{pressure gradient} = 4 \times (V_2^2 - V_1^2)$$

where V_2 is the peak velocity distal to the obstruction and V_1 is the peak velocity proximal to the obstruction.

Peak velocities through the aorta or pulmonary artery may be reduced when there is poor ventricular function or contractility, e.g. dilated cardiomyopathy. Other Doppler measurements of systolic ventricular function include peak and mean flow acceleration, and stroke volume and cardiac output determination (Goldberg *et al.*, 1988). Diastolic dysfunction appears more difficult to quantify; the reader is referred to Danford *et al.* (1986) and Nishimura *et al.* (1989). Ventricular inflow velocities normally result in a passive filling phase (E wave) and atrial contraction phase (A wave), where the E wave is greater than the A wave. When the ventricle becomes non-compliant, e.g. in hypertrophic cardiomyopathy, then the E wave is reduced, and the A wave increased (Fig. 6.15a). Thus the A:E wave ratio may become reversed (Fig. 6.16). Other variables used to quantify diastolic dysfunction include changes in the time–velocity interval, prolongation of early diastolic acceleration and deceleration times, and half-times. Accurate recording of inflow velocities is particularly important in the interpretation of absolute values.

Contrast echocardiography

Non-selective contrast echocardiography is achieved by injecting a suspension of microbubbles into a peripheral vein and observing the 2-D image for the presence of shunts. The microbubbles can be created by pushing intravenous fluid (e.g. saline or Haemaccel) rapidly to-and-fro between two syringes connected by a three-way tap. When a suspension of bubbles has been produced, the three-way tap is opened to a previously placed intravenous canula and the fluid injected. Only a small amount of fluid is required, e.g. 5–10 ml for a medium-sized dog. The microbubbles are quickly seen to opacify the right atrium, ventricle and pulmonary artery. The presence of right-to-left shunts can been seen as the microbubbles shunt into the left side of the heart. If there is a left-to-right shunt, negative contrast may sometimes be seen. Occasionally bubbles may pass through the pulmonary circulation, to return to the left side of the heart, which may potentially be confused with the presence of a shunt. This technique requires an additional assistant to perform the injection, while the echocardiographer maintains adequate visualization of the area of interest. The difficulty in obtaining good visualization of the right heart complicates the procedure. It is recommended that the procedure is recorded on video, so that repeat viewings may be studied.

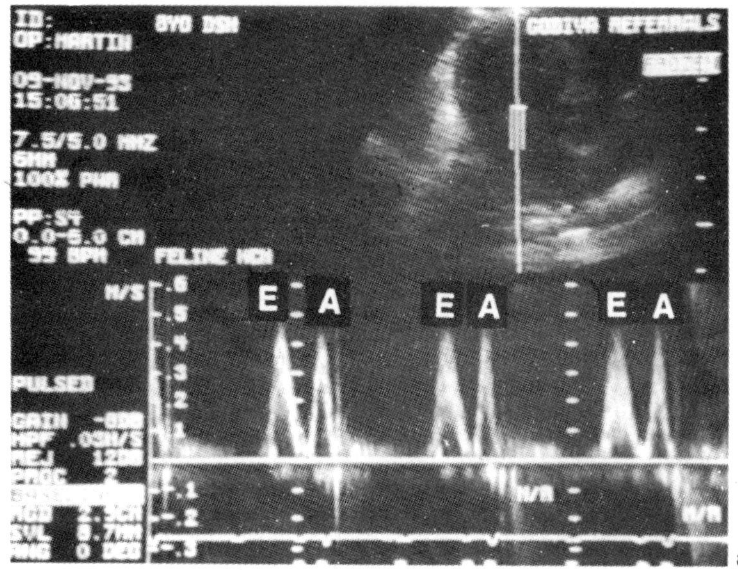

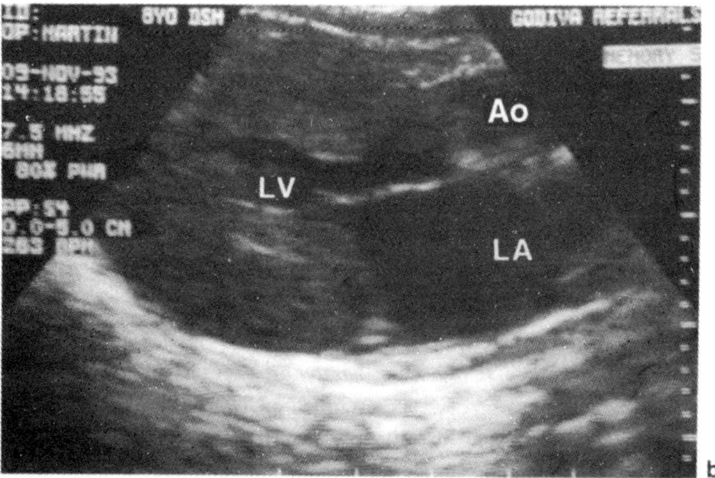

Fig. 6.15. (a) Doppler spectral velocity display obtained from the mitral valve of a cat with idiopathic hypertrophic cardiomyopathy, showing left ventricular inflow velocities (also Fig. 6.17b). Note that the A wave is now equal to the E wave, indicating a reduction in left ventricular compliance, i.e. diastolic dysfunction (cf. Fig. 6.16). **(b)** Two-dimensional echocardiogram (right parasternal long-axis view) from the same cat. Note the marked left ventricular hypertrophy and left atrial dilation. (Scale on the right: smaller divisions = 2 mm; larger divisions 10 mm.) LA = left atrium; LV = left ventricle; Ao = aorta.

Clinical applications

Pericardial disease

2-D and M-mode echocardiography are the methods of choice for the identification of pericardial effusion, being superior to radiography or

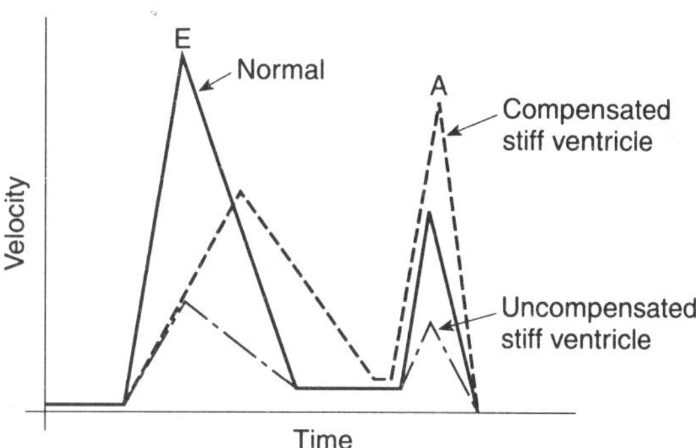

Fig. 6.16. Schematic illustration of the ventricular inflow spectral velocity display for a normal ventricle and for a poorly compliant, stiff ventricle, with and without physiological compensation. Reproduced with kind permission from Danford *et al.* (1986). Copyright (1986) Futura Publishing Company Inc.

electrocardiography. The typical echocardiographic features have been described (Berg and Wingfield, 1984). A large anechoic area is seen between the pericardium and the myocardium, and the right ventricle is easily visualized away from the thoracic wall (Fig. 6.17a). Clots or strands of fibrin are occasionally seen within this space. With large effusions, the heart can be seen to swing within the pericardium. Differentiation from pleural effusion is usually not a problem, due to the easily identified pericardium. A method for estimating the volume of pericardial effusion in humans using echocardiography has been proposed by Horowitz *et al.* (1974). The compression of the right atrium and ventricle may be visualized when tamponade is present. The detection of cardiac masses by 2-D echocardiography is often possible (Thomas *et al.*, 1984) and should be performed before and after pericardial drainage. Cardiac tumours may be seen as a mass around the right atrium (haemangiosarcoma) or attached to the ascending aorta. The identification of pericardial thickening due to pericarditis, a rare condition in small animals, is likely to be difficult.

Myocardial diseases

The echocardiographic features of dilated cardiomyopathy (DCM) have been described in a number of reports (Soderberg *et al.*, 1983; Calvert and Brown, 1986; Gooding *et al.*, 1986). Doxorubicin-induced cardiomyopathy, myocarditis and DCM produce similar echocardiographic findings. These diseases result in a primary systolic dysfunction of one or both ventricles, more commonly the left, which itself leads to additional secondary changes. On 2-D echocardiography the left ventricle appears dilated and hypocontractile (Figs 6.18a and 6.18b). M-mode measurements confirm the presence of increased systolic and diastolic chamber dimensions and reduced FS, usually to less than 15–20%. The ventricular wall thicknesses (septum and posterior wall) may be reduced or normal if

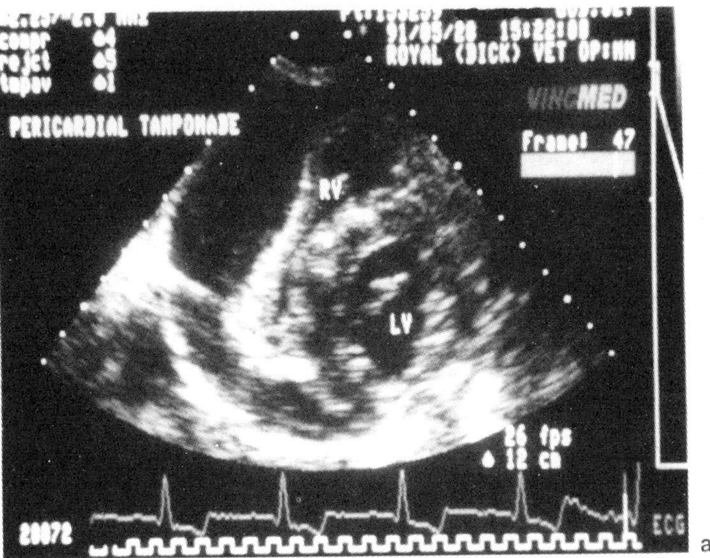

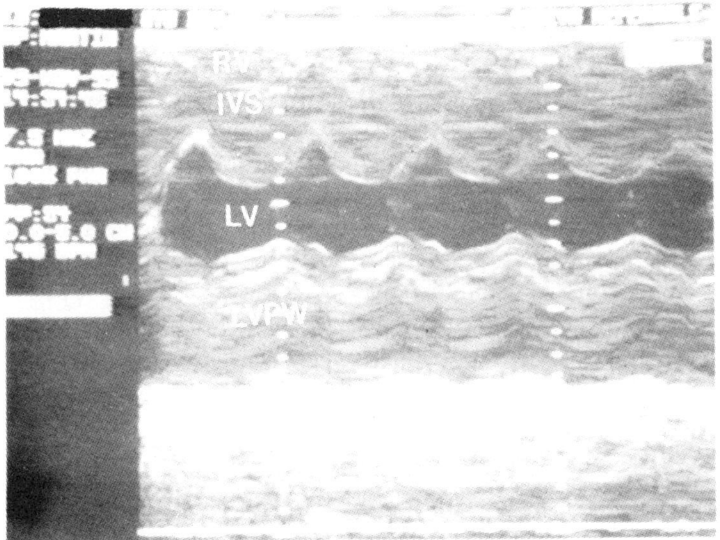

Fig. 6.17. (a) Two-dimensional echocardiogram obtained from the right parasternal short-axis view (at the mitral valve level) from a dog with pericardial tamponade. Note how the pressure due to the pericardial effusion is causing compression of the right ventricle in diastole. Pericardial effusion can be distinguished from pleural effusion by identifying the pericardium, seen in the left lower quadrant of this echocardiogram. The orientation here is not standard and should be reversed from left to right. **(b)** M-mode echocardiogram (right parasternal short-axis view at the level of the chordae tendineae) from the same cat as in Fig. 6.15. (Scale: small divisions = 2 mm.) Note that the interventricular septum is approximately 7 mm thick and there is a relatively slow rate of diastolic relaxation (cf. Fig. 6.2b). RV = right ventricle; LV = left ventricle; IVS = interventricular septum; LVPW = left ventricular posterior wall.

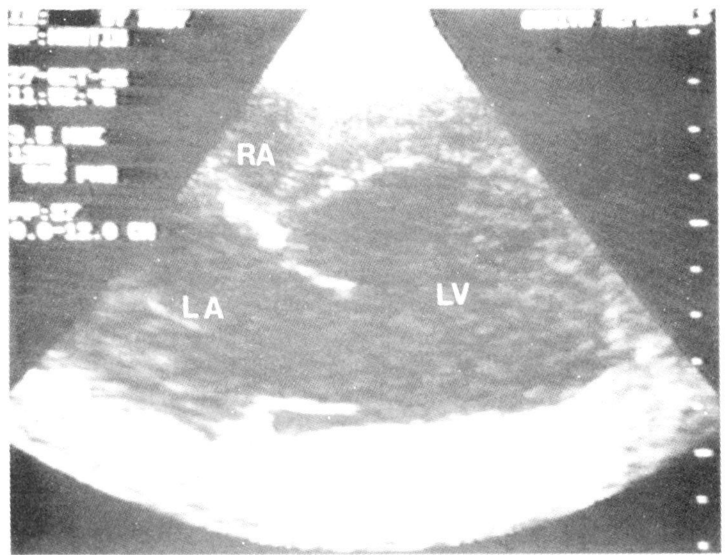

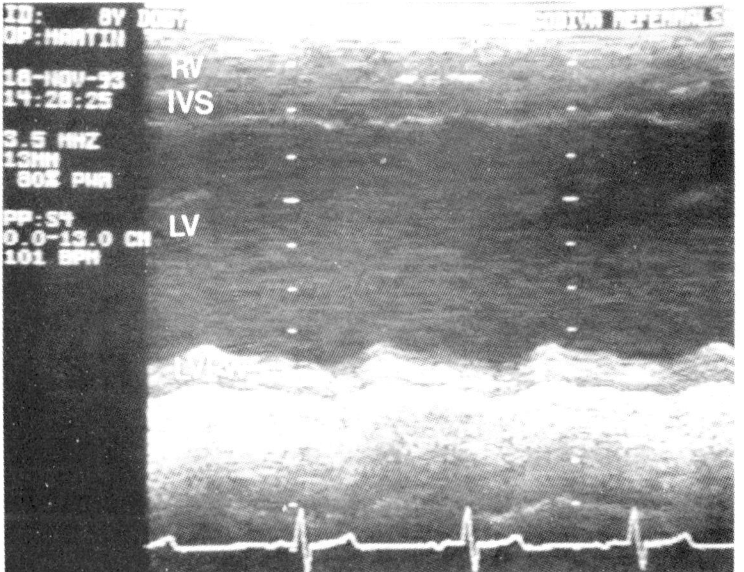

Fig. 6.18. (a) Two-dimensional echocardiogram (right parasternal long-axis view) from an eight-year-old Dobermann with idiopathic dilated cardiomyopathy. The left ventricle and left atrium are dilated, although this is not properly appreciated on a photographic still. The orientation here is not standard and should be reversed from left to right. **(b)** M-mode echocardiogram (right parasternal short-axis view at the level of the chordae tendineae) from the same dog. The left ventricle is dilated and contractility is extremely poor. Fractional shortening in this dog is approximately 5%. LA = left atrium; RA = right atrium; LV = left ventricle; RV = right ventricle; IVS = interventricular septum; LVPW = left ventricular posterior wall.

there is a compensatory hypertrophy (eccentric hypertrophy). It should be noted that in the normal Dobermann pinscher, many of these measurements are less than in other breeds (Smucker *et al.*, 1990). The EPSS is increased and a 'B' shoulder may be seen on the M-mode of the mitral valve. Doppler echocardiography will reveal reduced systolic function, e.g. reduced aortic or pulmonic velocities. Dilation of the atrio-ventricular (A-V) valve annulus occurs as a result of the ventricular dilation, leading to A-V valve regurgitation, and consequently atrial dilation. The atrial dilation can be seen on 2-D echocardiography and left atrial dilation quantified by M-mode (increased LA:Ao ratio). A-V valve regurgitation can be demonstrated by Doppler echocardiography, and the transvalvular pressure gradient is usually reduced as a result of poor ventricular systolic function, or the ventricle's inability to generate normal systolic pressures.

Hypertrophic cardiomyopathy (HCM), which is most commonly seen in the cat, may be primary (i.e. idiopathic) or secondary (e.g. hyperthyroidism). On 2-D echocardiography (Fig. 6.15b) there is the appearance of a thick-walled left ventricle with a small chamber diameter (Moise *et al.*, 1986; Bright *et al.*, 1992). This subjective appearance should always be confirmed by more accurate M-mode measurements (Fig. 6.17b). If the interventricular septum and/or the left ventricular posterior wall are thicker than 6 mm in diastole, this is considered significant in cats. Often there is asymmetric septal hypertrophy, i.e. septal thickness/left ventricular posterior wall thickness >1.3. Other causes of left ventricular hypertrophy should be excluded, e.g. hypertension secondary to renal failure or congenital aortic stenosis. There may be normal to increased indices of systolic function. M-mode examination of the mitral valve may reveal systolic anterior motion (SAM), due to dynamic left ventricular outflow tract obstruction (hypertrophic obstructive cardiomyopathy, HOCM) or early systolic closure and/or fluttering of the aortic valve (cf. subaortic stenosis). Dilation of the atria often occurs as a result of the poor ventricular compliance and reduced ventricular filling. A left atrial ball thrombus may be seen in the left atrium of some cats. Doppler echocardiography may reveal abnormal ventricular inflow velocities (increased A/E ratio; Fig. 6.15a) and A-V valve regurgitation with normal to increased transvalvular pressure gradients.

Echocardiographic findings in cats with HCM secondary to hyperthyroidism are considered distinctive from those seen in cases of idiopathic HCM; there is left ventricular hypertrophy with normal end-systolic but dilated end-diastolic chamber dimensions and an elevated FS (Bond *et al.*, 1988).

Restrictive cardiomyopathy may appear similar to HCM, although with less ventricular hypertrophy and an irregular shaped left ventricle with irregular echogenicities in the myocardium and endocardium. There is less ventricular wall motion and the FS may be less. There may be more severe atrial dilation than in HCM, and the Doppler indices of diastolic dysfunction may be more severe.

Excessive left ventricular moderator bands, which may cause heart failure in cats, may be seen on 2-D echocardiography.

Diseases of the atrio-ventricular valves

Diseases of the A-V valves may be congenital, e.g. dysplasia or stenosis, or acquired, e.g. endocardiosis or endocarditis. The result of valvular disease is an incompetent valve, allowing retrograde regurgitation of blood into the atria. Doppler echocardiography is therefore required to document the regurgitation (Plate 5, frontispiece). 2-D echocardiography may demonstrate a variable degree of thickening of the valve, most commonly seen on the anterior leaflet in mitral valve disease, or abnormal location, shape, movement or chordae attachment in congenital dysplasia. The valve may appear to bulge retrogradely into the atria (prolapse), or, if there is chordae tendineae rupture, then complete inversion of the valve may be seen (flail valve). On M-mode echocardiography there may be an abrupt posterior, or downward, motion (greater than 5 mm) of the valve in late systole.

As a consequence of the regurgitation, atrial dilation ensues, which can be seen and measured on 2-D and M-mode. The pulmonary veins or caudal vena cava may also appear dilated. Mapping of the regurgitant jet by Doppler echocardiography can give an indication of severity, and measurement of the transvalvular pressure gradient can give an indication of ventricular function. As A-V valve regurgitation progresses and volume overload develops, dilation of the ventricle is also seen. Ventricular contractility is often not diminished until end-stage heart failure, and indices of systolic function may be normal until then. However, as the ventricle dilates in severely affected cases, the ventricular contractility (FS) reduces. Distinguishing severe primary mitral valve disease from dilated cardiomyopathy can occasionally be problematic.

Stenosis of an A-V valve rarely occurs, but can be recognized on an M-mode scan of the mitral valve as absence of the normal M shaped movement of the anterior cusp, i.e., no mid-diastolic closure and late diastolic opening with atrial contraction. On 2-D the valve often appears in a 'parachute' shape, and is abnormally thickened. Doppler documents continuous blood flow during diastole and absence of the normal E and A waves. The severity of the stenosis can be quantified from the Doppler spectral tracing, by measuring the pressure half-time (Feigenbaum, 1986).

Diseases of the semilunar valves

The semilunar valves, so called because of their appearance, may become incompetent as a result of bacterial endocarditis, or be stenotic due to a congenital abnormality. Aortic valve endocarditis may appear on 2-D echocardiography as irregularities, thickenings or vegetative type growths on the leaflets (Lombard and Buergelt, 1983; Bonagura and Pipers, 1983; Sisson and Thomas, 1984). Vegetations must be at least 3–4 mm in size to be seen on echocardiography. Prolapse of the aortic valve may occasionally be seen with valvular endocarditis or a ventricular septal defect. The regurgitation can be documented by Doppler echocardiography. The regurgitant jet often causes fluttering of the anterior mitral valve, and premature closure of the valve, seen on M-mode. The regurgitation leads to left ventricular volume overload, which can be seen on 2-D echocardiography, with an apparent increase in FS. A mild degree of pulmonic valve regurgitation, or backflow, is commonly seen in the normal dog during a Doppler examination, but is usually very brief (Yuill and O'Grady, 1991). Pulmonic regurgitation is commonly seen with congenital valvular stenosis, and may be seen with dirofilariasis or patent ductus arteriosus with pulmonary hypertension. If a pulmonic regurgitant jet can be documented with pulmonary hypertension, the transvalvular pressure gradient (from pulmonary artery to right ventricle) at the start of diastole will be elevated.

Aortic stenosis is commonly of the subvalvular type in the dog (Plate 6, frontispiece), comprising a fibrous ring which may be visualized (Wingfield *et al.*, 1983; O'Grady *et al.*, 1989). Pulmonic stenosis is more usually valvular, with thickening and increased echogenicity of the valves evident on 2-D echocardiography (Fingland *et al.*, 1986; Martin *et al.*, 1992). Valvular and supravalvular aortic stenosis have been reported in the dog and cat. Moderate to severe cases will develop ventricular hypertrophy and a post-stenotic bulge. Doppler echocardiography is able to quantify the severity of the stenosis and regurgitation is commonly found with both lesions. In severe cases, hypertrophy of the outflow tracts may lead to a dynamic outflow obstruction, occurring during systole, and can be recognized by a characteristic spectral velocity display which documents an increasing acceleration to peak velocity (cf. HOCM). Mid-systolic closure and fluttering of the aortic valve are sometimes seen with subaortic stenosis (cf. HOCM) but not with valvular stenosis. Transvalvular pressure gradients of less than 50 mmHg are considered mild, and the animal is likely to live a normal life. However, gradients greater than 75 mmHg in aortic stenosis and 100 mmHg in pulmonic stenosis are considered severe lesions, and the animal is likely to develop clinical signs and/or die early. Cases of pulmonic stenosis with marked ventricular hypertrophy frequently develop tricuspid valve regurgitation. This may be as a result of distortion of the tricuspid valve apparatus by the hypertrophy. Consequently, tricuspid regurgitation and dilation of the right atrium is often seen in cases of pulmonic stenosis, in contrast to cases of aortic stenosis where mitral valve incompetence is uncommon.

Cardiac shunts

The more commonly seen shunts (atrial septal defect (ASD), ventricular septal defect (VSD) and patent ductus arteriosus (PDA)), normally produce left-to-right shunting. Thus contrast echocardiography is unlikely to be diagnostic in these cases. ASDs and VSDs can be visualized on 2-D (Figs 6.19a and 6.19b). Unfortunately, echo-dropout in these areas can result in false positive diagnoses. When a true defect exists, an interface is created between the edge of the communication and blood, which results in a very echogenic border, sometimes referred to as a 'matchstick' sign (Figs 6.19a and 6.19b).

VSDs usually occur high in the ventricular septum, just below the aortic valve (Fig. 6.19b). Doppler echocardiography is able to document a high-velocity jet through the VSD (Plate 7). Increased velocities are also seen in the right ventricular outflow tract. In large shunts, the right ventricular pressure increases and the transventricular pressure gradient decreases, thus the peak measured velocity reduces. Some dogs with a VSD also have aortic regurgitation due to prolapsing of an aortic cusp into the VSD.

ASDs occur low (primum) or high (secundum) in the septal wall. ASDs result in volume overload of the right heart, and thus dilation of the atrium and ventricle

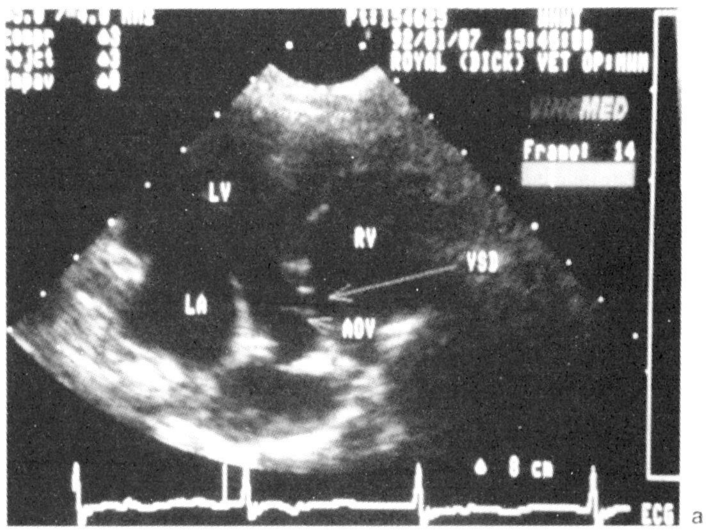

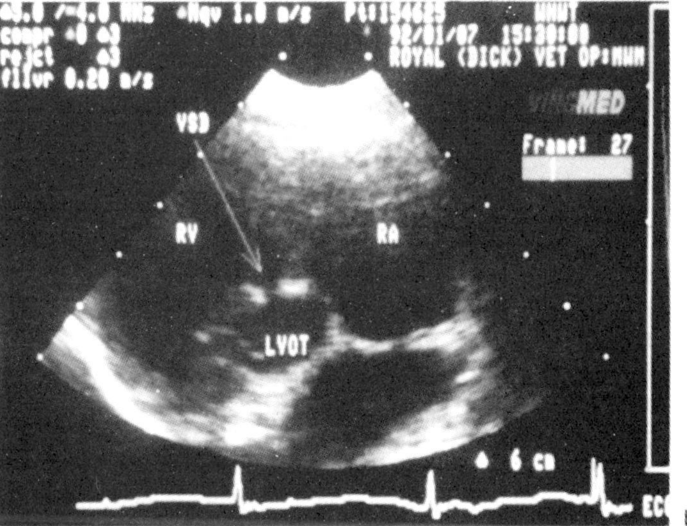

Fig. 6.19. (a) Two-dimensional echocardiogram (left caudal parasternal long-axis view) from a West Highland White puppy (see also Plate 7, frontispiece) with a ventricular septal defect. The presence of a 'hole' can be seen (arrowed) in the membranous portion of the interventricular septum, just below the aortic valve. Note how there is an increased echogenicity to the edges of the septal membrane due to the soft tissue/fluid interface ('matchstick' sign). **(b)** Two-dimensional echocardiogram (right parasternal short-axis view) from the same dog. The presence of the defect can again be seen (arrowed) in the membranous portion of the interventricular septum, just below the aortic valve. The orientation here is not standard and should be reversed from left to right. AO = aortic valve; LA = left atrium; LV = left ventricle; RV = right ventricle; RA = right atrium; LVOT = left ventricular outflow tract; VSD = ventricular septal defect.

may be seen in severe cases. However, most cases do not cause clinical problems, and are an incidental finding. Spectral velocity displays are often difficult to obtain across an ASD, due to the proximity of inflow velocities from the caudal vena cava. Increased velocities will be found in the pulmonary artery.

PDA is difficult to visualize on 2-D echocardiography, but occasionally may be seen in the left cranial parasternal short-axis view, optimized for the pulmonary artery and not to be confused with the left and right branches of the pulmonary artery. Doppler echocardiography documents a continuous flow pattern characteristic for PDA, in the pulmonary artery (Plate 8, frontispiece). The left ventricle often appears hyperdynamic, and the FS may be increased. Dilation of the left atrium and mitral regurgitation are often found.

Acknowledgement

Many of the sonograms reproduced in this chapter were obtained by the author during his period as Resident in Veterinary Cardiology at the Royal (Dick) School of Veterinary Studies, University of Edinburgh. This post was partly funded by the Royal College of Veterinary Surgeons Trust Fund for which the author is grateful.

References

Berg, R.J. and Wingfield, W.E. (1984) Pericardial effusion in the dog: a review of 42 cases. *Journal of the American Animal Hospital Association*, 20, 721–730.

Bonagura, J.D. and Pipers, F.S. (1983) Echocardiographic features of aortic valve endocarditis in a dog, a cow, and a horse. *Journal of the American Veterinary Medical Association*, 182, 595–599.

Bonagura, J.D., O'Grady, M.R. and Herring, D.S. (1985) Echocardiography: principles of interpretation. *Veterinary Clinics of North America: Small Animal Practice*, 15, 1177–1194.

Bond, B.R., Fox, P.R., Peterson, M.E. and Skavaril, R.V. (1988) Echocardiographic findings in 103 cats with hyperthyroidism. *Journal of the American Veterinary Medical Association*, 192, 1546–1549.

Boon, J., Wingfield, W.E. and Miller, C.W. (1983) Echocardiographic indices in the normal dog. *Veterinary Radiology*, 24, 214–221.

Bright, J.M., Golden, A.L. and Daniel, G.B. (1992) Feline hypertrophic cardiomyopathy: variations on a theme. *Journal of Small Animal Practice*, 33, 266–274.

Brown, D.J., Knight, D.H. and King, P.R. (1991) Use of pulsed-wave Doppler echocardiography to determine aortic and pulmonary velocity and flow variables in clinically normal dogs. *American Journal of Veterinary Research*, 52, 543–550.

Calvert, C.A. and Brown, J. (1986) Use of M-mode echocardiography in the diagnosis of congestive cardiomyopathy in Doberman pinschers. *Journal of the American Veterinary Medical Association*, 189, 293–297.

Danford, D.A., Huhta, J.C. and Murphy, D.J. (1986) Doppler echocardiographic approaches to ventricular diastolic function. *Echocardiography: A Review of Cardiovascular Ultrasound*, 3, 33–40.

Darke, P.G.G., Bonagura, J.D. and Miller, M. (1993) Transducer orientation for Doppler echocardiography in dogs. *Journal of Small Animal Practice*, 34, 2–8.

DeMadron, E., Bonagura, J.D. and O'Grady, M.R. (1985) Normal and paradoxical ventricular septal motion in the dog. *American Journal of Veterinary Research*, 46, 1832–1841.

Feigenbaum, H. (1986) *Echocardiography*, 4th edn. Lea and Febiger, Philadelphia.

Fingland, R.B., Bonagura, J.D. and Myer, C.W. (1986) Pulmonic stenosis in the dog: 29 cases (1975–1984). *Journal of the American Veterinary Medical Association*, 189, 218–226.

Goldberg, S.J., Allen, H.D., Marx, G.R. and Donnerstein, R.L. (1988) *Doppler Echocardiography*, 2nd edn. Lea and Febiger, Philadelphia.

Gooding, J.P., Robinson, W.F., Wyburn, R.S. and Cullen, L.K. (1986) A cardiomyopathy in the English cocker spaniel: a clinico-pathological investigation. *Journal of Small Animal Practice*, 23, 133–149.

Henry, W.L., DeMaria, A., Gramaik, R., King, D.L., Kisslo, J.A., Popp, R.L., Sahn, D.J., Schiller, N.B., Tajik, A., Teichhilz, L.E. and Weyman, A.E. (1980) Report of the American Society of Echocardiography Committee on nomenclature and standards in two-dimensional echocardiography. *Circulation*, 62, 212–217.

Horowitz, M.S., Schultz, C.S., Stinson, E.B., Harrison, D.C. and Popp, R.L. (1974) Sensitivity and specificity of echocardiographic diagnosis of pericardial effusion. *Circulation*, 50, 239–247.

Jacobs, G. and Knight, D.H. (1985) M-mode echocardiographic measurements in non-anaesthetized healthy cats: effects of body weight, heart rate, and other variables. *American Journal of Veterinary Research*, 46, 1705–1711.

Lombard, C.W. (1984) Normal values of the canine M-mode echocardiogram. *American Journal of Veterinary Research*, 44, 2015–2018.

Lombard, C.W. and Buergelt, C.D. (1983) Vegetative bacterial endocarditis in dogs; echocardiographic diagnosis and clinical signs. *Journal of Small Animal Practice*, 24, 325–339.

Martin, M.W.S., Godman, M., Luis Fuentes, V., Clutton, R.E., Haihg, A. and Darke, P.G.G. (1992) Assessment of balloon pulmonary valvuloplasty in six dogs. *Journal of Small Animal Practice*, 33, 443–449.

Moise, N.S., Dietze, A.E., Mezza, L.E., Strickland, D., Erb, H. and Edwards, N.J. (1986) Echocardiography, electrocardiography and radiography of cats with dilation cardiomyopathy, hypertrophic cardiomyopathy, and hyperthyroidism. *American Journal of Veterinary Research*, 47, 1476–1486.

Morrison, S.A., Moise, S., Scarlett, J., Mohammed, H. and Yeager, A.E. (1992) Effect of breed and body weight on echocardiographic values in four breeds of dogs of differing somatotype. *Journal of Veterinary Internal Medicine*, 6, 220–224.

Nishimura, R.A., Abel, M.D., Hatle, L.K. and Tajik, A.J. (1989) Assessment of diastolic function of the heart: background and current applications of Doppler echocardiography. Part II. Clinical studies. *Mayo Clinic Proceedings*, 64, 181–204.

O'Grady, M.R., Bonagura, J.D., Powers, J.D. and Herring, D.S. (1986) Quantitative cross-sectional echocardiography in the normal dog. *Veterinary Radiology*, 27, 34–49.

O'Grady, M.R., Holmberg, D.L., Miller, C.W. and Cockshutt, J.R. (1989) Canine congenital aortic stenosis: A review of the literature and commentary. *Canadian Veterinary Journal*, 30, 811–815.

O'Rourke, R.A., Hanrath, P., Henry, W.N., Hugenholtz, P.G., Pisa, Z., Roelandt, J. and Tanaka, M. (1984) Report of the Joint International Society and Federation of Cardiology/World Health Organization Task Force on recommendations for standardization of measurements from M-mode echocardiograms. *Circulation*, 69, 854–857.

Sahn, D.J., DeMaria, A., Kisslo, J. and Weyman, A. (1978) Recommendations regarding quantitation in M-mode echocardiography: results of a survey of echocardiographic measurements. *Circulation*, 58, 1072–1083.

Schnittger, I., Gordon, E.P., Fitzgerald, P.J. and Popp, R.L. (1983) Standardized intracardiac measurements of two-dimensional echocardiography. *Journal of the American College of Cardiology*, 2, 934–938.

Sisson, D. and Thomas, W.P. (1984) Endocarditis of the aortic valve in the dog. *Journal of the American Veterinary Medical Association*, 184, 570–577.

Smucker, M.L., Kaul, S., Woodfield, J.A., Keith, J.C., Manning, S.A. and Gascho, J.A. (1990) Naturally occurring cardiomyopathy in the Doberman pinscher: a possible large animal model of human cardiomyopathy? *Journal of the American College of Cardiology*, 16, 200–206.

Soderberg, S.F., Boon, J.A., Wingfield, W.E. and Miller, C.W. (1983) Echocardiography as a diagnostic aid for feline cardiomyopathy. *Veterinary Radiology*, 24, 66–73.

Thomas, W.P., Sisson, D., Bauer, T.G. and Reed, J.R. (1984) Detection of cardiac masses in dogs by two-dimensional echocardiography. *Veterinary Radiology*, 25, 65–72.

Thomas, W.P. (1984) Two-dimensional real-time echocardiography in the dog. *Veterinary Radiology*, 25, 50–64.

Wingfield, W.E., Boon, J.A. and Miller, C.W. (1983) Echocardiographic assessment of congenital aortic stenosis. *Journal of the American Veterinary Medical Association*, 183, 673–676.

Yuill, C.D.M. and O'Grady, M.R. (1991) Doppler-derived velocity of blood flow across the cardiac valves in the normal dog. *Canadian Journal of Veterinary Research*, 88, 352–356.

7 # Equine Reproductive Ultrasonography

P.G. Griffin

Lone Oak Veterinary Clinic Inc.,
34775 Road 132, Visalia, California CA 93291, USA

Introduction

Diagnostic real-time ultrasonography provides equine practitioners with a non-invasive and nondisruptive means to directly image the reproductive tract and its contents. An extensive amount of information can be gained from even a single examination, including determination of ovarian and uterine status (luteal or follicular dominance), detection and monitoring of ovarian and uterine pathology, monitoring the post-partum mare, detection of twins and detection of ovulation. When first introduced, the use of ultrasonography was primarily limited to early pregnancy diagnosis; as technology, knowledge and interpretive skills have improved, it is apparent that diagnostic ultrasonography has a much wider application in reproduction. Its use has become a prerequisite for, and a standard procedure in, reproductive work, augmenting transrectal palpation, uterine culture and cytology, and endometrial biopsy as mainstays in the diagnostic and management armamentarium. Clinical applications of ultrasonography in equine reproduction have been reviewed in detail since the advent of its use in the early 1980s, and the reader is guided to these sources for a thorough treatment of the subject and additional detailed information (Ginther, 1986, 1988a; McKinnon *et al.*, 1987a, b; Squires *et al.*, 1988; Fontijne and Hennis, 1989; McKinnon and Carnevale, 1993). This chapter is intended as a brief review of the basics of reproductive ultrasonography in the equid, emphasizing its applications in the mare.

Technique

Transrectal scanning is the most common approach to ultrasonic examination of the mare's reproductive tract. The intimate anatomical relationship between the rectum and the uterus and ovaries allows the use of high-frequency transducers, resulting in the acquisition of detailed images. The most commonly used transducer frequencies are 3.5, 5.0 and 7.5 MHz, the choice being dependent upon the size and location of the structures of interest. The higher the transducer frequency, the better the image resolution and the shallower the depth of penetration. Therefore, for routine examination of relatively small structures located close to the rectal wall (e.g. ovaries, non-gravid or early pregnant uterus), the use of a 5.0 or 7.5 MHz transducer is indicated. In contrast, for examination of large structures (e.g. the mid- to late gestation fetus and uterus, or early post-partum uterus) the use of a 3.5 MHz transducer is advantageous, as the depth of penetration is more important than a detailed image. The linear array transducer is the most commonly used transducer design, producing a rectangular, two-dimensional image on the ultrasound screen. Less commonly, sector and convex array transducers are employed. All the images shown in this chapter were obtained using a 5.0 MHz linear array transducer.

Preparations and precautions for transrectal scanning are as for transrectal palpation. Whenever possible, examining conditions should be optimized (e.g. ultrasound screen close to eye level, external light minimized, mare well restrained in stocks). A coupling medium (e.g. carboxymethylcellulose) should be used both as a lubricant and to provide contact and eliminate air between the rectal mucosa and the transducer face.

Transabdominal scanning (e.g. through the skin of the inguinal region) can be used in the mare, primarily for examination and evaluation of the late-term fetus and placental membranes and fluids (Pipers and Adams-Brendemuehl, 1984; Adams-Brendemuehl and Pipers, 1987). Hair and excessive subcutaneous fat are obstacles to obtaining a detailed and diagnostically meaningful image with this approach.

Artifacts are commonly encountered during imaging of the reproductive tract, due to the presence of many fluid-filled structures (e.g. embryonic vesicle, ovarian follicles) and the close proximity of gas-filled bowel and the bones of the pelvis. These artifacts are discussed in detail elsewhere (Ginther, 1986). Artifactual echoes can complicate the diagnostic and interpretive process, and are easily mistaken for normal or pathological structures or changes. As with any diagnostic technique, interpretation becomes increasingly sophisticated as experience is gained by the clinician.

When using a linear array transducer, the cervix and uterine body are generally viewed in longitudinal section, while the uterine horns are imaged in transverse section or cross-section. Because the equine ovary is essentially free to rotate about its mesovarial attachment, it can be viewed in longitudinal, transverse, or oblique section. A systematic and thorough approach to examination is essential and should be developed individually and used consistently so that important, and sometimes obvious, information is not overlooked. The following approach has been described (Ginther, 1986) and is found by the author to maximize the information gained during a given scan. First, longitudinal sections of the cervix and uterine body are obtained upon entering the rectum. Next, the uterine bifurcation is identified and the right uterine horn is imaged in sequential cross-section until the tip of the horn is reached. The right ovary can then be imaged by moving the transducer in a cranio-lateral direction. At times, the ovary can become trapped by the broad ligament or in a loop of bowel, and manual repositioning is necessary to obtain an adequate image. After imaging the ovary, the transducer is moved back down the right horn, again obtaining cross-sectional views. The left uterine horn and ovary are then imaged in an analogous fashion. The scan is completed by again obtaining longitudinal images of the uterine body and cervix as the transducer is withdrawn.

Ovaries

Ultrasonic anatomy

The ultrasonic anatomy of the ovaries has been described in detail (Ginther and Pierson, 1984a, b; Ginther, 1988a). Follicles appear as black (i.e. nonechogenic), circumscribed structures which are spherical to irregular in shape (Fig. 7.1). The irregular shapes are attributable to compression by adjacent follicles and luteal structures or the ovarian stroma (Ginther, 1988a). Follicles as small as 2 to 3 mm

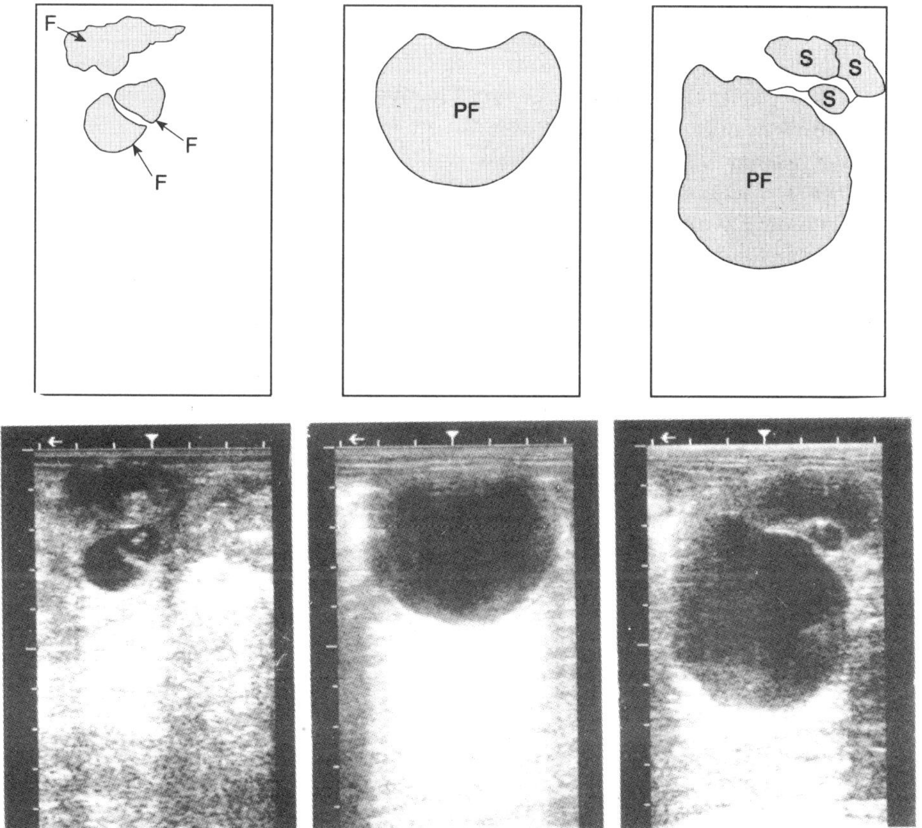

Fig. 7.1. Ovarian follicles. Left, multiple small follicles. Middle and right, large preovulatory follicles. F = follicles, PF = preovulatory follicles, S = satellite follicles.

can be detected with a high frequency transducer; follicle diameter ranges up to 40–50 mm (i.e. preovulatory follicles). The number and sizes of follicles on a given ovary will vary widely and are dependent upon the time of year and stage of the oestrous cycle or pregnancy. (See Ginther, (1992) for a review.)

Preovulatory follicle

The ultrasonic characteristics of the preovulatory follicle have been studied extensively (Ginther, 1992). The preovulatory follicle grows at an average rate of approximately 3 mm per day during oestrus (Pierson and Ginther, 1985a). The size of the follicle on the day prior to ovulation varies considerably, but in two studies, no follicle ovulated prior to reaching 35 mm in single ovulating mares (Ginther, 1988a). Changes in follicle shape from spherical to nonspherical (flattened, pear-shaped or irregular) occur as the interval to ovulation decreases (Pierson and Ginther, 1985a). The shape changes occur coincidentally with an increase in the ultrasonically determined thickness of the follicle wall, and probably in conjunction with a reduction in follicular tone (Carnevale *et al.*, 1988).

Ovulation

The disappearance of a previously detected preovulatory-sized follicle is an indication of recent ovulation. The subsequent formation and identification of a corpus luteum confirms ovulation. In most cases, the ovulation site (i.e. the developing luteal gland) can be visualized on the day of ovulation (Ginther, 1988a). The extent and pattern of follicular fluid release during the course of ovulation has been well-characterized (Townson and Ginther, 1987, 1989a). Two patterns of follicular evacuation were reported: (1) an abrupt loss of follicular fluid in which the majority of fluid (>90%) disappeared within one minute and (2) a slow, gradual loss of follicular fluid in which 80% of the fluid disappeared within approximately four minutes. Apparent breaks or rents in the follicular wall towards the ovulation fossa (Carnevale *et al.*, 1988) and apparent extraovarian fluid collections in the area of the fossa (Townson and Ginther, 1989a) have been detected prior to, or in association with, follicular evacuation. Additionally, pronounced changes in shape of adjacent nonovulatory follicles presaged or occurred in conjunction with evacuation of the ovulatory follicle (Townson and Ginther, 1989a).

Corpus luteum

The corpus luteum is generally detectable with a 5 MHz transducer for approximately 17 days after ovulation (Pierson and Ginther, 1985b). There are two distinct luteal morphologies in the mare (Pierson and Ginther, 1985b; Fig. 7.2). Approximately 50% of corpora lutea are uniformly echogenic throughout their period of detectability (i.e. centrally echogenic corpora lutea). That is, they have no, or a very small, central nonechogenic cavity. The remaining 50% develop a centrally located, nonechogenic area representative of a blood clot (i.e. centrally nonechogenic corpora lutea). In corpora lutea which form a central clot, the aver-

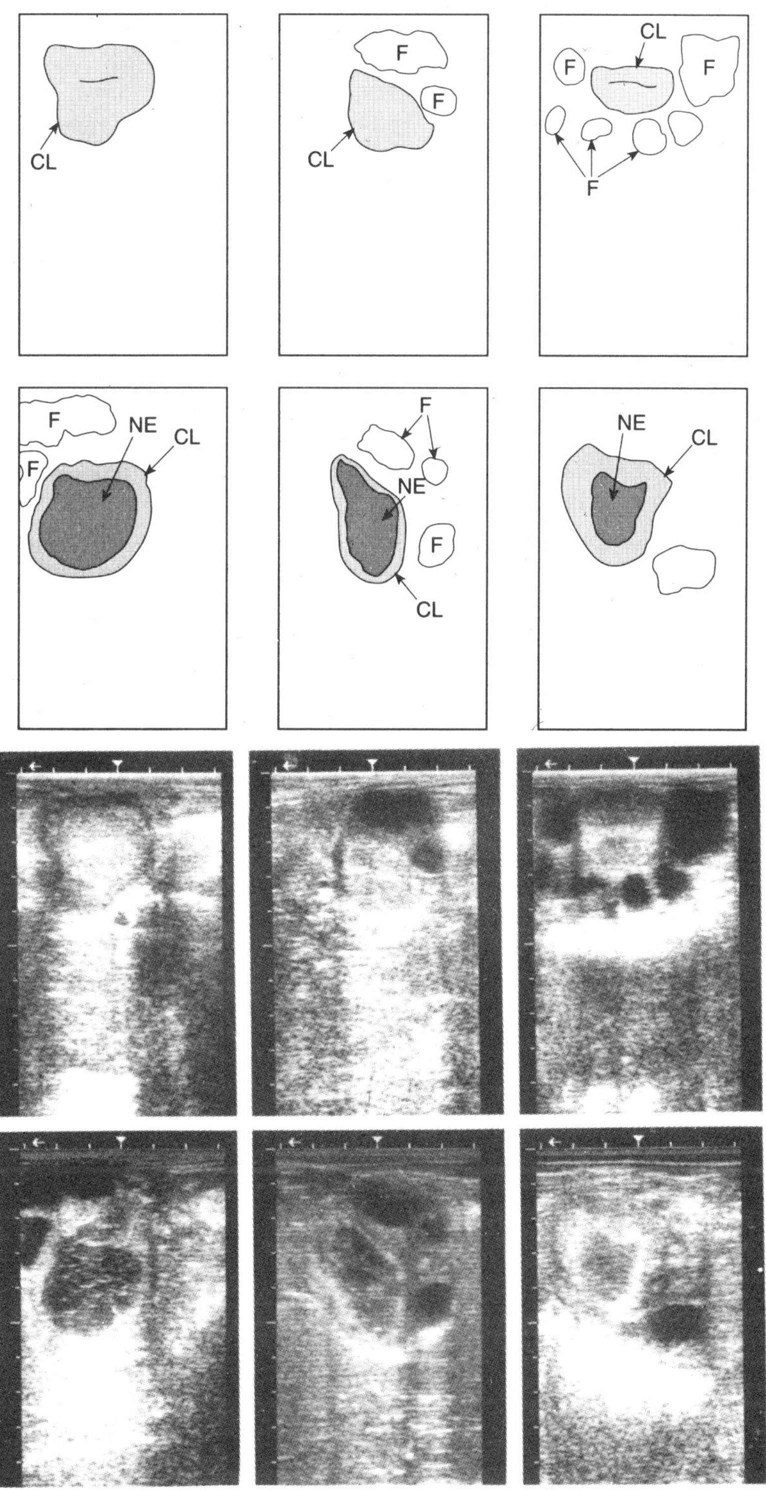

Fig. 7.2. Corpora lutea. Upper series, centrally echogenic corpora lutea. Lower series, centrally nonechogenic corpora lutea. Note differences in overall luteal size, size of the nonechogenic central cavities, and luteal echogenicity. CL = corpus luteum, NE = nonechogenic centre, F = follicle.

age time to first detection of the clot is approximately 30 hours after ovulation; the size of the central area gradually increases and reaches a maximum at two to five days postovulation (Townson and Ginther, 1988). Subsequently, the size of the central area decreases over the period of luteal detectability (Pierson and Ginther, 1985b). There are no functional differences between the two types of luteal glands; plasma progesterone concentrations were not significantly different between morphologies (Townson and Ginther, 1989b). As a result of these findings, the well-ingrained notion (Ginther, 1979) of a consistent formation of a corpus haemorrhagicum in the mare prior to the development of a mature corpus luteum can no longer be accepted as dogma.

Echogenicity or brightness of the corpus luteum is greatest during the 24 to 48 hours following its formation (Townson and Ginther, 1989c). Subsequently, echogenicity decreases until the end of the luteal phase, when it increases again (Ginther, 1986). The dynamics in echogenicity are thought to be reflective of changes in luteal haemodynamics (Ginther, 1986). Among other applications, the identification of a corpus luteum can be used to determine if a filly has reached puberty or if a mare has entered the ovulatory season.

Plasma progesterone concentrations in heifers and llamas are highly correlated with ultrasonically-determined luteal size (see Griffin and Ginther (1992) for a review). Similarly, progesterone concentrations in pregnant mares closely paralleled observed changes in cross-sectional area of the corpus luteum, as determined by ultrasonography, in temporal association with the initial release of equine chorionic gonadotropin on approximately day 35 (Bergfelt *et al.*, 1989). While not yet definitive in the mare, the observed close relationship between luteal size and progesterone concentration indicates that ultrasonic measurement of the equine corpus luteum may be a valuable and immediate adjunct to plasma progesterone assay as an index of luteal function, as has been suggested for the cow (Kastelic *et al.*, 1990). Awareness of this relationship can aid the clinician in the sometimes difficult decision regarding exogenous progesterone supplementation, particularly early (e.g. after day 15 or 16) in pregnancy. Ultrasonic assessment of the corpus luteum may also be useful in evaluating the suitability of potential embryo transfer recipients (Squires, 1993).

Uterus

Ultrasonic anatomy

The ultrasonic echotexture or characteristic image of the uterus changes dynamically during the oestrous cycle and early pregnancy (Ginther and Pierson, 1984c; Hayes *et al.*, 1985; Griffin and Ginther, 1991b). Changes in uterine echotexture are primarily the result of changes in the degree of oedema of the longitudinal endometrial folds (Ginther and Pierson, 1984c; Hayes *et al.*, 1985). During oestrus, there is marked oedematous expansion of the folds and echotexture is characterized by alternating and intertwining areas of hyper- and hypoechogenicity (Fig. 7.3). The hyperechoic (white) areas are attributable to the dense connective tissue core of the folds, while the hypoechoic (dark) areas are attributable

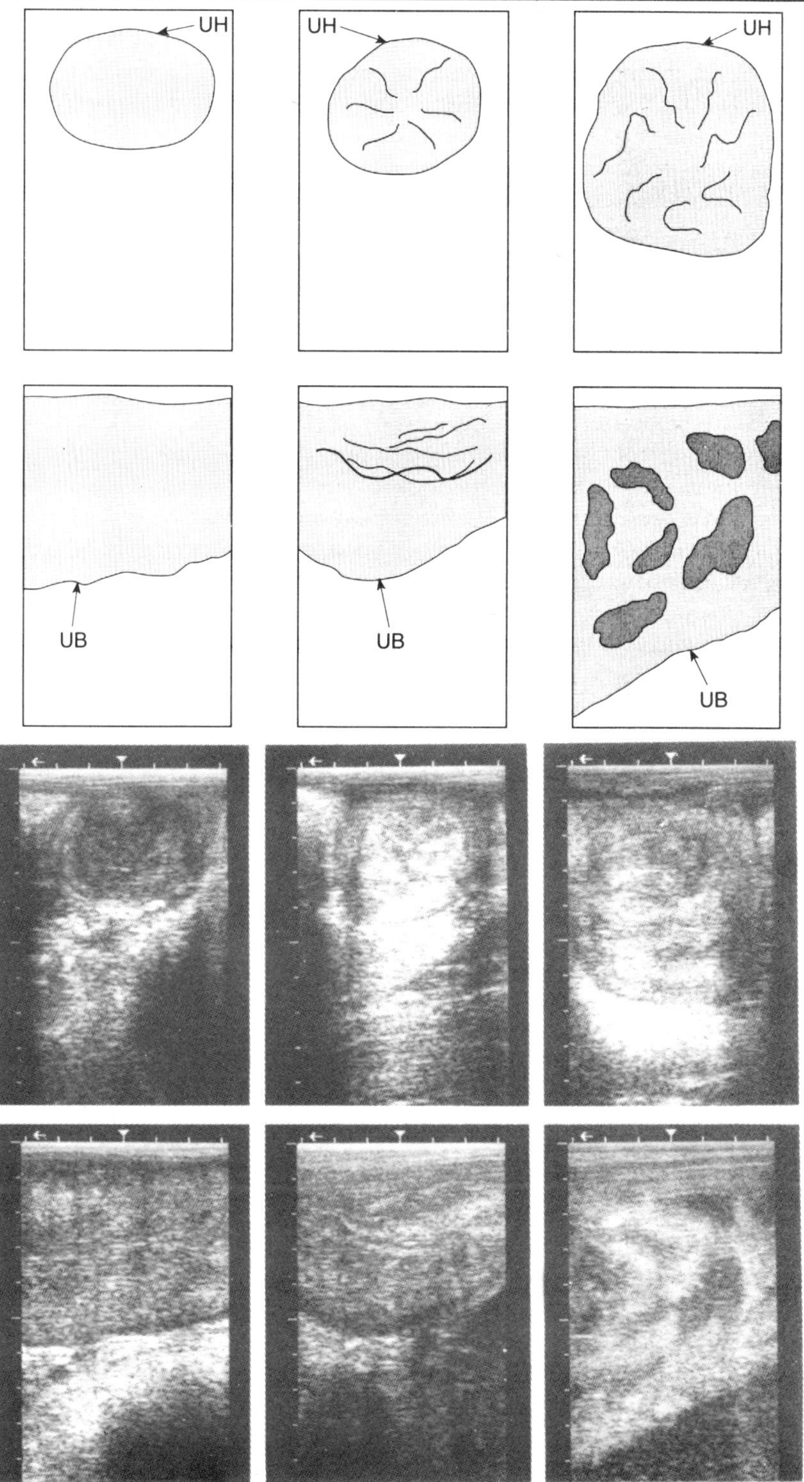

Fig. 7.3. Uterus. Upper series, cross-sections of the uterine horns. Lower series, longitudinal sections of the uterine body. From left to right, images from mid-dioestrus, early oestrus, and mid-oestrus, respectively. Note differences in uterine echotexture at different stages of the oestrous cycle. In particular, note intertwining areas of white and black in the oestrous images on the right, representing extensive endometrial folding. UH = uterine horn, UB = uterine body.

to the oedematous outer portion of the folds (Ginther and Pierson, 1984c). In contrast, during dioestrus, echotexture is marked by minimal discernible endometrial folding; the dioestrous image is relatively homogeneous grey in appearance (Fig. 7.3). Because of the marked differences in echotexture at different stages of the oestrous cycle, the nature of the uterine image provides, in effect, an instant indicator of the prevailing hormonal status of a mare (oestrogen or progesterone dominance). During anoestrus (i.e. the anovulatory season), there is a lack of endometrial folding and a dioestrous-like echotexture prevails.

The pattern of change in uterine echotexture during the oestrous cycle closely parallels the pattern of change in the intensity of oestrous behaviour (Hayes *et al.*, 1985). Oestrous behaviour is attributable to oestrogen exposure (Ginther, 1992) and this relationship indicates that uterine echotexture provides a sensitive indication of oestrogen exposure (Hayes *et al.*, 1985). In this regard, in 98% of follicular phases examined in one study (Ginther and Pierson, 1989), a uterine echotexture characteristic of oestrus, or intermediate between oestrus and dioestrus, was detected on at least one day in the three days preceding ovulation. Consequently, partitioning the mare's oestrous cycle into follicular (oestrus) and luteal (dioestrus) phases based on uterine echotexture and luteal detectability is an accurate tool for estimation of the stage of the oestrous cycle (Ginther and Pierson, 1989). In some breeding management schemes (e.g. utilizing artificial insemination), ultrasonic assessment of uterine echotexture and ovarian status may alleviate the need for an extensive teasing programme. At the very least, ultrasonography can be an invaluable adjunct to an existing teasing programme, particularly when dealing with a population of mares in which it can be difficult to elicit a definitive behavioural response (e.g. post-partum mares with foal at foot or maiden mares).

During early pregnancy, echotexture is similar to that of dioestrus until approximately day 15 or 16, after which an increase in endometrial folding can, at times, be detected (Ginther, 1986; Griffin and Ginther, 1991a, b). Importantly, while this increase in folding is a normal phenomenon, it may be an indication of impending embryonic loss and a return to oestrus; identification and assessment of the corpus luteum is important in differentiating these two possibilities, in addition to consideration of other clinical findings (i.e. flaccid uterine tone).

Uterine pathology

Diagnostically, one of the most important applications of ultrasonography in reproduction is in the detection and monitoring of uterine abnormalities. The two most common forms of uterine pathology observed ultrasonically are intrauterine fluid collections and uterine cysts. Additionally, fetal remnants and/or retained endometrial cups can occasionally be imaged following abortion.

Intrauterine fluid collections are ultrasonically detectable as mobile, free, nonechogenic (i.e. fluid-filled) areas with poorly defined borders within the uterine lumen (Ginther, 1986; Fig. 7.4). They can range in size from several mm on the ultrasound screen to greater than the width and height of the screen (e.g. greater than 50 × 100 mm). Echogenicity of the fluid can also vary considerably from nonechogenic (i.e. black) to hyperechogenic (i.e. white; frank pyometra). Fluid

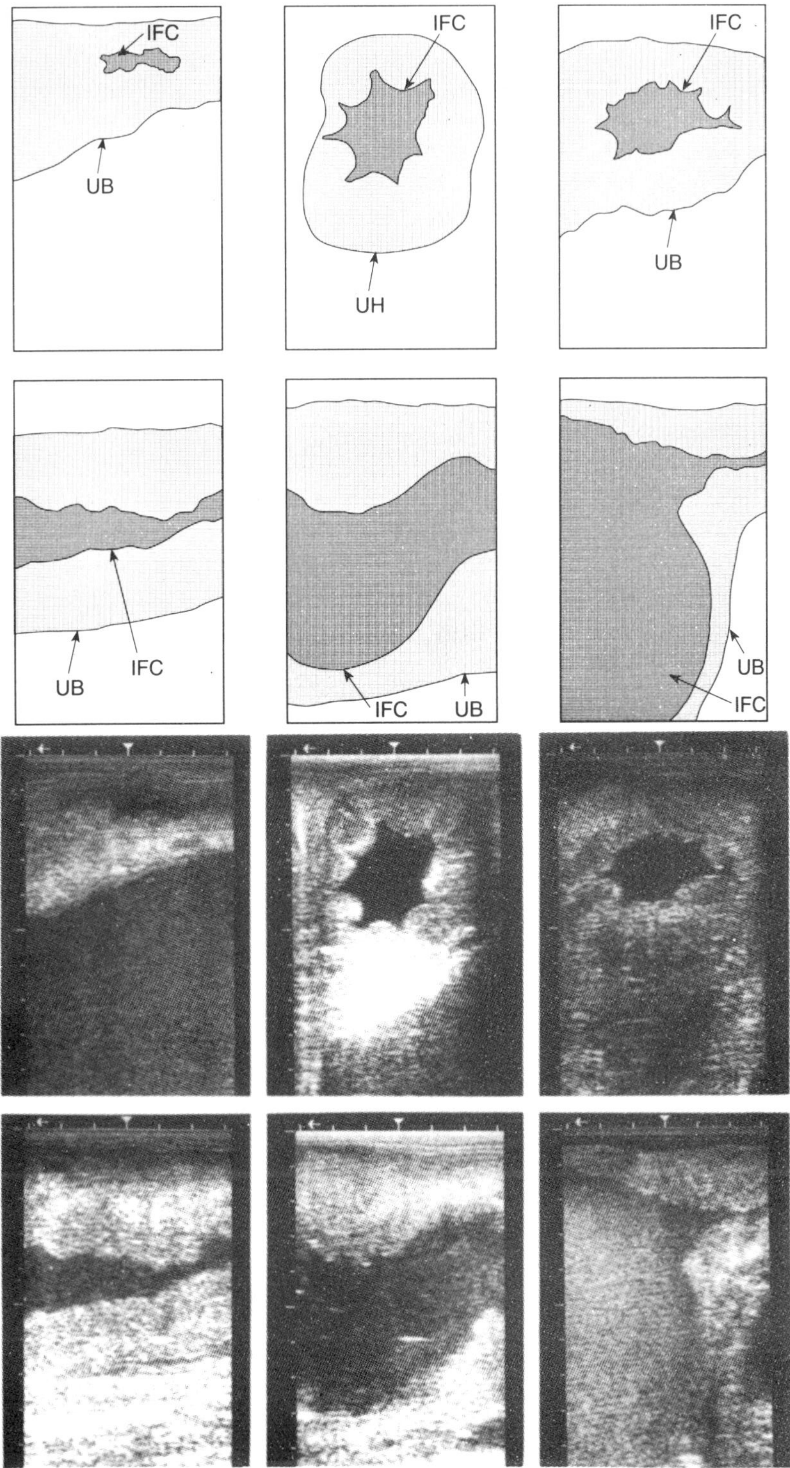

Fig. 7.4. Intrauterine fluid collections. Note variations in the amount of fluid and echogenicity (shades of grey). Bottom right, example of frank pyometra. IFC = intrauterine fluid collection, UH = uterine horn, UB = uterine body.

echogenicity is apparently dependent upon the amount of inflammatory cells and debris within the fluid (McKinnon *et al.*, 1988a). A system for grading echogenicity (e.g. grades I to IV, hyperechogenic to nonechogenic; McKinnon *et al.*, 1988b) is helpful in documenting the severity of an inflammatory condition, as well as a means of monitoring the response to therapy.

Collections of ultrasonically-detectable intrauterine fluid in mares under progesterone dominance (i.e. during dioestrus) are strong indications for the presence of an active inflammatory process. In this regard, dioestrous fluid collections have been associated with histological evidence of endometrial inflammation, premature luteolysis and an abbreviated interovulatory interval, decreased pregnancy rates at day 11, and an increased embryonic loss rate between days 11 and 20 (Adams *et al.*, 1987). Similarly, in another study, mares with a history of embryonic loss on days 11 to 15 and mares with a history of small intrauterine fluid collections during dioestrus had several similarities: reduced pregnancy rates, reduced progesterone concentrations at days 7 and 11, shortened interovulatory intervals, and repeatability of the conditions within individual mares (Ginther *et al.*, 1985; Ginther, 1986). In effect, the presence of dioestrous fluid collections provides an immediate indication of endometritis. The efficacy and effectiveness of various intrauterine treatment regimens can be monitored ultrasonically (Adams and Ginther, 1989), as can the individual response to therapy.

The clinical importance of intrauterine fluid during oestrus is unclear. While it has been suggested that the presence of fluid during oestrus is associated with reduced fertility in nonlactating mares (McKinnon *et al.*, 1988a), controlled research has apparently not been conducted to support this conclusion. Clinical impressions suggest that relatively small amounts (e.g. 10 to 15 mm in size) of nonechogenic fluid during oestrus may be normal and may not be detrimental to the establishment and maintenance of pregnancy.

Uterine cysts are ultrasonically visible as immobile, usually compartmentalized, nonechogenic structures with well-defined borders (Ginther and Pierson, 1984c; Fig. 7.5). They can be located in any portion of the uterus (Ginther, 1986) and can be internal (confined to the uterine lumen), external (associated with the uterine serosa), or transmural (extending through the uterine wall). They can be found singly or in association with other cysts, often in a compartmentalized fashion (i.e. cystic complex; Ginther and Pierson, 1984c). Mares with a large number and/or size of cysts tended to have a reduced pregnancy rate at day 40 (Adams *et al.*, 1987). In another study (Chevalier-Clement, 1989), the embryonic loss rate in mares with uterine cysts was increased compared to unaffected mares. However, as cysts are more common in older mares (Adams *et al.*, 1987), the relationship between cysts and fertility is likely to be confounded by age and further work is necessary before definitive conclusions can be reached in this regard. Ultrasonic imaging has provided a much needed means for noninvasively identifying uterine cysts, assessing the need for intervention (e.g. surgical extirpation) based upon uterine location and severity, and for monitoring their formation and progression from breeding season to breeding season.

Fetal remnants (e.g. fetal bones, mummified fetuses) are ultrasonically detectable as highly echogenic structures within the uterine lumen (Ginther and

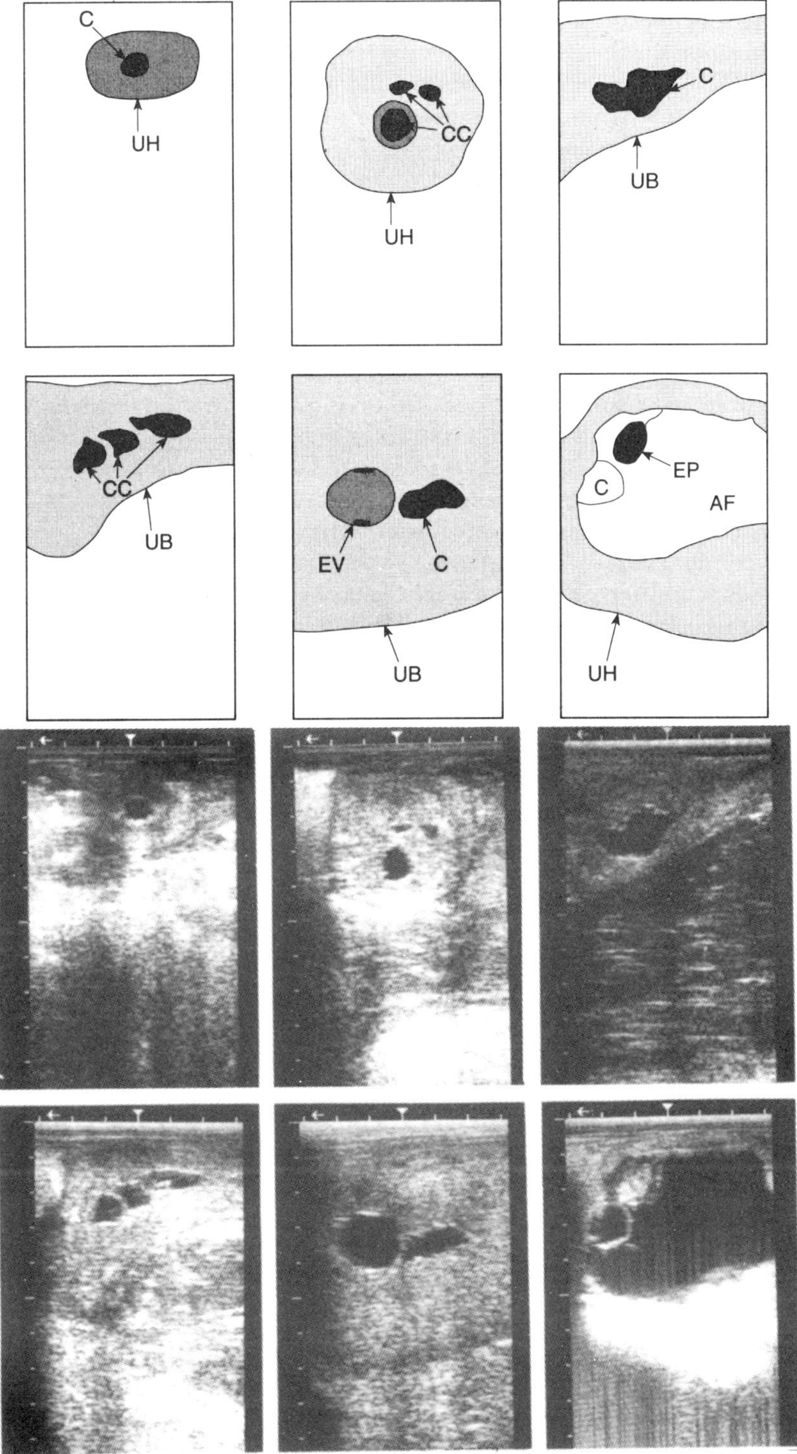

Fig. 7.5. Uterine cysts. Upper left, small cyst in a uterine horn, easily confused with a day 10 or 11 embryonic vesicle. Upper middle and right, cysts in a uterine horn and body, respectively. Lower left, cystic complex in the uterine body. Lower middle, day 12 embryonic vesicle next to a cyst in the uterine body. Lower right, cyst impinging upon a day 40 embryonic vesicle at the base of one uterine horn. C = cyst, CC = cystic complex, UB = uterine body, UH = uterine horn, EV = embryonic vesicle, EP = embryo proper, AF = allantoic fluid.

Pierson, 1984c). Many smaller bone remnants are difficult to detect by transrectal palpation and their identification and removal is greatly facilitated by ultrasonography. At times, remnants of the endometrial cups are recognizable as hyperechogenic structures at, or near, the uterine bifurcation. Their detection is evidence of abortion (fetal loss after 35–40 days) and is helpful in explaining a failure of regular cyclicity in a mare due to the systemic presence of equine chorionic gonadotropin (eCG) (Ginther,1992).

Post-partum uterus

The ultrasonic morphology of the post-partum uterus in mares has been described (Ginther and Pierson, 1984c; Griffin and Ginther, 1991a) and the ultrasonic progression of uterine involution characterized (McKinnon *et al.*, 1988b; Griffin and Ginther, 1991a). Based on ultrasonic measurements of the uterine horns, involution in the first study was complete in a mean of 23 days, with the previously gravid horn recognizable as the larger horn for a mean of 21 days. In the second study, involution was complete by day 27 post-partum (previously nongravid horn) and by day 31 (previously gravid horn).

A bright, fern-like pattern of hyperechogenicity outlining the endometrial folds was observed for an average of approximately two days following parturition (Griffin and Ginther, 1991a). The regularity and echogenicity of this pattern decreased over time, probably reflecting the stage of involution. Oestrus-like echotexture (i.e. prominent endometrial folding) was detected in post-partum mares at a time corresponding to the onset of behavioural oestrus following parturition (i.e. foal heat; see Ginther, (1992) for a review).

In the studies cited above, the number of post-partum mares with ultrasonically detectable intrauterine fluid collections decreased as the interval from parturition increased; no fluid was detected after day 15 or 16 post-partum in any apparently normal mare. The echogenicity of the fluid collections decreased between days 3 and 15 post-partum (McKinnon *et al.*, 1988b). Importantly, pregnancy rates in mares with detectable intrauterine fluid during their first post-partum ovulatory period (i.e. during their foal heat) were significantly lower than those of mares without detectable fluid during that time. Ultrasonography, therefore, is a valuable tool to use when reaching a decision on whether to breed a mare during her first post-partum ovulatory period, or to delay (e.g. hormonally) or postpone breeding until subsequent ovulations. This decision should, in part, be based on the perceived degree of uterine involution (size and echotexture) and the presence, amount and character (i.e. echogenicity) of detectable intrauterine fluid.

Conceptus

Ultrasonic anatomy

The equine embryonic vesicle can first be detected ultrasonically on day 9 or 10 after ovulation (2–3 mm in diameter) with a high frequency transducer and under optimal conditions (Ginther, 1986). Its identification is facilitated by the visualization of two artifactual, hyperechogenic reflections (specular echoes; Ginther, 1986) located at the dorsal and ventral aspects of the early vesicle. When first detected, the vesicle is a circular, nonechogenic, fluid-filled structure (Fig. 7.6). It maintains its spherical shape until approximately day 17 or 18, when it begins to become irregular in outline (Ginther, 1986). It is important to recognize that this irregularity in shape is a normal phenomenon and is not an indication of impending embryo loss. Until approximately day 16, the vesicle grows at a rate of 3 to 4 mm per day (Ginther, 1986). From day 16 to day 28, there is a plateau in the growth of the vesicle when measured in cross-section, presumably due to longitudinal expansion of the vesicle towards the tip of the uterine horn and increasing uterine tone (Ginther, 1986). After this time, its cross-sectional diameter increases at a rate of approximately 2 mm per day.

The embryo proper can be imaged by day 20 or 21 and its heart-beat can be visualized by day 22 (Ginther, 1984a, 1986). Beginning on approximately days 20 to 24, a gradual transition in placentation begins to occur (i.e. regression of the yolk sac and expansion of the allantoic sac; see Ginther (1992) for a review). As this transition occurs, the embryo proper is lifted off the floor of the vesicle and gradually ascends to reach the top, or dorsal aspect, of the vesicle by approximately day 40 (Fig. 7.6). By this time, the yolk sac has been functionally and anatomically replaced by the allantochorion. Subsequently, the umbilicus forms and begins to elongate, and the embryo proper slowly descends towards the floor of the allantoic sac, resting there by approximately day 50. The size and shape of the early vesicle and the ascent and descent of the embryo proper are diagnostically important in estimating the age of a conceptus, particularly when breeding dates are unknown or when the mare is examined on a one-time-only basis.

When examining the pregnant mare before day 25, the clinician must be aware of the early embryo–uterus interactions which characterize equine pregnancy (see Ginther (1985a) for a review). Specifically, the phenomena of equine embryo mobility, fixation, and orientation must be considered for purposes of diagnosis and interpretation. The conceptus is highly mobile within the uterine lumen from the time it is first detected with ultrasonography until day 15 or 16, at which time it becomes fixed in the caudal aspect of one of the uterine horns (Ginther, 1983a, b). Some time after fixation, but prior to visualization of the embryo proper (e.g. day 21), the vesicle becomes orientated or rotated so that the embryo proper, when first imaged, is located in a ventral, antimesometrial position (Fig. 7.6). Awareness of these phenomena is important both diagnostically and prognostically. In this regard, in making an early pregnancy diagnosis (before day 15 or 16), it is essential that the entire uterus is scanned, as the vesicle can be located anywhere within the uterine lumen during its mobility phase. As well, detection of an embryonic vesicle that is still mobile within the lumen after day 17 or 18 (i.e. fixation has not occurred, or the vesicle has become dislodged) may be an indication that embryonic loss is imminent (Ginther *et al.*, 1985; see next section). Orientation of the vesicle so that the embryo proper is not in the expected position when first imaged occurs occasionally (Fig. 7.7); the clinical importance of this is unclear but seems to be negligible.

Twinning

Ultrasonography has been used extensively in the past several years for the characterization of the nature of twinning in mares (see Ginther (1986; 1989a, b)

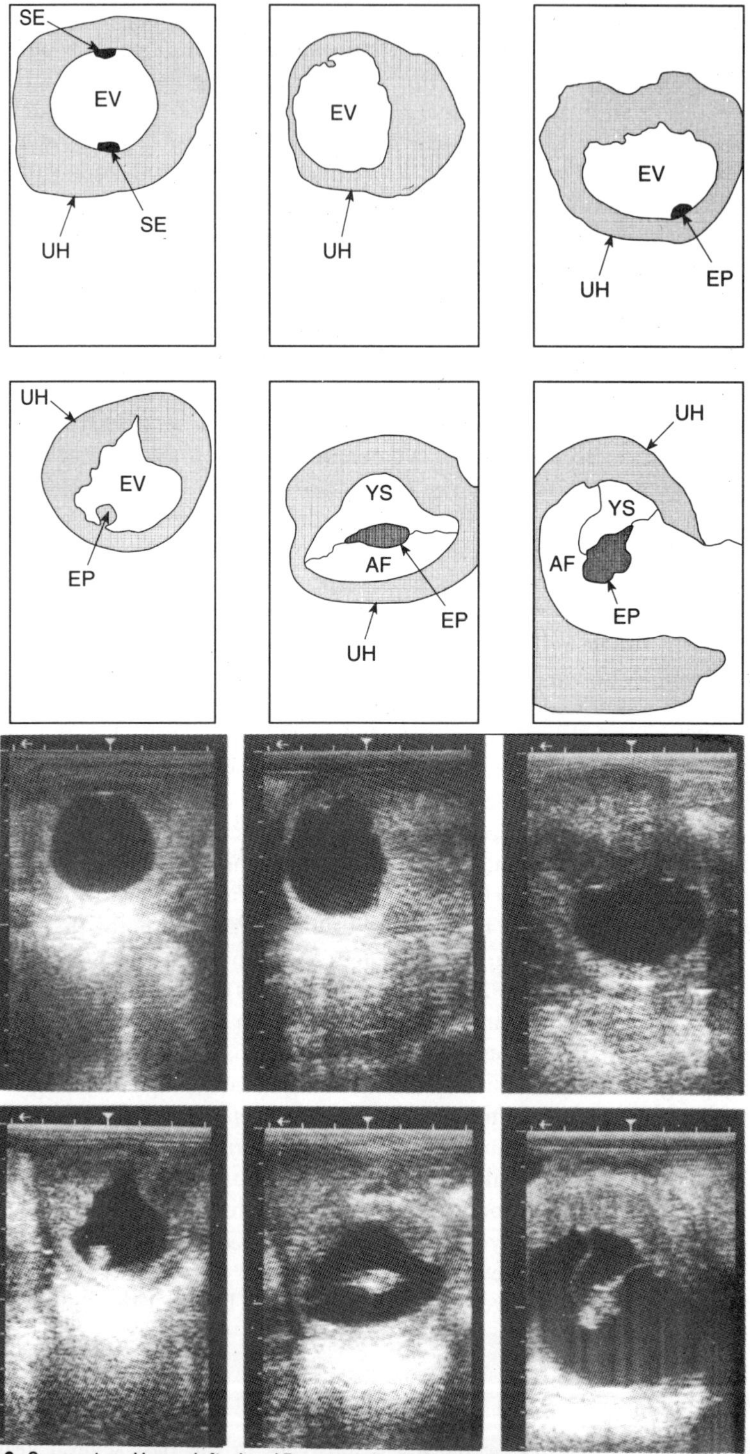

Fig. 7.6. Conceptus. Upper left, day 15, note spherical shape and specular echoes on the dorsal and ventral aspects of the vesicle. Upper middle, day 18, note irregular shape of the vesicle. Upper right, day 21, embryo proper is just visible. Lower series, left to right, days 23, 28 and 38, respectively. Note ascent of embryo proper within the vesicle as early pregnancy progresses. EV = embryonic vesicle, EP = embryo proper, AF = allantoic fluid, YS = yolk sac fluid, UH = uterine horn, SE = specular echoes.

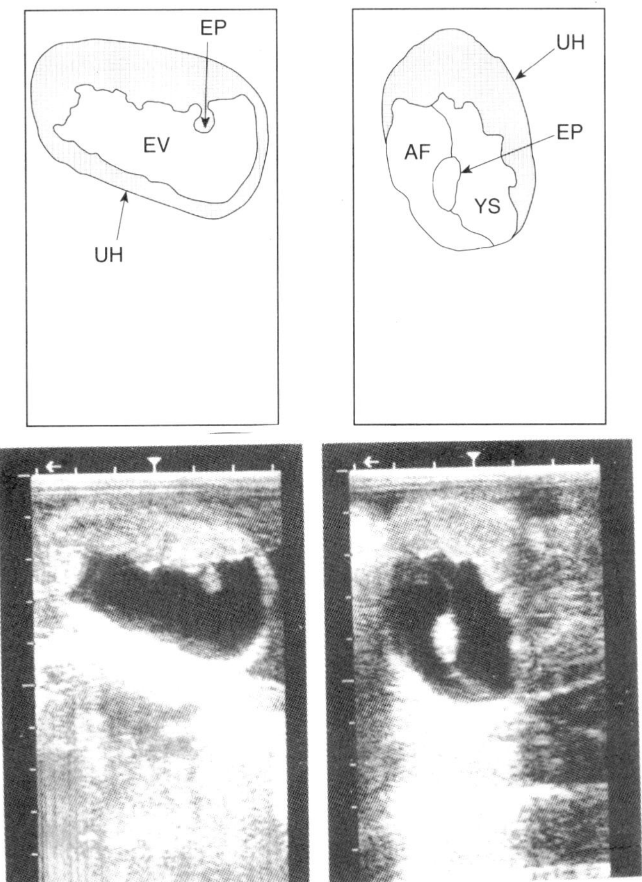

Fig. 7.7. Disorientation of the embryonic vesicle. Left, the embryo proper on day 23 is located dorsally. Right, note vertical orientation of the membranes between the allantoic sac and yolk sac; normally membranes are orientated horizontally. Compare these images with those in Fig. 7.6. EV = embryonic vesicle, EP = embryo proper, AF = allantoic fluid, YS = yolk sac fluid, UH = uterine horn.

for reviews). These investigations clarified the origin of twins (Ginther, 1987; Pascoe *et al.*, 1987; Ginther and Bergfelt, 1988), characterized the growth and development of twin embryos (Ginther, 1984c; 1987), discovered the embryo-uterine interactions involved in the twin embryo phenomenon (Ginther, 1984c, 1987, 1989c), and calculated the probability and timing of embryo reduction (natural elimination by the mare of one member of a twin set) under specific conditions of relative size and location of the two embryos (Ginther, 1984b, 1988b, 1989c). The details of the twinning phenomenon are beyond the scope of this text, and the reader is guided to the above sources for an in-depth discussion. From a practical standpoint, ultrasonography is an essential tool for effectively managing twin pregnancies, particularly in regards to detection of multiple ovulations (Fig. 7.8), early detection of a twin set (preferably during the mobility phase), manual elimination of one member of a twin set (locating the twin to be

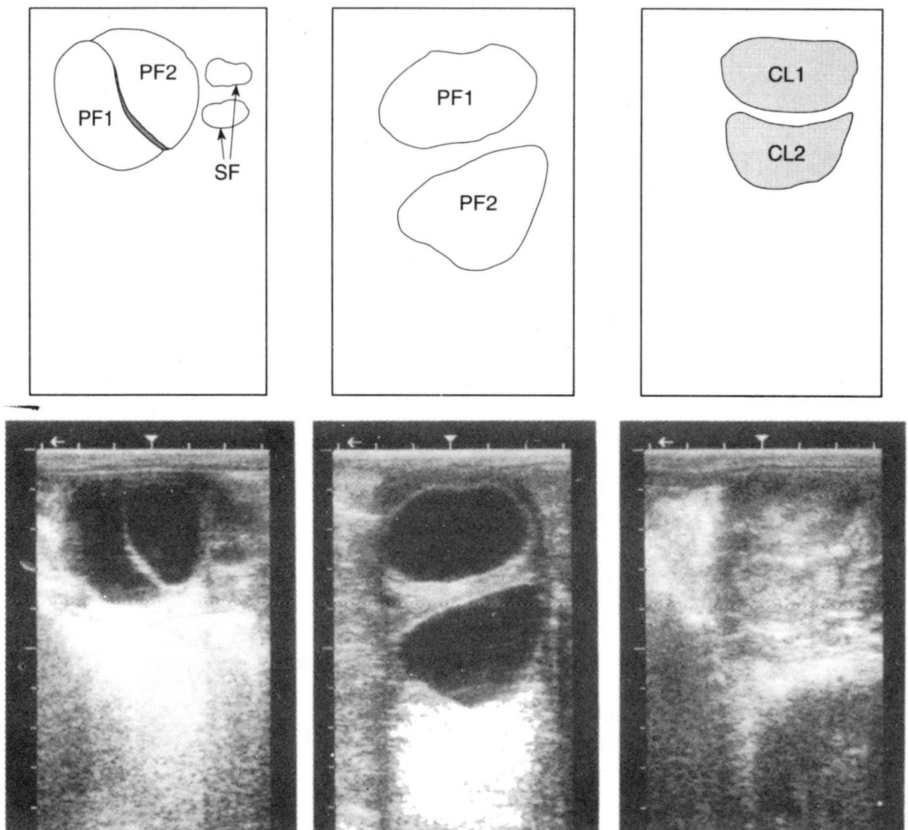

Fig. 7.8. Multiple follicles and corpora lutea. Left, two preovulatory follicles early in oestrus. Middle, two preovulatory follicles on the day prior to ovulation. Right, two corpora lutea resulting from ovulation of the follicles shown in the middle image. Examples are from unilateral (same ovary) double ovulations. Double ovulations also occur bilaterally (from opposite ovaries). PF1 = preovulatory follicle 1, PF2 = preovulatory follicle 2, SF = satellite follicles, CL1 = corpus luteum 1, CL2 = corpus luteum 2.

eliminated), and determining if natural embryo reduction has occurred in a previously diagnosed twin set in which intervention was not attempted (determining the number of embryos entering the fetal stage; Fig. 7.9).

Fetus

In horse mares, growth profiles for the fetal eye socket, cranium, ribs, stomach, and trunk have been developed using ultrasonography (Kähn and Leidl, 1987). Until breed differences are accounted for, the utility of these measurements in determining fetal age or in assessing fetal well-being is limited. Transabdominal scanning has been used to image the late-gestation fetus, and it has been suggested that fetal and placental imaging may be useful for prenatal evaluation (Pipers and Adams-Brendemuehl, 1984; Adams-Brendemuehl and Pipers, 1987). To date, the normal database for fetal and placental parameters has not been well established, and further research is needed before this potentially valuable application of ultrasonography in the mare can be fully utilized.

A recent application of ultrasonography in equine reproduction is the development of a highly accurate technique for the diagnosis of fetal sex (Curran and Ginther, 1989). Diagnosis is based upon the determination of the relative location of the genital tubercle (forerunner of the penis or clitoris). In males, the tubercle migrates from its neutral position between the hind limbs towards the umbilical cord. In females, it migrates towards the tail. Ultrasonically, the tubercle is visible as a highly echogenic structure, characteristically bi-lobed in appearance. The optimal time for sex diagnosis based on the position of the tubercle is days 59 to 68 (Curran and Ginther, 1989). The reader is guided to the cited study for a detailed description of this technique.

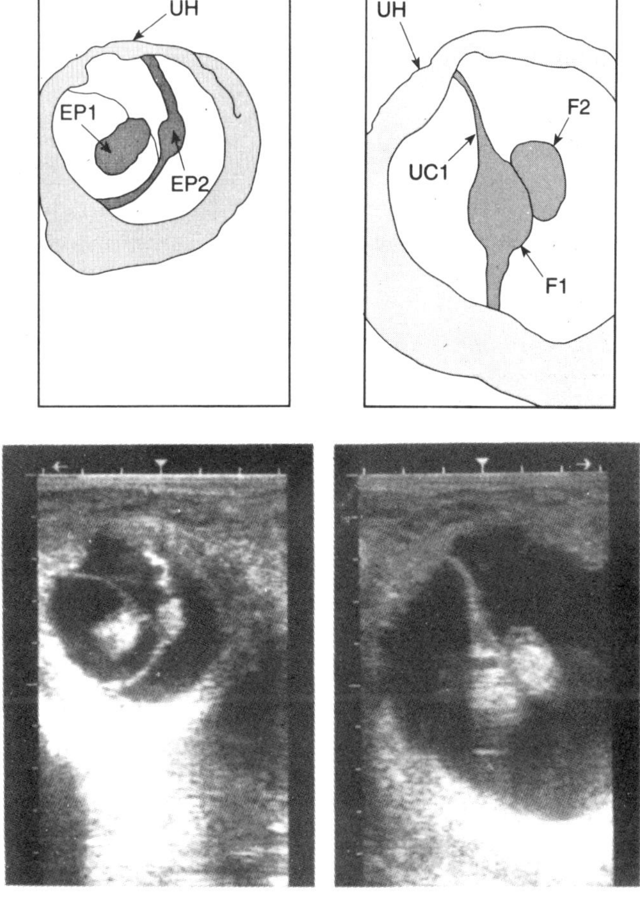

Fig. 7.9. Twins. Twin set fixed in the caudal aspect of one uterine horn (unilateral fixation). Left, day 32, note the disorientation of the vesicles. Right, same twin set on approximately day 45. Natural embryo reduction did not occur. EP1 = embryo proper 1, EP2 = embryo proper 2, F1 = fetus 1, F2 = fetus 2, UH = uterine horn, UC1 = umbilical cord 1.

Embryonic loss

The ability to detect and monitor the equine embryo from a very early stage (day 9 or 10) has enabled critical study of early embryonic loss (see Ginther (1986) for a review). The ultrasonic morphology of spontaneous and induced embryonic loss in mares has been described (Ginther *et al.*, 1985; Ginther, 1985b). Early losses (prior to the detection of an embryo proper) generally occur without ultrasonic indications of impending loss (Ginther *et al.*, 1985). However, some early losses are presaged by the development of small collections of ultrasonically-detectable intrauterine fluid outside the embryonic vesicle. Ultrasonic indicators of loss at later stages include a failure of fixation or dislodgement after fixation (i.e. continued mobility), absence of heart-beat, an echogenic ring or mass floating in a collection of fluid, an echogenic area in the dead embryo proper, and an apparent gradual decrease in the amount of placental fluid, with a disorganization of placental membranes.

Conclusions

Real-time ultrasonography is a diagnostic tool which, when fully utilized, provides the clinician with a wide array of information on the reproductive status of the mare, the health of the reproductive tract, and the viability of the conceptus. Interpretation of findings requires experience and an understanding of the anatomy and physiology of the mare's reproductive tract. Its use, in combination with other more traditional diagnostic techniques, has become a standard practice in equine reproduction.

References

Adams, G.P. and Ginther, O.J. (1989) Efficacy of intrauterine infusion of plasma for treatment of infertility and endometritis in mares. *Journal of the American Veterinary Medical Association*, 194, 372–378.

Adams, G.P., Kastelic, J.P., Bergfelt, D.R. and Ginther, O.J. (1987) Effect of uterine inflammation and ultrasonically detected uterine pathology on fertility in the mare. *Journal of Reproduction and Fertility*, (supplement), 35, 445–454.

Adams-Brendemuehl, C.S. and Pipers, F.S. (1987) Antepartum evaluation of the equine fetus. *Journal of Reproduction and Fertility* (supplement), 35, 565–573.

Bergfelt, D.R., Pierson, R.A. and Ginther, O.J. (1989) Resurgence of the primary corpus luteum during early pregnancy in the mare. *Animal Reproduction Science*, 21, 261–270.

Carnevale, E.M., McKinnon, A.O., Squires, E.L. and Voss, J.L. (1988) Ultrasonographic characteristics of the preovulatory follicle preceding and during ovulation in mares. *Journal of Equine Veterinary Science*, 8, 428–431.

Chevalier-Clement, F. (1989) Pregnancy loss in the mare. *Animal Reproduction Science*, 20, 231–244.

Curran, S. and Ginther, O.J. (1989) Ultrasonic diagnosis of equine fetal sex by location of the genital tubercle. *Journal of Equine Veterinary Science*, 9, 77–83.

Fontijne, P. and Hennis, C. (1989) The use of ultrasonography in the reproductive management of mares in the field. In: Taverne, M.A.M. and Willemse A.H., (eds) *Diagnostic Ultrasound and Animal Reproduction.* Kluwer Academic Publishers, The Netherlands, pp. 11–19.

Ginther, O.J. (1979) *Reproductive Biology of the Mare: Basic and Applied Aspects.* Equiservices, Cross Plains, Wisconsin, USA.

Ginther, O.J. (1983a) Mobility of the early equine conceptus. *Theriogenology,* 19, 603–611.

Ginther, O.J. (1983b) Fixation and orientation of the early equine conceptus. *Theriogenology,* 19, 613–623.

Ginther, O.J. (1984a) Ultrasonic evaluation of the reproductive tract of the mare: The single embryo. *Journal of Equine Veterinary Science,* 4, 75–81.

Ginther, O.J. (1984b) Postfixation embryo reduction in unilateral and bilateral twins in mares. *Theriogenology,* 22, 213–223.

Ginther, O.J. (1984c) Mobility of twin embryonic vesicles in mares. *Theriogenology,* 22, 83–95.

Ginther, O.J. (1985a) Dynamic physical interactions between the equine embryo and uterus. *Equine Veterinary Journal* (supplement), 3, 41–47.

Ginther, O.J. (1985b) Embryonic loss in mares: nature of loss after experimental induction by ovariectomy or prostaglandin $F_2\alpha$. Theriogenology, 24, 87–98.

Ginther, O.J. (1986) *Ultrasonic Imaging and Reproductive Events in the Mare.* Equiservices, Cross Plains, Wisconsin, USA.

Ginther, O.J. (1987) Relationships among number of days between multiple ovulations, number of embryos, and type of embryo fixation in mares. *Journal of Equine Veterinary Science,* 7, 82–88.

Ginther, O.J. (1988a) Ultrasonic imaging of equine ovarian follicles and corpora lutea. *Veterinary Clinics of North America: Equine Practice,* 4, 197–213.

Ginther, O.J. (1988b) Using a twinning tree for designing equine twin-prevention programs. *Journal of Equine Veterinary Science,* 8, 101–107.

Ginther, O.J. (1989a) Twin embryos in mare. I. From ovulation to fixation. *Equine Veterinary Journal,* 21, 166–170.

Ginther, O.J. (1989b) Twin embryos in mares. II. Post fixation embryo reduction. *Equine Veterinary Journal,* 21, 171–174.

Ginther, O.J. (1989c) The nature of embryo reduction in mares with twin conceptuses: deprivation hypothesis. *American Journal of Veterinary Research,* 50, 45–53.

Ginther, O.J. (1992) *Reproductive Biology of the Mare: Basic and Applied Aspects,* 2nd edn. Equiservices, Cross Plains, Wisconsin, USA.

Ginther, O.J. and Bergfelt, D.R. (1988) Embryo reduction before Day 11 in mares with twin conceptuses. *Journal of Animal Science,* 66, 1727–1731.

Ginther, O.J. and Pierson, R.A. (1984a) Ultrasonic anatomy of equine ovaries. *Theriogenology,* 21, 471–483.

Ginther, O.J. and Pierson, R.A. (1984b) Ultrasonic evaluation of the reproductive tract of the mare: ovaries. *Journal of Equine Veterinary Science,* 4, 11–16.

Ginther, O.J. and Pierson, R.A. (1984c) Ultrasonic anatomy and pathology of the equine uterus. *Theriogenology,* 21, 505–516.

Ginther, O.J. and Pierson, R.A. (1989) Regular and irregular characteristics of ovulation and the interovulatory interval in mares. *Journal of Equine Veterinary Science,* 9, 4–12.

Ginther, O.J., Bergfelt, D.R., Leith, G.S. and Scraba, S.T. (1985) Embryonic loss in mares: incidence and ultrasonic morphology. *Theriogenology,* 24, 73–86.

Griffin, P.G. and Ginther, O.J. (1991a) Uterine morphology and function in postpartum mares. *Journal of Equine Veterinary Science,* 11, 330–339.

Griffin, P.G. and Ginther, O.J. (1991b) Dynamics of uterine diameter and endometrial morphology during the estrous cycle and early pregnancy in mares. *Animal Reproduction Science,* 25, 133–142.

Griffin, P.G. and Ginther, O.J. (1992) Research applications of ultrasonic imaging in reproductive biology. *Journal of Animal Science*, 70, 953–972.

Hayes, K.E.N., Pierson, R.A., Scraba, S.T. and Ginther, O.J. (1985) Effects of estrous cycle and season on ultrasonic uterine anatomy in mares. *Theriogenology*, 24, 465–477.

Kähn, W. and Leidl, W. (1987) Ultrasonic measurement of the equine fetus *in utero* and sonographic imaging of fetal organs. *Deutsche Tierärztliche Wochenschrift*, 94, 509–515.

Kastelic, J.P., Bergfelt, D.R. and Ginther, O.J. (1990) Relationship between ultrasonic assessment of the corpus luteum and plasma progesterone concentration in heifers. *Theriogenology*, 33, 1269–1278.

McKinnon, A.O. and Carnevale, E.M. (1993) Ultrasonography. In: McKinnon A.O., and Voss, J.L. (eds) *Equine Reproduction*. Lea and Febiger, Philadelphia, pp. 211–220.

McKinnon, A.O., Squires, E.L. and Voss, J.L. (1987a) Ultrasonic evaluation of the mare's reproductive tract – Part I. *Compendium on Continuing Education for the Practicing Veterinarian*, 9, 335–345.

McKinnon, A.O., Squires, E.L. and Voss, J.L. (1987b) Ultrasonic evaluation of the mare's reproductive tract – Part II. *Compendium on Continuing Education for the Practicing Veterinarian*, 9, 472–482.

McKinnon, A.O., Squires, E.L. and Pickett, B.W. (1988a) Uterine pathology. In: *Equine Reproductive Ultrasonography*. Colorado State University-ARL. Bulletin No. 04, pp. 31–40.

McKinnon, A.O., Squires, E.L., Harrison, L.A., Blach, E.L. and Shideler, R.K. (1988b) Ultrasonographic studies on the reproductive tract of mares after parturition: effect of involution and uterine fluid on pregnancy rates in mares with normal and delayed first postpartum ovulatory cycles. *Journal of the American Veterinary Medical Association*, 192, 350–353.

Pascoe, R.R., Pascoe, D.R. and Wilson, M.C. (1987) Influence of follicular status on twinning rate in mares. *Journal of Reproduction and Fertility* (supplement), 35, 183–189.

Pierson, R.A. and Ginther, O.J. (1985a) Ultrasonic evaluation of the preovulatory follicle in the mare. *Theriogenology*, 24, 259–268.

Pierson, R.A. and Ginther, O.J. (1985b) Ultrasonic evaluation of the corpus luteum in the mare. *Theriogenology*, 23, 795–806.

Pipers, F.S. and Adams-Brendemuehl, C.S. (1984) Techniques and applications of trans-abdominal ultrasonography in the pregnant mare. *Journal of the American Veterinary Medical Association*, 185, 766–771.

Squires, E.L. (1993) Progesterone. In: McKinnon, A.O. and Voss, J.L. (eds) *Equine Reproduction*. Lea and Febiger, Philadelphia, pp. 57–64.

Squires, E.L., McKinnon, A.O. and Shideler, R.K. (1988) Use of ultrasonography in reproductive management of mares. *Theriogenology*, 29, 55–70.

Townson, D.H. and Ginther, O.J. (1987) Duration and pattern of follicular evacuation during ovulation in the mare. *Animal Reproduction Science*, 15, 131–138.

Townson, D.H. and Ginther, O.J. (1988) The development of fluid-filled luteal glands in mares. *Animal Reproduction Science*, 17, 155–163.

Townson, D.H. and Ginther, O.J. (1989a) Ultrasonic characterization of follicular evacuation during ovulation and fate of the discharged follicular fluid in mares. *Animal Reproduction Science*, 20, 131–141.

Townson, D.H. and Ginther, O.J. (1989b) Characterization of plasma progesterone concentrations for two distinct luteal morphologies in mares. *Theriogenology*, 32, 197–204.

Townson, D.H. and Ginther, O.J. (1989c) Ultrasonic echogenicity of developing corpora lutea in pony mares. *Animal Reproduction Science*, 29, 143–153.

8 Equine Abdominal Ultrasonography

C.M. Marr

Valley Equine Hospital, Upper Lambourn Road, Lambourn, Berkshire RG16 7QG, UK

Equipment and Examination Technique

Ultrasonography is used to investigate hepatic, renal, splenic, umbilical and certain gastrointestinal diseases, and for fetal assessment in the mare. It is the technique of choice for characterizing abdominal masses and can be used very effectively to facilitate biopsy of organs or masses. In the absence of ultrasonographic imaging, the horse's abdomen is relatively inaccessible to the clinician because palpation is confined to the caudal abdomen, radiography has limited penetration and exploratory laparotomy, although certainly feasible, is a major undertaking. The technique is well-tolerated by the horse and noninvasive. Instruments are portable and relatively inexpensive, and thus ultrasonography is an ideal tool.

Transducer selection is dependent on the particular site or organ under investigation. Table 8.1 lists appropriate transducers for various abdominal applications. Sector transducers are most appropriate for abdominal imaging because they allow a large area to be imaged from a small point of contact; barriers created by the ribs, lungs and intestinal gas are not a major problem. The transducer's frequency determines both its depth of penetration and its resolution. The highest possible frequency that provides images of the entire area of interest should be selected. Often, more than one transducer is required, and it is usually helpful to start with a high frequency transducer to optimize resolution and change to lower frequencies until the complete area of interest has been examined. Image quality can be maximized by careful preparation of the skin. In most horses the hair coat must be clipped and the skin should be cleaned thoroughly and echolucent gel applied.

Examination of the caudal abdomen and intrapelvic structures is achieved *per rectum*. In this situation, linear array transducers have the advantage that they are usually smaller and easier to manipulate. Sector transducers specially designed for rectal examination (0–90° transducers) have their ultrasound beam offset by

Table 8.1. Selection of transducers for equine abdominal ultrasonography.

Application	Transducer
Adult	
Liver and spleen	5 then 3.5 MHz sector
Right kidney	5 MHz sector
Left kidney (transcutaneous)	3.5 then 2.5 MHz sector
Left kidney (rectal)	5 MHz sector or linear
Body wall and peritoneal fluid	7.5 MHz sector or linear with a stand-off
Fetus and uterus (transcutaneous)	2.5 MHz sector
Bladder (rectal)	5 MHz sector or linear
Abdominal aorta (rectal)	7.5 or 5 MHz 0–90° sector or linear
Foal	
Liver, kidney, spleen	7.5 then 5 MHz sector
Umbilical structures	7.5 MHz sector with stand-off, linear array allows partial visualization
Gastrointestinal tract	7.5 MHz sector or linear with stand-off then 7.5 and 5 MHz sector

45° so that it can be orientated to image cranioventrally or craniodorsally within the confines of the rectum (Fig. 8.1).

Organs and lesions are usually imaged in at least two planes if possible. Transverse and longitudinal (sagittal) images are made by orientating the sound

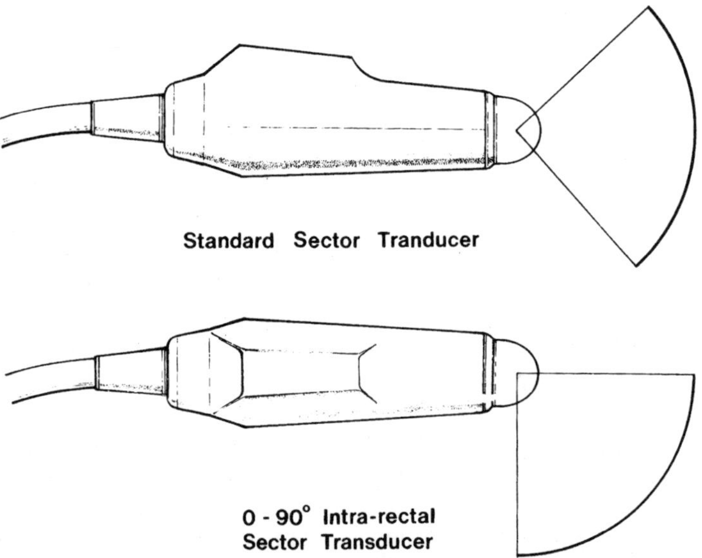

Fig. 8.1. Ultrasound beams which are produced by different sector transducers. A standard transducer has a beam which is orientated straight forwards. The 0–90° intrarectal transducer has a beam which is angled at 45° and can be orientated cranioventrally or craniodorsally, for ease of manipulation in the rectum.

beam along the appropriate axis of the body. Multiple oblique images can be made by rotating the transducer. It is helpful to adopt standardized image orientations so that records are consistent. The images should be displayed with cranial to the right in longitudinal sonograms and dorsal to the right in transverse sonograms. In images made from the ventral midline, the horse's right side should be to the right of the sonogram.

The Liver

The horse's liver is composed of right and left lobes and lies immediately caudal to the diaphragm. The entire organ cannot be visualized in horses because the lung overlies it. Two windows are used to examine the liver in adult horses (Figs 8.2 and 8.3). On the left side, the liver is imaged from the seventh to ninth intercostal spaces, ventral to the lung margins, lateral to the spleen and medial to the

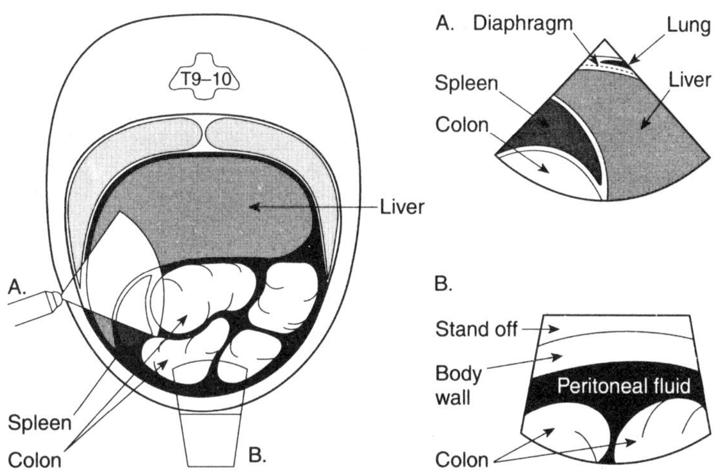

Fig. 8.2. The transverse cross-sectional anatomy of the horse at the level of the ninth and tenth thoracic vertebrae, illustrating windows used to examine the spleen, left lobe of the liver and to identify peritoneal fluid. Corresponding sonograms are illustrated in Figs. 8.4a and 8.4b.

body wall and diaphragm which lies parallel to the body wall (Fig. 8.2). On the right side, the liver is imaged from the sixth to the fifteenth intercostal spaces, ventral to the lung margins and immediately deep to the diaphragm and body wall (Fig. 8.3). In young foals, portions of the liver can be seen from the ventral midline extending beyond the sternum.

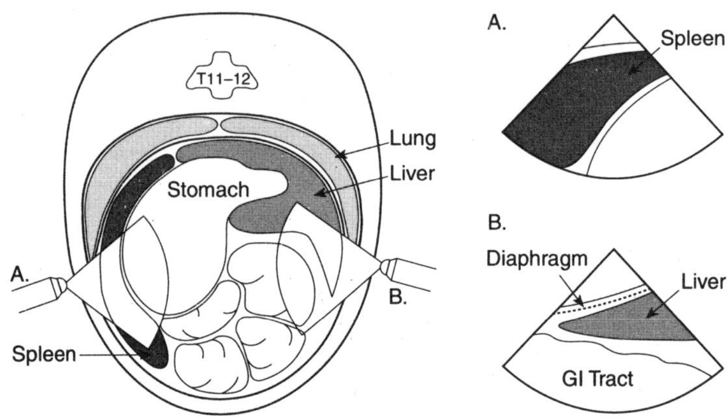

Fig. 8.3. The transverse cross-sectional anatomy of the horse at the level of the 11th to 12th thoracic vertebrae, illustrating windows used to examine the spleen and right liver lobe. Corresponding sonograms are illustrated in Figs 8.4c and 8.4d.

In most adult horses the accessible portions of liver are visualized successfully with a 5 MHz transducer, because they have a relatively superficial location. An impression of liver size can be gained by evaluating the amount of liver visible beyond the lung margins. However, caution must be exercised in estimating liver size in this way. Many older horses undergo atrophy of the right liver lobe as a normal ageing change. Although liver size cannot be determined precisely, its shape can be assessed by examination of the liver's edges. Both increases and decreases in liver size change the contours of the liver and this is recognized by rounding of the edge of the liver which, on the right side, should have a sharp point (Figs 8.4 and 8.5).

Normal liver has a coarse echotexture with even, mid-level echogenicity. Since the echogenicity of an organ is dependent on machine settings, comparing organs within the same horse proves valuable. The liver is usually more echogenic than the kidney and less echogenic than the spleen. Hepatic and portal vessels are visible within the liver. Portal vessels are distinguished by their bright walls which are absent in hepatic vessels (Fig. 8.4).

Fibrosis, seneciosis and hepatic necrosis decrease the liver size and fatty infiltration and cholangiohepatitis increase the liver size, and alter its echogenicity. In fibrosis and seneciosis the echogenicity is usually increased, whereas in acute hepatitis or necrosis it is decreased (Fig. 8.5). However, these changes are not always consistent, and biopsy is required for definitive categorization of hepatic pathology.

Localized hepatic lesions such as neoplasms or abscesses are uncommon in horses, while cholelithiasis occurs more frequently. The ultrasonographic features of cholelithiasis have been described by several authors (Rantanen, 1986a; Johnston *et al.*, 1989; Reef *et al.*, 1990). Mineralized choleliths are readily identified as hyperechoic foci with strong acoustic shadows (Fig. 8.5). There can be

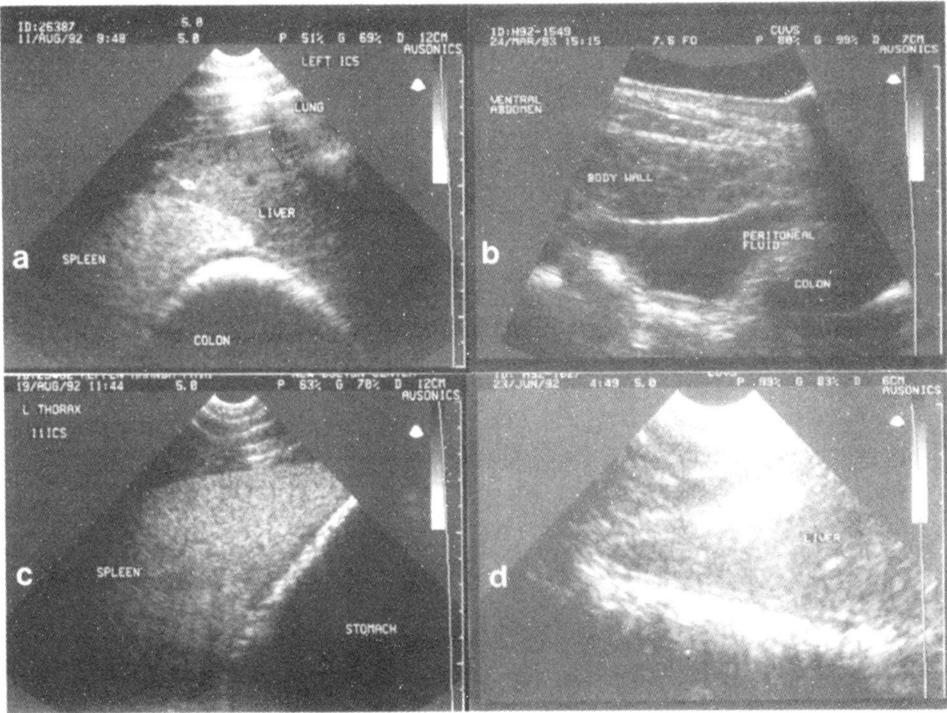

Fig. 8.4. Sonograms of the structures in the cranial and mid-abdomen in the horse (**a** and **b** correspond to the diagrams in Fig. 8.2, and **c** and **d** to the diagrams in Fig. 8.3). **(a)** In this transverse view, obtained from the left seventh intercostal space, the periphery of the lung is visible in the dorsal part of the image. Beneath it is the striated diaphragm and within the abdomen the spleen lies medial to the liver. Notice that the liver is less echogenic than the spleen and vessels are visible within it. **(b)** In this transverse sonogram, obtained from the cranioventral midline, a pocket of anechoic peritoneal fluid lies between the body wall and the colon indicating that this would be a suitable site for paracentesis abdominis. This sonogram was obtained with a 7.5 MHz sector transducer with a built-in fluid stand-off. **(c)** In this transverse sonogram, obtained from the left 11th intercostal space, the spleen lies lateral to the stomach. The wall of the stomach is a thin hypoechoic band and the gas within it produces a hyperechoic curve with an acoustic shadow behind it. Notice that the texture of the spleen is smooth and evenly echogenic. **(d)** In this transverse sonogram, obtained from the right 12th intercostal space, the edge of liver is pointed and the echogenicity of the liver is granular and less than that of the spleen. The sonograms in **a**, **c** and **d** were obtained with a 5 MHz sector transducer, and in **b** with a 7.5 MHz sector transducer (Opus One, Ausonics Pty Ltd, Sydney, Australia; Universal Medical Ltd, NY, USA; BCF Technology Ltd, Livingstone, Scotland).

varying degrees of hepatic enlargement and dilation of the biliary tree. Biliary obstruction is recognized by an increased number of ducts within the liver which are often straighter than hepatic blood vessels and often run parallel to a blood vessel (Fig. 8.5) (Reef *et al.*, 1990). There is often an accompanying cholangiohepatitis and the echogenicity of the liver can be increased. The prognosis in cholelithiasis is variable but some horses respond well to medical management. Repeated ultrasonographic examinations will confirm reduction in numbers of choleliths and resolution of the biliary obstruction if the condition improves.

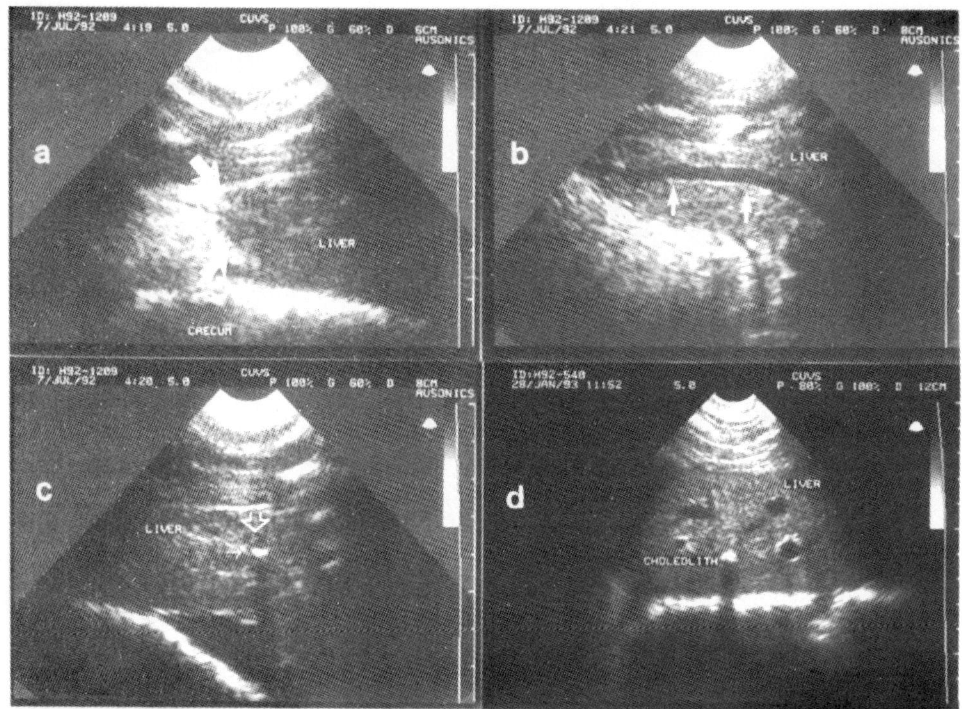

Fig. 8.5. Sonograms of equine hepatic diseases. Sonograms **a–c** were obtained from an aged pony presenting with signs of hepatic encephalopathy, cholelithiasis and hepatic fibrosis. **(a)** A sonogram, obtained from the right 12th intercostal space, in which the ventral edge of the liver is rounded (arrows) and its echogenicity is irregular. **(b)** A transverse sonogram, obtained from the right 11th intercostal space, in which a dilated bile duct is visible (arrows). **(c)** A transverse sonogram, obtained from the right 11th intercostal space, in which a cholelith (arrow) is visible within a bile duct (open arrow). The cholelith is extremely echogenic, producing a strong acoustic shadow. **(d)** A transverse sonogram, in which a cholelith is visible, obtained from the right 15th intercostal space of a nine-year-old riding horse with a history of recurrent colic and raised serum concentrations of gamma glutamyl transferase. In contrast to the pony in Figs 8.5 **a–c**, the hepatic parenchyma has a normal appearance, and this was confirmed by liver biopsy. These sonograms were obtained with a 5 MHz sector transducer (Opus One, Ausonics Pty Ltd, Sydney, Australia; Universal Medical Ltd, NY, USA; BCF Technology Ltd, Livingstone, Scotland).

The Spleen

The equine spleen primarily occupies the left abdomen, lying immediately deep to the body wall in all but the most cranial abdomen where it usually lies medial to the liver (Figs 8.2, 8.3 and and 8.6). It is examined using a 5 MHz sector transducer, although a lower frequency is required occasionally. The spleen is the most echogenic abdominal organ. It has a smooth, even echotexture and blood vessels are visible within it (Fig. 8.4). In older horses, small echogenic foci with acoustic shadowing, consistent with mineralization, can be present on the capsule of the spleen, but these do not appear to have any clinical significance. Equine splenic disease is uncommon. Solitary splenic lymphosarcoma, abscesses and haemato-

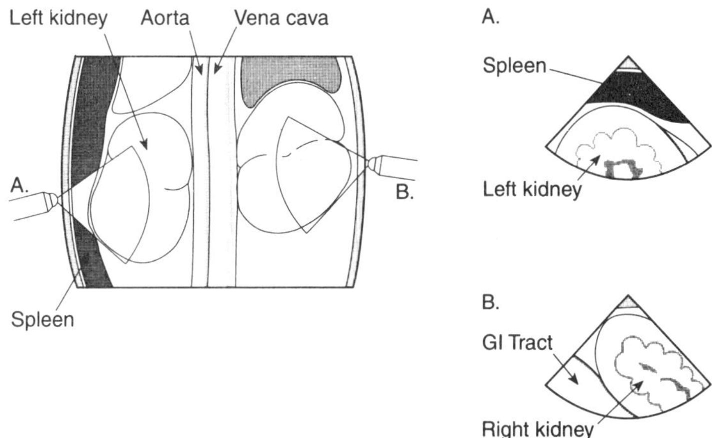

Fig. 8.6. The longitudinal cross-sectional anatomy of the caudodorsal abdomen of the horse, illustrating windows used to examine the kidneys. Corresponding sonograms are presented in Fig. 8.7.

mas result in localized masses, and the spleen can be involved in generalized lymphosarcoma, granulomatous disease or other infiltrative conditions which can be demonstrated ultrasonographically (Rantanen, 1986b; Spier *et al.*, 1986; Marr *et al.*, 1989). Mild to moderate splenomegaly does not appear to be a specific finding.

The Kidneys

The right kidney lies in the retroperitoneal space, from the 14th to 16th intercostal spaces (Fig. 8.6). The left kidney is more mobile, but it is usually imaged in the caudodorsal abdomen deep to the spleen from the 15th intercostal space and sublumbar fossa (Fig. 8.6). The right kidney can usually be imaged with a 5 MHz sector transducer, but a 3.5 or 2.5 MHz transducer is needed to image the left kidney transcutaneously. The left kidney can also be imaged from the rectum with a 5 MHz sector or linear transducer. The right kidney cannot routinely be imaged *per rectum* unless it is massively enlarged. The kidneys should be imaged in both longitudinal and transverse planes and a rough guide to their size can be obtained by measuring their length; most normal horses have kidneys which measure less than 16 cm in length (Fig. 8.7). In normal horses the kidneys are less echogenic than the spleen and liver (Fig. 8.7). The cortex, medulla, renal pelvis, renal artery and ureter can be distinguished ultrasonographically. The cortex is slightly more echogenic than the medulla and at the corticomedullary junction arcuate vessels may be represented as pinpoint echogenic foci with acoustic shadows. Fat associated with the renal pelvis produces central hyperechoic areas (Fig. 8.7).

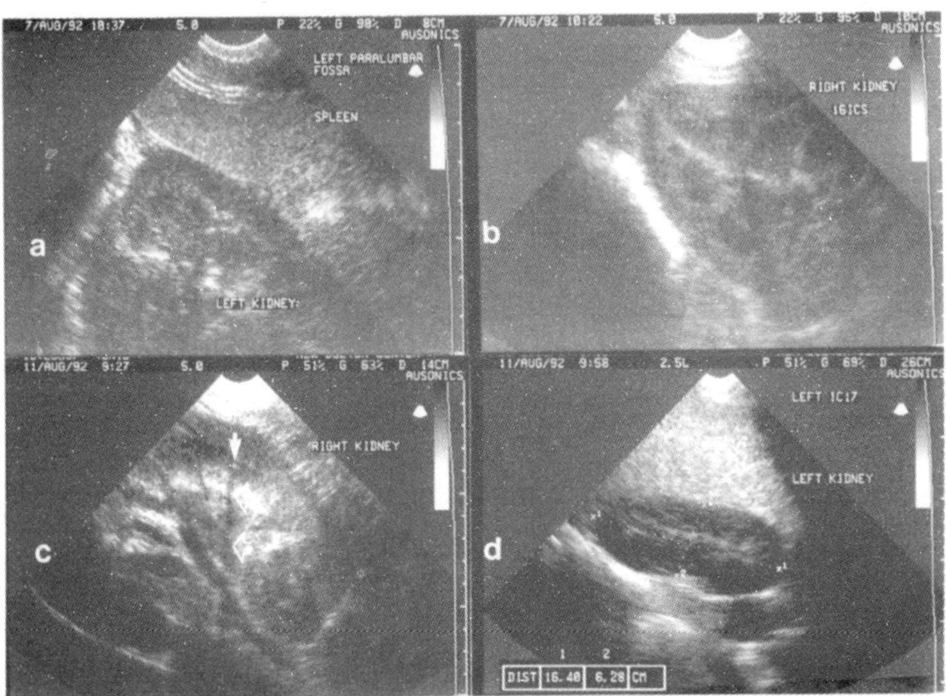

Fig. 8.7. Sonograms of normal equine kidneys (**a** and **b** correspond to the diagrams in Fig. 8.6). **(a)** In this longitudinal image, obtained from the left sublumbar fossa, the spleen is uniformly echogenic. The cortex and medulla of the left kidney can be distinguished. Notice that by using a 5 MHz transducer the resolution is good but not all of the left kidney can be visualized. **(b)** In this longitudinal image, obtained from the right 16th intercostal space, the right kidney is visible. **(c)** In this oblique image of the right kidney, obtained from the right 15th intercostal space, the renal artery is visible in the centre of the kidney. At the corticomedullary junction there are pinpoint echogenic foci (arrow) with associated acoustic shadowing (open arrows) representing arcuate vessels. The echogenic areas in the centre of the kidney are due to pelvic fat. **(d)** In this longitudinal sonogram of the left kidney, obtained from the left 17th intercostal space, the left kidney (between crosses) is visible medial to the spleen. This image is used to measure the length of the kidney. The sonograms in **a**, **b** and **c** were obtained with a 5 MHz sector transducer, and in **d** with a 2.5 MHz sector transducer (Opus One, Ausonics Pty Ltd, Sydney, Australia; Universal Medical Ltd, NY, USA; BCF Technology Ltd, Livingstone, Scotland).

Renal ultrasonography is most helpful in horses with localized lesions such as nephroliths, neoplasia, or cysts although these diseases are relatively uncommon (Penninck *et al.*, 1986; Ehnen *et al.*, 1990; Hillyer *et al.*, 1990; Kiper *et al.*, 1990). Cystic masses can be distinguished from solid ones very easily because of the absence of echoes within a fluid-filled structure (Fig. 8.8). However cysts, particularly hydatid cysts, are usually an incidental finding.

Nephrolithiasis is a disease which appears to be increasing in prevalence (Ehnen *et al.*, 1990). Like choleliths, nephroliths are extremely echogenic, producing marked acoustic shadowing. Care should be taken not to misinterpret fat and fibrous tissue at the renal pelvis which can also produce an acoustic shadow,

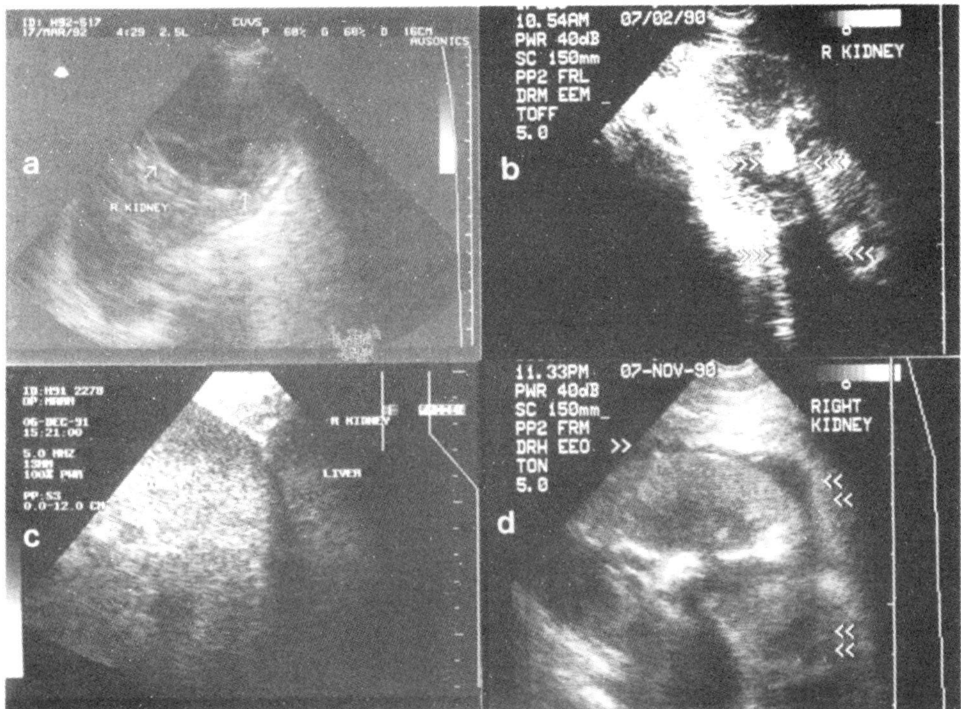

Fig. 8.8. Sonograms of equine renal diseases. **(a)** A longitudinal sonogram of the right kidney from a pony with a hydatid cyst which was of no clinical significance. There is a well-circumscribed cystic structure (arrows) containing some echogenic tissue visible within the kidney. This sonogram was obtained from the right 15th intercostal space with a 2.5 MHz sector transducer (Opus One, Ausonics Pty Ltd, Sydney, Australia; Universal Medical Ltd, NY, USA; BCF Technology Ltd, Livingstone, Scotland). **(b)** A sonogram of the right kidney from a horse with urolithiasis and chronic renal failure. Within the renal pelvis the urolith is an extremely echogenic structure casting an acoustic shadow (between arrowheads). The echogenicity of the kidney is increased and it has a nodular contour. This sonogram was obtained from the right 15th intercostal space with a 5 MHz sector transducer (Microimager 2000, Ausonics Pty Ltd, Sydney, Australia; Universal Medical Ltd, NY, USA; BCF Technology Ltd, Livingstone, Scotland). **(c)** A sonogram of the right kidney from an aged pony with generalized lymphosarcoma and renal infiltration, in which the echogenicity of the kidneys is increased compared to the liver. The internal structure of the kidney has been disrupted and the corticomedullary junction is no longer visible. The sonogram was obtained from the right 14th intercostal space with a 5 MHz sector transducer (Interspec XL, Siel Imaging Equipment Ltd, Aldermaston, Berks, UK). **(d)** An oblique sonogram of the right kidney from a horse with acute vasomotor renal failure secondary to anterior enteritis and endotoxaemia, in which there is a distinct anechoic layer of perirenal oedema (arrowheads) surrounding the kidney. This sonogram was obtained from the right 14th intercostal space with a 5 MHz sector transducer (Microimager 2000, Ausonics Pty Ltd, Sydney, Australia; Universal Medical Ltd, NY, USA; BCF Technology Ltd, Livingstone, Scotland).

mimicking a nephrolith. The clinical significance of nephroliths is variable since some horses are asymptomatic while, in others, nephroliths are associated with chronic renal failure. Therefore, it is important that ultrasonographic findings are considered in the light of other clinical and clinicopathological data. If there is urinary obstruction, the renal pelvis and/or ureter become dilated. Dilated ureters and ureteral uroliths can be imaged most easily *per rectum*.

The renal neoplasms, adenoma, adenocarcinoma, squamous cell carcinoma and lymphosarcoma, are fairly uncommon in horses (Penninck *et al.*, 1986; Rantanen, 1986c). Neoplastic infiltration leads to disruption of the renal architecture and contour, enlargement and changes in echogenicity (Fig. 8.8). A biopsy is required to confirm the precise nature of any tumour. Ultrasonography is invaluable in guiding renal biopsy, which can be hazardous if performed blind. Ideally a biopsy gun should be used because the kidney tends to move during manual biopsy procedures.

The aetiology of renal failure is varied, but in horses renal failure is most commonly the result of toxicity or vasomotor mechanisms (Bayly *et al.*, 1986). Clinical signs can arise in the acute stages or, in chronic renal failure, the onset is often more insidious with severe signs appearing only when the majority of the nephrons have been lost. Ultrasonography is only an adjunctive, rather than definitive, diagnostic aid in horses with renal failure. However, it may have some value in differentiating acute from chronic renal failure (Bayly *et al.*, 1986; Rantanen, 1986c). In acute renal failure the kidneys are usually enlarged with a layer of perirenal oedema, but the internal renal architecture often appears unremarkable (Fig. 8.8) (Bayly *et al.*, 1986; Rantanen, 1986c). In chronic renal fibrosis, the echogenicity of the kidney is most often increased and the kidneys are shrunken and nodular (Fig. 8.8) (Ehnen *et al.*, 1990).

The Gastrointestinal Tract and Peritoneal Fluid

In the adult horse, ultrasonographic access to the gastrointestinal tract is limited by gas in the colon and stomach. Ultrasonography can be helpful in certain specific diseases such as gastric squamous cell carcinoma, faecal peritonitis, ileocaecal intussusception and caecocolic intussusception, particularly in young horses or small ponies where rectal examination is impossible (McGladdery, 1992). However, in the majority of adult horses with signs of acute abdominal crisis, abdominal ultrasonography will provide little useful data.

In foals, because the colon has not fully developed, more of the gastrointestinal tract is visible sonographically and abdominal ultrasonography is an important tool, particularly in small intestinal disease which is common in young foals. The major aim in gastrointestinal ultrasonography is to rule out or confirm specific disorders. It is impossible to definitely differentiate forms of mechanical obstruction in which the specific lesion cannot be visualized (e.g. atresia coli, small intestinal torsion) from functional obstructions (e.g. ileus due to enterocolitis or peritonitis) based on ultrasonography alone. In these foals, ultrasonography should be used in conjunction with other techniques such as paracentesis abdominis, survey and contrast radiography, and laparotomy.

The foal's gastrointestinal tract is first examined using a 7.5 MHz transducer with a stand-off to ensure that the most superficial areas are imaged adequately. Subsequently 7.5 and 5 MHz transducers without a stand-off are used to image the deeper portions of the abdomen. Sector transducers are ideal, although images of the ventral abdomen can be obtained satisfactorily with linear transducers. Because fluid-filled, oedematous or intussuscepted portions of small intestine are heavy and fall to the dependent areas of the abdomen, small intestinal abnormalities can be readily detected. Also, for this reason, it is important to image from the most dependent portion of the abdomen if the foal is recumbent, as intestinal structures will move depending on the foal's position.

Normal small intestine is fairly empty but motile. The intestine can become distended with fluid in foals with both enterocolitis and mechanical obstructions. In enterocolitis, the bowel can be either hypermotile or hypomotile with generalized or segmental thickening of the wall (Fig. 8.9) (Reef, 1993). Large quantities of fluid in the stomach should prompt immediate nasogastric intubation to

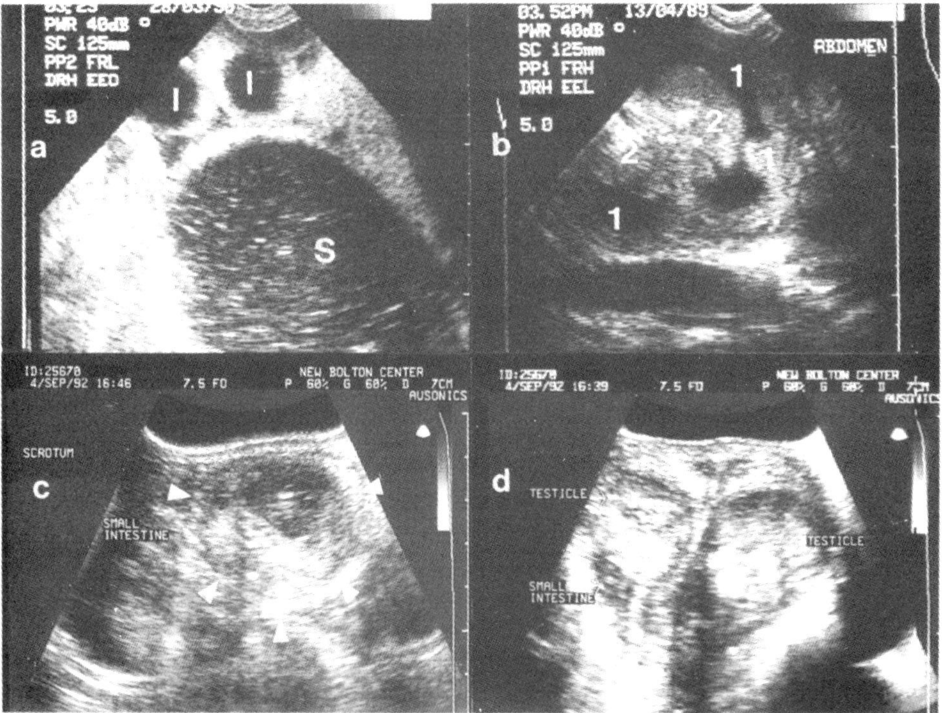

Fig. 8.9. Sonograms of gastrointestinal diseases in foals. **(a)** This transverse sonogram was obtained from the cranioventral midline of a foal with enterocolitis and ileus. Beneath the body wall there are two circular fluid-filled loops of small intestine (i) with thickened walls, and dorsal to them there is a large quantity of fluid containing some echogenic particles of ingesta within the stomach (s) which should be removed by nasogastric intubation. **(b)** An oblique sonogram which was obtained from the ventral midline of a foal with a small intestinal intussusception. Notice the loop of intestine (1) containing an intussusception (2). The loop is folded on itself so that the scanning plane has transected it in two places. **(c)** A sonogram which was obtained from the lateral aspect of the scrotum of a foal with an inguinal hernia. A small loop of intestine (arrowheads) with a thickened, oedematous wall is visible. **(d)** A sonogram which was obtained from the ventral aspect of the scrotum of a foal with an inguinal hernia. Small intestine is visible within the scrotum, dorsolateral to the testicles, which contain echogenic foci, suggesting that they are damaged. The sonograms in **a** and **b** were obtained with a 5 MHz sector transducer (Microimager 2000, Ausonics Pty Ltd, Sydney, Australia; Universal Medical Ltd, NY, USA; BCF Technology Ltd, Livingstone, Scotland), and those in **c** and **d** with a 7.5 MHz sector transducer with an built-in fluid stand-off (Opus One, Ausonics Pty Ltd, Sydney, Australia; Universal Medical Ltd, NY, USA; BCF Technology Ltd, Livingstone, Scotland).

allow decompression. In small intestinal intussusception there are characteristic ultrasonographic findings: the intussuscepted portion of intestine is visible within another loop of small intestine (Fig. 8.9) (Bernard *et al.*, 1989; Reef, 1991, 1993). Ultrasonography can be used to demonstrate intraluminal obstructions such as meconium and ascarid impactions, to confirm the presence of and assess the viability of loops of small intestine within hernias and, in scrotal hernias, to evaluate the testicles (Fig. 8.9) (Reef, 1991, 1993).

Ultrasonography can be used to identify and quantify peritoneal fluid. This is useful in peritonitis, intestinal rupture and uroperitoneum (Reef, 1991; McGladdery, 1992; Reef, 1993). It can also be invaluable in paracentesis abdominis. In adult horses in which the standard technique has been unrewarding, ultrasonography is a simple way to identify pockets of peritoneal fluid for sampling (Fig. 8.4). In foals with marked small intestinal distention, there is a risk of laceration of the intestine during paracentesis abdominis and, ideally, ultrasonography should be performed first to identify a suitable site and minimize this risk.

The Umbilical Structures

The umbilical structures can be imaged ultrasonographically in foals of up to two months of age. Thereafter they normally atrophy and are no longer visible (Reef, 1991, 1993). However, abnormal umbilical structures can be identified in older foals (Collatos *et al.*, 1989). The internal umbilical remnants consist of the umbilical vein, two umbilical arteries and the urachus. They are examined using a 7.5 MHz transducer with a stand-off. Ideally a sector transducer should be used. However, adequate images can be produced with a linear transducer, except in the inguinal region where body contact may be limited with these larger transducers.

The umbilical vein lies just dorsal to the linea alba. It is identified near the external umbilical remnant and followed cranially to the liver. It is an oval or round structure with thin walls and an anechoic lumen or an echogenic core associated with clot formation (Fig. 8.10). In normal foals it measures 6 ± 2 mm in diameter (Reef and Collatos, 1988). The umbilical arteries are identified immediately caudal to the external umbilical remnant, where they lie side by side, and can be followed caudally to the bladder's apex. Each one can then be examined separately alongside the bladder (Fig. 8.10). The arteries have thicker walls than the vein and usually contain an echogenic blood clot rather than fluid (Fig. 8.10). Together, at the bladder's apex, they should measure 17.5 ± 4 mm transversely (Reef and Collatos, 1988). Individually, at the side of the bladder, normal arteries measure 8.5 ± 2 mm. The normal urachus is not visible.

Umbilical infections are common, particularly in foals less than eight weeks old. They may occur in isolation, or accompany generalized septicaemia or localized infections such as pneumonia and septic arthritis. Palpation is not an accurate way to detect internal umbilical disease. Therefore, umbilical ultrasonography is recommended in all foals with signs of systemic infection (Reef *et al.*, 1989). Multiple infections may coexist and it is important not to overlook an

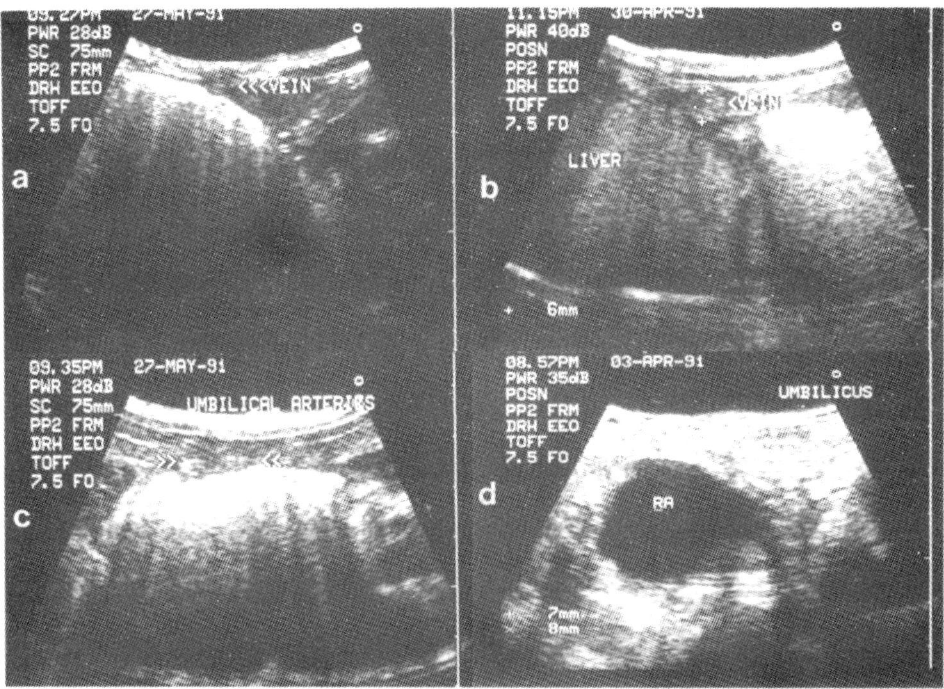

Fig. 8.10. Sonograms of internal umbilical structures in normal foals. **(a)** In this transverse sonogram, obtained from the ventral midline cranial to the external umbilical remnant, the umbilical vein is an oval structure lying immediately beneath the body wall. Beneath it there is a hyperechoic curved structure representing intestinal gas. **(b)** In this transverse sonogram, obtained from the ventral midline just caudal to the sternum, the umbilical vein is a round structure with a narrow anechoic lumen. In real time it could be followed into the adjacent liver. **(c)** In this transverse sonogram, obtained from the ventral midline caudal to the external umbilical remnant, the umbilical arteries are lying together in the midline (between arrowheads). They have thick walls and contain echogenic material (blood clots). Between them there is a small amount of hypoechoic tissue representing the closed urachus, and the hyperechoic curved structure dorsally represents intestinal gas. **(d)** In this transverse sonogram, obtained from the caudoventral midline, the bladder is anechoic and the right umbilical artery (between crosses) has hypoechoic walls and contains a hyperechoic blood clot. It measures 7–8 mm in diameter. These sonograms were obtained with a 7.5 MHz sector transducer with a built-in fluid stand-off (Microimager 2000, Ausonics Pty Ltd, Sydney, Australia; Universal Medical Ltd, NY, USA; BCF Technology Ltd, Livingstone, Scotland).

infected umbilicus in young foals with presenting signs localized to another area such as the joints.

Umbilical infections may involve one or more of the internal structures. Enlargement is a consistent finding in infection (Fig. 8.11). Purulent material within the arteries, vein or urachus varies in its echogenicity depending on its nature. Fluid contents are either completely or almost completely anechoic, and thicker pus is more echogenic (Fig. 8.11). The walls of the infected structure are often thickened, particularly if a localized abscess has formed. Occasionally, extremely bright echoes with acoustic shadowing, typical of gas reverberation echoes, are present (Reef *et al.*, 1989). Umbilical infections can be managed either

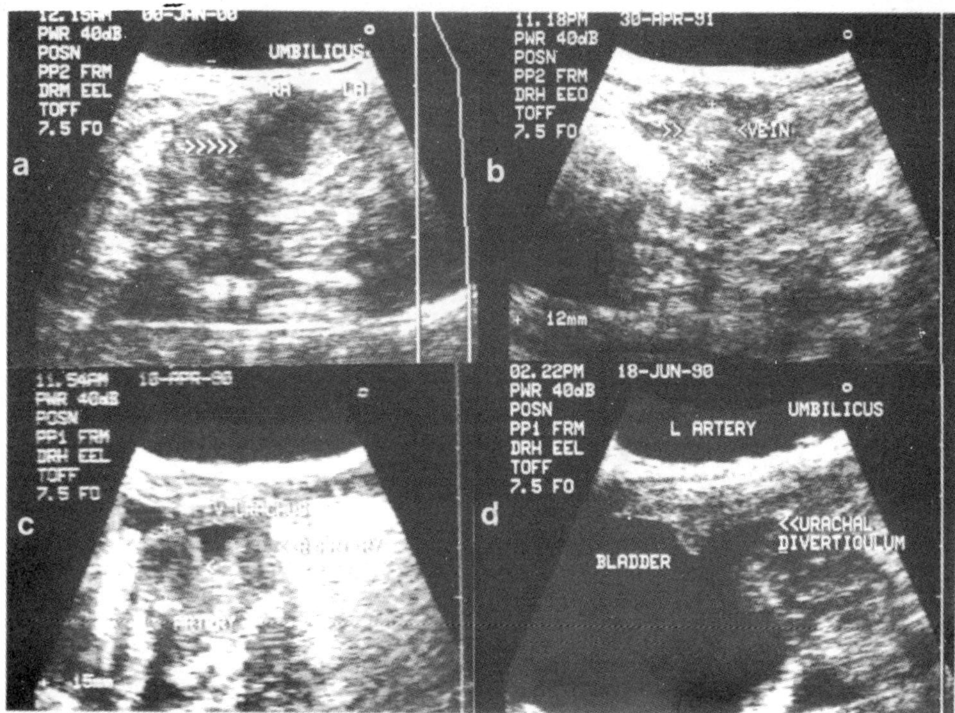

Fig. 8.11. Examples of umbilical abnormalities in foals. **(a)** In this transverse sonogram, obtained from the ventral midline caudal to the external umbilical remnant, from a foal with right omphaloarteritis, the right umbilical artery (arrowheads) is greatly enlarged, its walls are thickened and it contains fluid which is almost completely anechoic. The left umbilical artery which lies to the right of this image is normal. **(b)** In this transverse sonogram, obtained from the ventral midline cranial to the external umbilical remnant, from a foal with omphalophlebitis, the umbilical vein (between arrowheads and crosses) is enlarged. It measures 12 mm in diameter and contains hypoechoic, purulent material. **(c)** In this transverse sonogram, obtained from the ventral midline caudal to the external umbilical remnant, from a foal with omphaloarteritis both the left and right umbilical arteries are infected. They are enlarged with thickened walls. The left artery contains anechoic material and the right artery contains hypoechoic material. Between them, the patent urachus is filled with anechoic urine. **(d)** In this longitudinal sonogram, obtained from the caudoventral midline, from a foal with a urachal diverticulum, the bladder is anechoic and at its apex the diverticulum is seen extending cranially into the urachus. These sonograms were obtained with a 7.5 MHz sector transducer with a built-in fluid stand-off (Microimager 2000, Ausonics Pty Ltd, Sydney, Australia; Universal Medical Ltd, NY, USA; BCF Technology Ltd, Livingstone, Scotland).

surgically or medically, and ultrasonographic assessment can assist the clinician in determining the appropriate treatment plan. Surgery has been recommended in foals in which the infected structures are doubled in size or greater and/or multiple structures are involved (Reef, 1993). If medical treatment with broad-spectrum antibiotics is selected, ultrasonography is particularly helpful in monitoring the response to therapy. Examinations should be repeated at three- to five-day intervals to ensure that there is no further enlargement which may indicate the need for either a change in antibiotic or surgical intervention.

Ultrasonography is also indicated in foals presenting with persistent or patent urachus. In some of these foals, this is a congenital disorder resulting from excessive torsion on the umbilical cord *in utero* (Koterba and Madigan, 1990). However, in others, patent urachus is an acquired disorder associated with infection which can be detected ultrasonographically (Fig. 8.11). Urachal diverticulum is a less common problem causing urinary tenesmus in foals. In this condition, a small pocket of urine is visible in the caudal portion of the urachus (Fig. 8.11). This can also be an incidental ultrasonographic finding.

The Bladder

In adult horses the bladder is located within the pelvic canal and is examined *per rectum* by placing a 5 MHz sector or linear transducer directly over it, imaging ventrally or cranioventrally. Normal equine urine contains calcium carbonate crystals and mucoid material and, therefore, the adult horse's urine is often echogenic (Fig. 8.12). The ventral portions of the bladder usually contain the most echogenic urine and there may be two distinct layers, or swirling shapes may sometimes be visualized (Fig. 8.12). In foals, the bladder can usually be imaged from the caudoventral abdomen with a 7.5 or 5 MHz transducer. The foal's urine is less concentrated than the adult's and is usually anechoic.

Cystic calculi are the most common abnormality of the bladder in adult horses. These can be either single stones or sabulous (gelatinous) material (Divers, 1990). Solitary cystic calculi have a convex, highly echoic contour with strong acoustic shadowing, due to their mineralized structure. Ultrasonography allows confirmation of the diagnosis and assessment of calculi size to assist the surgeon in selecting the best approach for removal (Kaneps *et al.*, 1985).

In foals, ultrasonography is used to assess bladder size and integrity. Anuric renal failure can occur in association with prematurity, hypoxia and septicaemia. Equally, foals often do not urinate adequately if they are recumbent. Ultrasonographic examination is a quick, noninvasive method to differentiate anuric foals with renal failure from foals which are forming urine but not passing it and require catheterization (Fig. 8.12). Rupture of the bladder is a fairly common cause of colic, abdominal distension and depression in young foals. It occurs either during parturition or as a sequel to urinary tract infection (Adams *et al.*, 1988). The bladder usually contains some urine, but if it is ruptured, it has a compressed shape, the site of rupture may be visible and there are large quantities of anechoic or slightly echogenic free fluid within the peritoneal cavity, outlining the other abdominal contents (Fig. 8.12) (Reef, 1991).

Ultrasonography alone cannot definitively differentiate uroperitoneum from peritonitis and, therefore, analysis of the creatinine content of the free fluid is required to confirm the presence of urine if a bladder defect is not evident. An appropriate site for collection of fluid can be selected using ultrasonography.

The Aorta and its Branches

The terminal portions of the aorta, the iliac arteries and, in some horses, the cranial mesenteric arteries, can be examined *per rectum* using 5 or 7.5 MHz transducers. Diseases of the abdominal vasculature include cranial mesenteric arteritis,

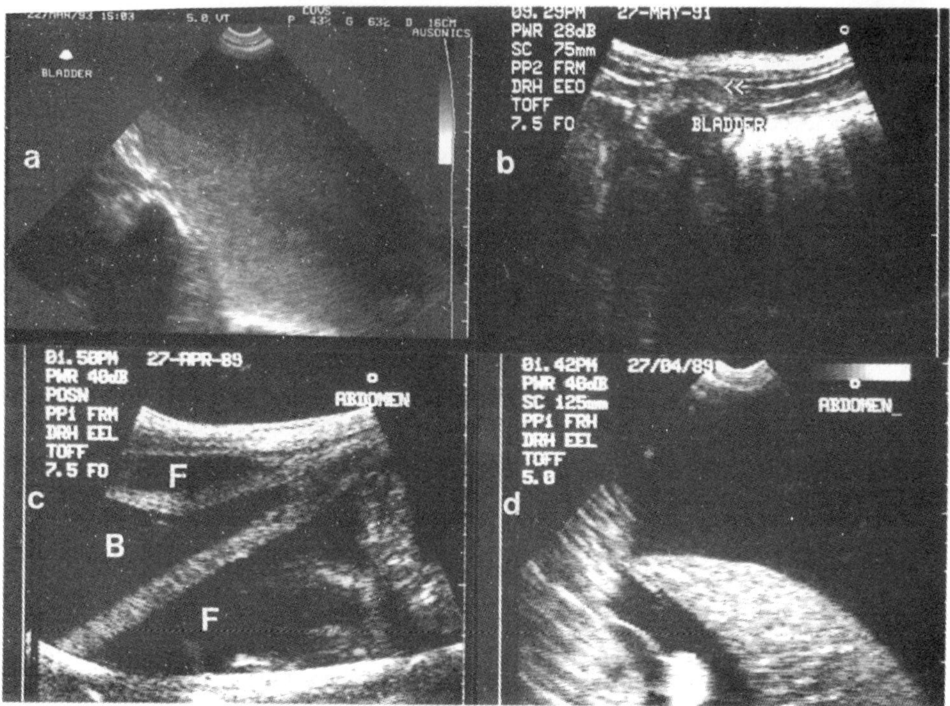

Fig. 8.12. Sonograms of the bladder. **(a)** In this longitudinal sonogram of the bladder in a normal adult horse the urine is echogenic, particularly in the ventral portions of the bladder, and there were irregular swirling shapes in the middle of the bladder as the urine moved. This sonogram was obtained with a 5 MHz 0–90° intrarectal sector transducer (Opus 1, Ausonics Pty Ltd, Sydney, Australia; Universal Medical Ltd, NY, USA; BCF Technology Ltd, Livingstone, Scotland). **(b)** In this transverse sonogram, obtained from the caudoventral abdomen, from a foal of approximately twelve hours of age which had never urinated, a tiny bladder is visible, confirming that there was failure of urine production associated with anuric renal failure rather than a micturition problem. The double arrowheads point to the umbilical arteries. **(c)** In this longitudinal sonogram, obtained from the caudoventral abdomen, from a foal with uroperitoneum, the bladder (B) is slightly collapsed and free fluid (F) surrounds it. **(d)** In this longitudinal sonogram, obtained from the cranioventral abdomen, from a foal with uroperitoneum, a portion of liver is outlined by anechoic free fluid. The sonograms in **b**, **c** and **d** were obtained with a 7.5 MHz sector transducer with a built-in fluid stand-off (Microimager 2000, Ausonics Pty Ltd, Sydney, Australia; Universal Medical Ltd, NY, USA; BCF Technology Ltd, Livingstone, Scotland).

aortic-iliac thrombosis and aortic aneurysms. The ultrasonographic abnormalities associated with cranial mesenteric arteritis have been described by Wallace *et al.* (1989). Aortic-iliac thrombosis is a disease of unknown aetiology affecting the terminal aorta and its quadrification, causing exercise-induced hindlimb lameness. The thrombus is usually an echogenic structure within the aorta. The level of echogenicity is related to the chronicity: progressive fibrosis increases echogenicity (Reef *et al.*, 1987). In normal peripheral vessels, blood is often echogenic and care must be taken not to mistake this for a thrombus. Careful examination will distinguish movement within normal vessels. Aortic aneurysms are uncommon and the presenting signs are variable, depending on the specific site involved.

In some horses the disease may not be suspected until the horse dies suddenly. However, this diagnosis should be considered if a mass is palpable in the region of the aorta. Ultrasonography confirms the vascular nature of the mass.

Abdominal Abscesses

Abdominal abscesses can arise in association with *Rhodococcus equi*, *Streptococcus equi*, and *Streptococcus zooepidemicus* and as a sequel to surgical procedures such as castration. If a mass is palpable *per rectum*, ultrasonography is the obvious next step. Abdominal ultrasonography should also be considered in horses presenting with weight loss, fever of unknown origin, leucocytosis and hyperfibrinogenaemia, particularly if peritoneal fluid analysis indicates an abdominal inflammatory process. The precise location of the abscess will determine if it can be imaged because intestinal gas can obscure some portions of the abdomen. Large masses within the mesentery will tend to fall towards the ventral abdomen. Masses palpable *per rectum* can be imaged by placing the transducer directly over them. It is unlikely that an abscess will be imaged *per rectum* if it is not palpable. The remainder of the abdomen is examined using the parenchymal organs as windows into deeper structures.

The ultrasonographic appearance of abscesses depends on their precise nature; they often have a very complex appearance (Fig. 8.13). Fluid-filled structures are completely or almost completely anechoic, pus of a custard-like consistency is fairly echogenic (although movement can often be detected), and caseous material can be very echogenic. Abscesses can be loculated and frequently contain echogenic clots of fibrin and cellular debris. Anaerobic organisms produce gas which tends to accumulate in dorsal gas caps (Fig. 8.13). Reliable indicators that a mass is an abscess are a fluid component, particularly if it looks cellular (echogenic), and the presence of gas and fibrin clots. In addition to confirming the diagnosis, ultrasonography is used to measure the abscess and define its relationship to other structures, and can be used to assess the feasibility of and approach to drainage, and to monitor the response to medical treatment.

Abdominal Neoplasia

Lipoma and lymphosarcoma are the most common neoplasms of the equine abdomen. Gastric squamous cell carcinoma and granulosa thecal cell tumours appear to occur fairly frequently, while other neoplasms such as metastatic melanomas and renal, ovarian and hepatic adenocarcinomas occur sporadically. Strangulating lipoma leads to abdominal crisis and ultrasonography can contribute nothing to its diagnosis. Similarly, the alimentary form of lymphosarcoma is investigated with other techniques. For other neoplasms, however, ultrasonography is extremely helpful, particularly if masses can be palpated *per rectum*. The role of ultrasonography in abdominal neoplasia is to identify the exact location and distribution of abdominal neoplasm and, depending on the specific site, it can facilitate a percutaneous biopsy. Ultrasonography cannot be used as a substitute for histological diagnosis as most solid neoplasms are indistinguishable ultrasonographically.

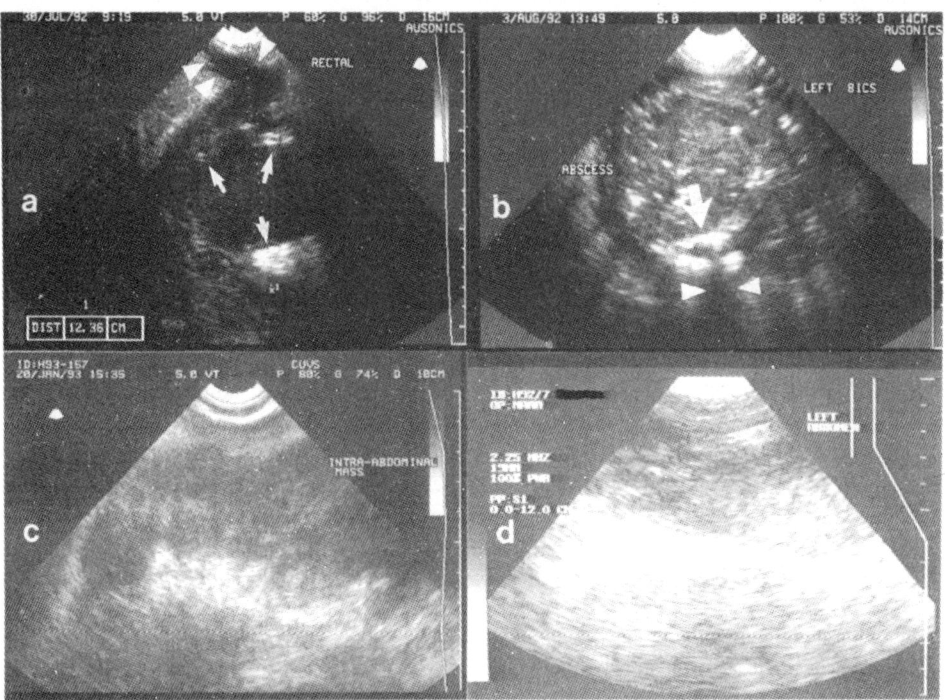

Fig. 8.13. Sonograms of intra-abdominal masses. **(a)** A longitudinal sonogram, obtained *per rectum* from a mare with an abscess ventral to the rectum and dorsal to the uterus as a sequel to rectal perforation (arrowheads). The contents of the abscess, measuring 12.4 cm from dorsal to ventral (between crosses), are almost hypoechoic with some echogenic clots of fibrin (arrows) and debris. Precise demonstration of the position and size of the abscess allowed a successful transvaginal surgical approach to be adopted. **(b)** In this transverse sonogram, obtained from the cranioventral abdomen, from a weanling with an abdominal abscess due to *Rhodococcus equi* infection, the abscess has a complex appearance with echogenic fluid contents, hyperechoic clots and a dorsal gas cap (arrow) with associated acoustic shadowing (between arrowheads). **(c)** In this longitudinal oblique sonogram, obtained *per rectum* from an aged pony with generalized lymphosarcoma, there is a large multilobular mass with fairly uniform echogenicity, consistent with a solid neoplasm such as a lymphosarcoma. **(d)** In this transverse sonogram, obtained from the left seventh intercostal space from a horse with gastric squamous cell carcinoma, a solid mass with a heterogeneous echogenicity is overlying the stomach in a position normally occupied by the spleen. This sonogram was obtained with a 2.25 MHz sector transducer (Interspec XL, Siel Medical Imaging Ltd, Aldermaston, Berks, UK). The sonograms in **a** and **c** were obtained with a 0–90° 5 MHz sector transducer, and in **b** with a 5 MHz sector transducer (Opus One, Ausonics Pty Ltd, Sydney, Australia; Universal Medical Ltd, NY, USA; BCF Technology Ltd, Livingstone, Scotland).

Generalized lymphosarcoma can affect multiple abdominal organs and lymph nodes. Typically, these masses have uniform echogenicity of a level similar to that of the abdominal organs (Fig. 8.13). However, there can be anechoic or hypoechoic areas within them, particularly if the tumour contains foci of necrosis (Marr *et al.*, 1989).

Granulosa thecal cell tumours are often multicystic and this is reflected in their ultrasonographic appearance of multiple anechoic areas (White and Allen,

1985; Gatewood *et al.*, 1990). However, they can be solid. Gastric squamous cell carcinoma causes weight loss, recurrent colic, anaemia and, occasionally, ptyalism in middle-aged and older horses. Ultrasonographic examination of the cranial abdomen reveals a solid mass with fairly uniform echogenicity associated with the stomach, displacing the spleen caudally and ventrally (Fig. 8.13).

The Fetus and Uterus

In early gestation the fetus is evaluated *per rectum* (see Chapter 7) but, after around 80 days of gestation, it can be imaged from the ventral body wall using a 2.5 MHz transducer with a field of view of 27.5–30 cm. The main indications are to confirm the presence of twins and destroy one if possible, and, in later gestation, to identify fetal distress and uterine and placental disease. Ultrasonography can also be used to guide amniocentesis although this procedure is currently only used for research rather than clinical purposes. One study has shown that one pair of twins can be removed successfully in approximately 50% of cases following a lethal injection of potassium chloride administered under ultrasound guidance (Rantanen and Kincaid, 1988). Alternatively, an injection of penicillin/streptomycin in aqueous suspension has been recommended (McKinnon *et al.*, 1993). If successful, these procedures lead to mummification of one twin and delivery of a live foal at term. However, loss of both fetuses is common (Rantanen and Kincaid, 1988; McKinnon *et al.*, 1993).

Bradycardia, tachycardia and cardiac arrhythmias are indicators of fetal distress. The aortic root diameter correlates with birth weight (Pipers and Adams-Brendermuel, 1984). The fetal thorax is easily identified because of the characteristic appearance of the ribs, and the heart can be seen beating within it. Heart rate and aortic diameter are best determined using M-mode imaging (Fig. 8.14). Recent work has been directed at the development of a biophysical profile for assessment of fetal health and distress in late gestation, using fetal heart rate, aortic diameter, quality of fetal fluid, utero-placental contact, utero-placental thickness and fetal activity indices (V.B. Reef, Pennsylvania, 1994, personal communication). In mares with placentitis, the uterus and placenta are thickened and the echogenicity of the fetal fluids is increased.

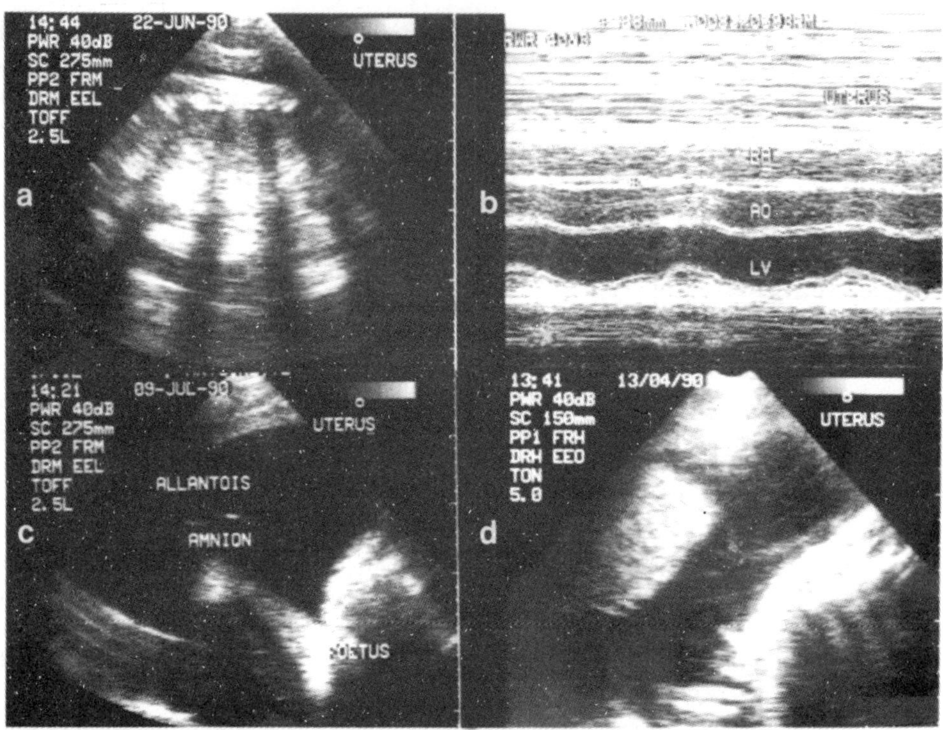

Fig. 8.14. Sonograms of the fetus and uterus. **(a)** A sonogram, obtained from the ventral abdomen, from a mare at around 320 days of gestation, in which the fetal thorax can be identified by the characteristic appearance of the ribs which are echogenic and cast acoustic shadows. **(b)** An M-mode sonogram, obtained from the ventral abdomen, from a mare at around 320 days of gestation, in which the M-mode cursor has been placed through the fetal heart so that the aortic diameter (AO) and heart rate can be measured. (The heart rate can be calculated from any image of the cardiac structures provided that several cardiac cycles are observed.) **(c)** A sonogram, obtained from the ventral abdomen, from a mare at around 320 days of gestation, in which allantoic fluid (allantois) and amniotic fluid (amnion) are separated by the allantoamnoin. Parts of the fetus's forelimb are visible. **(d)** A sonogram, obtained from the ventral abdomen, from a mare with placentitis at around 300 days of gestation, in which the amniotic fluid is echogenic and contains echogenic particles, and the uteroplacental unit is thickened. At this point the fetus was alive but it was aborted within a few days. The sonograms were obtained with a 2.5 MHz sector transducer with a 27.5 cm field of view (Microimager 2000, Ausonics Pty Ltd, Sydney, Australia; Universal Medical Ltd, NY, USA; BCF Technology Ltd, Livingstone, Scotland).

References

Adams, R., Koterba, A.M., Cudd, T. and Baker, W.A. (1988) Exploratory celiotomy for suspected urinary tract disruption: a review of 18 cases. *Equine Veterinary Journal*, 20, 13–17.

Bayly, W.M., Elfers, R.S., Liggitt, H.D., Brobst, D.F., Gavin, P.R. and Reed, F.M. (1986) A reproducible means of studying acute renal failure in the horse. *Cornell Veterinarian*, 76, 287–298.

Bernard, W.V., Reef, V.B., Reimer, J.M., Humber, K.A. and Orsini, J.A. (1989) Ultrasonographic diagnosis of small-intestinal intussusception in three foals. *Journal of the American Veterinary Medical Association*, 194, 395–397.

Collatos, C., Reef, V.B. and Richardson, D.W. (1989) Umbilical cord remnant abscess in a yearling colt. *Journal of the American Veterinary Medical Association*, 195, 1252–1254.

Divers, T.J. (1990) Diseases of the renal system. In: Smith, B.P. (ed.) *Large Animal Internal Medicine.* CV Mosby Co., St Louis, pp. 872–900.

Ehnen, S.J., Divers, T.J., Gillette, D. and Reef, V.B. (1990) Obstructive nephrolithiasis and ureterolithiasis associated with chronic renal failure in horses: eight cases (1981–1987). *Journal of the American Veterinary Medical Association*, 197, 249–253.

Gatewood, D.M., Douglass J.P., Cox, J.H., DeBowes, R.M. and Kennedy, G.A. (1990) Intra-abdominal haemorrhage associated with a granulosa-thecal cell neoplasm in a mare. *Journal of the American Veterinary Medical Association*, 196, 1827–1828.

Hillyer, M.H., Mar, T.S. and Lucke, V.H. (1990) Bilateral renal calculi in an adult horse. *Equine Veterinary Education*, 2, 117–120.

Johnston, J.K., Divers, T.J., Reef, V.B. and Acland, H. (1989) Cholelithiasis in horses: ten cases (1982–1986). *Journal of the American Veterinary Medical Association*, 194, 405–409.

Kaneps, A.J., Shires, G.M.H. and Watrous, B.J. (1985) Cystic calculi in two horses. *Journal of the American Veterinary Medical Association*, 187, 737–739.

Kiper, M.L., Traub-Dargatz, J.L. and Wrigley, R.H. (1990) Renal ultrasonography in horses. *Compendium of Continuing Education for the Practising Veterinarian*, 12, 993–999.

Koterba, A.M. and Madigan, J.E. (1990) Manifestations of disease in the neonate. In: Smith, B.P. (ed.) *Large Animal Internal Medicine.* C.V. Mosby Co., St Louis, pp. 316–339.

Marr, C.M., Love, S. and Pirie, H.M. (1989) Clinical, ultrasonographic and pathological findings in a horse with splenic lymphosarcoma and pseudohyperparathyroidism. *Equine Veterinary Journal*, 21, 221–226.

McGladdery, A.J. (1992) Ultrasonography as an aid to the diagnosis of equine colic. *Equine Veterinary Education*, 4, 248–251.

McKinnon, A.O., Voss, J.L., Squires, E.L. and Carnevale, E.M. (1993) Diagnostic ultrasonography. In: McKinnon, A.O. and Voss, J.L. (eds) *Equine Reproduction.* Lea and Febiger, Malvern, pp. 266–302.

Penninck, D.G., Eisenberg, H.M., Teuscher, E.E. and Vrins, A. (1986) Equine renal ultrasonography: normal and abnormal. *Veterinary Radiology*, 27, 81–84.

Pipers, F.S. and Adams-Brendermuel, C.S. (1984) Techniques and applications of transabdominal ultrasonography in the pregnant mare. *Journal of the American Veterinary Medical Association*, 185, 766–771.

Rantanen, N.W. (1986a) Diseases of the liver. *Veterinary Clinics of North America (Equine Practice)*, 2, 105–114.

Rantanen, N.W. (1986b) Diseases of the abdomen. *Veterinary Clinics of North America (Equine Practice)*, 2, 67–88.

Rantanen, N.W. (1986c) Diseases of the kidneys. *Veterinary Clinics of North America (Equine Practice)*, 2, 89–103.

Rantanen, N.W. and Kincaid, B. (1988) Ultrasound guided fetal cardiac puncture: a method of twin reduction in the mare. *Proceedings of the American Association of Equine Practitioners*, 34, 173–179.

Reef, V.B. (1991) Equine paediatric ultrasonography. *Compendium of Continuing Education for the Practising Veterinary Surgeon*, 13, 1277–1284.

Reef, V.B. (1993) Diagnostic ultrasonography of the foal's abdomen. In: McKinnon, A.O. and Voss, J.L. (eds) *Equine Reproduction.* Lea and Febiger, Malvern, pp. 1088–1094.

Reef, V.B. and Collatos, C. (1988) Ultrasonography of umbilical structures in clinically normal foals. *American Journal of Veterinary Research*, 49, 2143–2146.

Reef, V.B., Roby, K.A., Richardson, D.W., Vaala, W.E., Johnston, J.K. (1987). Use of ultrasonography for the detection of aortic iliac thrombosis in horses. *Journal of the American Veterinary Medical Association*, 190, 286–288.

Reef, V.B., Collatos, C., Spencer, P.A., Orsini, J.A. and Sepesy, L.M. (1989) Clinical, ultrasonographic, and surgical findings in foals with umbilical remnant infections. *Journal of the American Veterinary Medical Association*, 195, 69–72.

Reef, V.B., Johnston, J.K., Divers, T.J. and Acland, H. (1990) Ultrasonographic findings in horses with cholelithiasis: eight cases (1985–1987). *Journal of the American Veterinary Medical Association*, 196, 1836–1840.

Spier, S., Carlson, G.P., Nyland, T.G., Snyder, J.R. and Fischer, P.E. (1986) Splenic haematoma and abscess as a cause of a chronic weight loss in a horse. *Journal of the American Veterinary Medical Association*, 189, 557–559.

Wallace, K.D., Selcer, B.A., Tyler, D.E. and Brown, J. (1989) Transrectal ultrasonography of the cranial mesenteric artery of the horse. *American Journal of Veterinary Research*, 50, 1699–1703.

White, R.A.S. and Allen, W.R. (1985) Use of ultrasound echography for the differential diagnosis of a granulosa cell tumour in a mare. *Equine Veterinary Journal*, 17, 401–402.

9 Scanning the Equine Limb

J.P.M. Main

O'Gorman, Slater and Main, Donnington Grove Veterinary Surgery, Oxford Road, Newbury, Berkshire RG13 2JB, UK

Introduction

Over the last ten years, real-time ultrasonography has developed to become an essential aid in the examination and diagnosis of soft tissue, tendon/ligament injury of the equine athlete. Structures that are routinely imaged include the flexor tendons, suspensory apparatus, inferior check ligament, posterior pastern, plantar ligament, peronius tertius and gastrocnemius tendon. However, many other soft tissue structures in the equine limb such as tendon sheaths, joint capsules, extensor tendons and bursae are also suitable for imaging. It is essential to be totally familiar with the normal anatomical features and relationship of structures within the equine limb. It is useful to remember that when imaging a structure the equivalent structure on the contralateral leg can be used for comparative purposes, although it must be remembered that a bilateral lesion may occasionally be seen.

Real-time ultrasonography is a noninvasive and painless technique which is safe to use, both for the operator and the patient, compared to other diagnostic aids such as radiography and scintography.

Most areas to be imaged should have a previously demonstrable clinical abnormality, whether it be pain, heat or swelling or more subtly identified by the use of nerve blocks, radiographs or scintography. Care should be taken to correlate ultrasonographic findings with clinical assessment and previous clinical history.

A basic understanding of the physics of ultrasound helps in the interpretation of images and, importantly, the understanding of artifact formation. It also allows full use to be made of the modern, more sophisticated ultrasound machines.

Equipment Selection

There is a vast array of equipment available in the equine ultrasound market.

Choice in a veterinary practice is often a compromise, as other uses have to be taken into consideration. However, when considering equine limbs the main decision is whether to use a linear or a sector machine, or a combination. The sector mode probably has an advantage when used in the horizontal (cross-sectional) plane compared to the linear mode, whereas the converse is probably true when imaging in a vertical (sagittal) plane. The author feels that the horizontal plane is most diagnostic and therefore would probably recommend a sector machine. However, it is likely that very similar results can be achieved as long as the operator is totally familiar with the ultrasound machine, whether it be linear or sector. In the choice of ultrasound machines the following factors should be taken into consideration:

- The machine should be easily portable and robust
- It should fit into only one or two well designed containers (including the probe and printer)
- The probe connections should be simple and strong
- The probe lead should be reasonably supple and of adequate length (1.5–2 metres)
- The probe should have a suitable stand-off, either inbuilt or separate
- Good, simple controls with easy touch switching
- Advanced screen display: options include split-screen capability, measurement callipers with area calculation, multiple arrow pointers, multiple data display, ability to highlight and enlarge, contrast and brightness controls, freeze frame control (foot switch and frame storage)
- Good quality printer – thermal image or photograph
- Expense and finance options
- Back-up service and customer care.

Method

For the majority of equine ultrasound limb procedures, the limb to be examined should be in a weight-bearing position. For best results the procedure should be carried out in a quiet room with low light and without other distractions. The scanner is best placed on a wheel-based trolley and should be positioned where the operator can view the screen without having to alter his position in relation to the horse. If the horse is particularly fractious, sedation is probably the best means of restraint. A video recorder produces a permanent real-time recording which can allow for more detailed analysis at a later date. The level of contrast and brightness should be adjusted as necessary according to the level of light in the examination room. Whenever possible, ultrasound examination should not be carried out in bright daylight, as important detail on the screen can be lost due to a lack of contrast. A 7.5 MHz probe should be used for most tendon work.

Preparation of limbs

The area to be scanned should be clipped with number 40 clipper blades, possibly followed by close shaving (a disposable razor lends itself to this purpose). The author has found that shaving the skin leaves the area prone to reaction and chafing and therefore often omits shaving, especially in thin-skinned, non-hairy animals. The area should be thoroughly soaked in warm water and then a liberal coating of ultrasound gel applied. It is beneficial to massage the gel into the area for several minutes as this greatly improves skin conductivity. Preparation of the skin area before setting up the machine allows further time for the gel to soak in.

Normal Ultrasonic Anatomy

The metacarpus

For the purpose of scanning, the metacarpus can be divided into six sections. This enables an accurate record of position of the probe to be made (Fig. 9.1). The probe may be placed so that it scans in a horizontal plane, producing a cross-sectional picture, or conversely in a vertical plane, producing a longitudinal picture. Generally the cross-sectional plane is most useful when looking for lesions within the metacarpus/tarsus. The longitudinal plane is most useful to assess

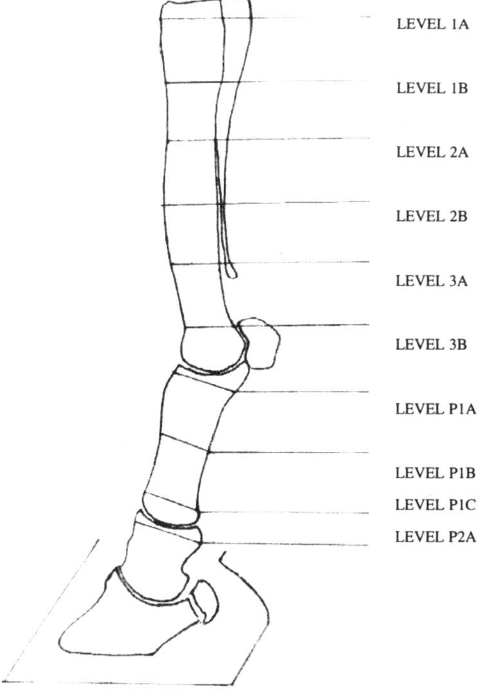

Fig. 9.1. Zonal division of metacarpus and pastern.

                                                      J.P.M. Main

Fig. 9.2. Sagittal view taken medial to accessory carpal bone though the metacarpus and medial sesamoid bone. **1** = superficial digital flexor tendon, **2** = deep digital flexor tendon, **3** = common flexor tendon carpal sheath, **4** = inferior check ligament, **5** = suspensory ligament, **6** = proximal annular ligament, **7** = digital sheath; **A** = radius, **B** = accessory carpal bone, **C** = radial carpal bone, **D** = third carpal bone, **E** = second carpal bone, **F** = third metacarpal bone, **G** = second metacarpal bone, **H** = medial proximal sesamoid bone, **I** = first phalange.

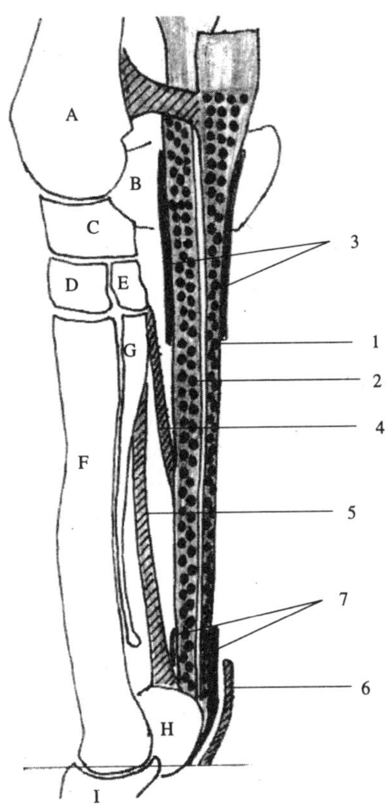

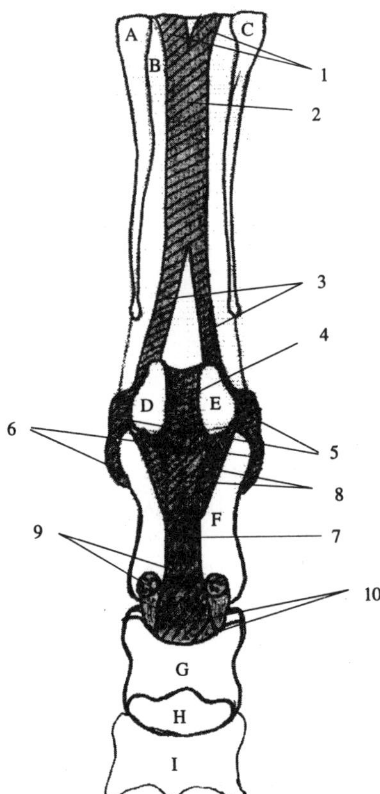

Fig. 9.3. Posterior view of the metacarpus and phalanges with flexor tendons removed. **1** = bifid origin of suspensory ligament, **2** = suspensory ligament, **3** = medial and lateral branches of suspensory ligament, **4** = intersesamoidian ligaments, **5** = collateral sesamoidian ligaments, **6** = medial and lateral extensor branches of suspensory ligament, **7** = straight sesamoidian ligaments, **8** = oblique sesamoidian ligaments, **9** = insertions of branches of superficial digital flexor tendon onto the distal first phalange, **10** = combined insertion of branches of superficial digital flexor tendon and straight sesamoidian ligament onto the proximal palmar prominence of the second phalange; **A** = second metacarpus, **B** = third metacarpus, **C** = fourth metacarpus, **D** = medial sesamoid bone, **E** = lateral sesamoid bone, **F** = first phalange, **G** = second phalange, **H** = navicular bone, **I** = third phalange.

tendon fibre quality and alignment, especially during the healing phases. The main structures to be imaged in the metacarpus are the superficial digital flexor tendon (S.D.F.T.), the deep digital flexor tendon (D.D.F.T.), the inferior check ligament (I.C.L.) and the suspensory ligament (S.L.). Schematic diagrams of the normal anatomy of the metacarpus are shown in Figs 9.2 and 9.3.

Zone 1A

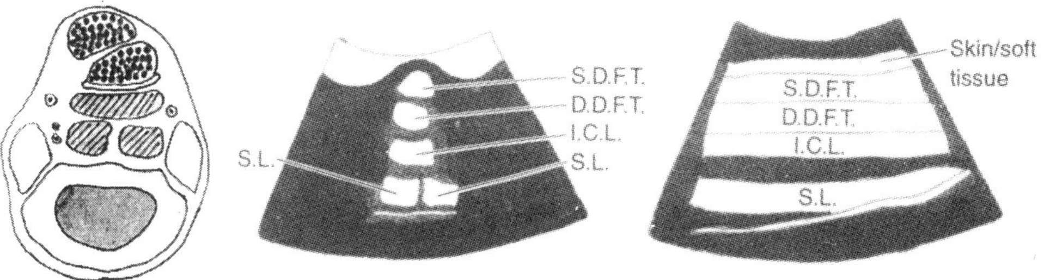

The S.D.F.T. is a crescent-shaped structure approximately 1.2 cm wide and 0.8 cm deep. It is of homogenous echogenicity with an obvious fibril pattern. The D.D.F.T. is a more rounded structure with a diameter of approximately 1 cm. It is of uniform echogenicity but always more echoic than the S.D.F.T. The I.C.L. originates from the palmar carpal ligaments forming an echoic, almost rectangular structure approximately 1.8 cm wide and 0.8 cm deep. It is of uniform echogenicity. The S.L. forms in the proximal part of Zone 1A arising from medial and lateral heads originating from the proximal posterior third of the metacarpus and the distal row of the carpal bones. It is a modified muscular structure (interossius muscle), and it should be noted that it contains some striated muscle fibres in its origin which are most obvious in younger horses. Therefore care must be taken in interpreting the proximal suspensory ligament: the ligament is not of uniform echogenicity at Zone 1A, and the two heads can often give the impression of one structure with an anechoic core in the middle. Hence it is very important to compare the structure in the contralateral leg.

Zone 1B

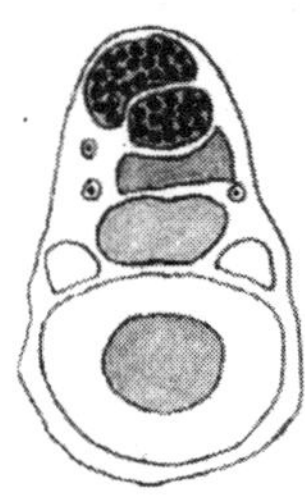
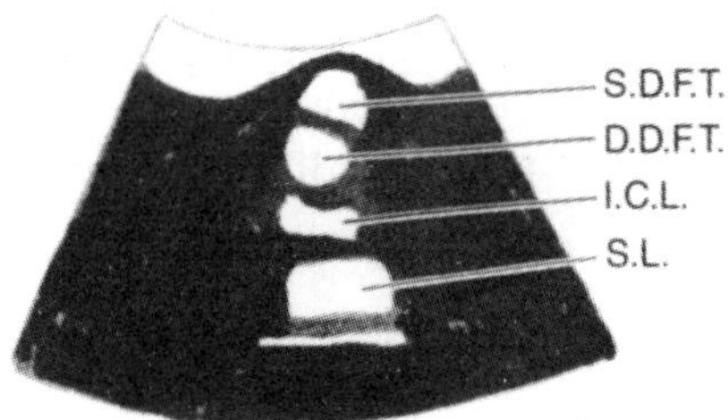

The S.D.F.T. tends to become wider and less deep as it continues distally, while the D.D.F.T. tends to become more circular. The I.C.L. attains maximum width and comes to lie closer to the D.D.F.T. It also tends to become less rectangular with the palmar edge demonstrating some curvature. The S.L. becomes more uniform and the two heads fuse to form one structure. Most of the anechoic muscle fibres have disappeared. Therefore the S.L. has a more uniform echoic appearance here than in Zone 1A.

Zone 2A

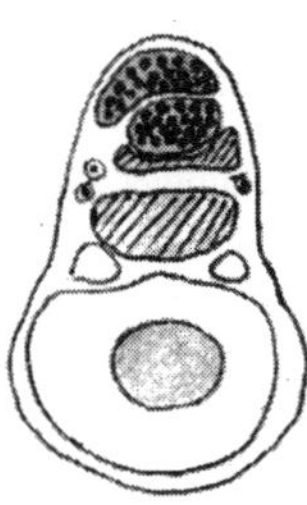
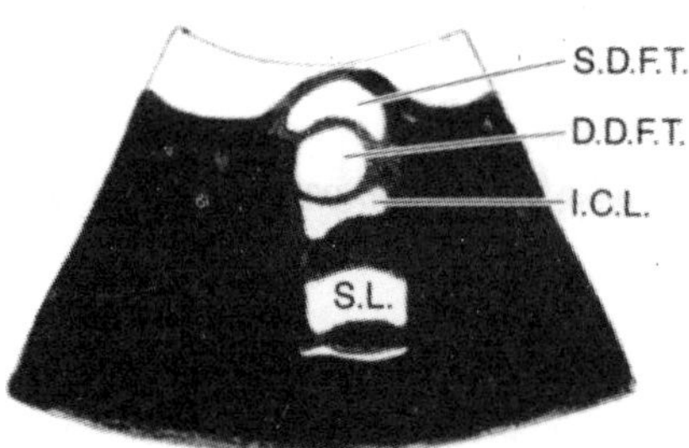

The I.C.L. comes to lie closer to the D.D.F.T. and has started to narrow, becoming less deep and more curved, complementing the curvature of the D.D.F.T.

Zone 2B

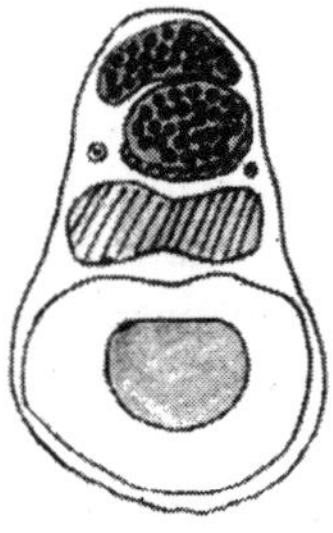
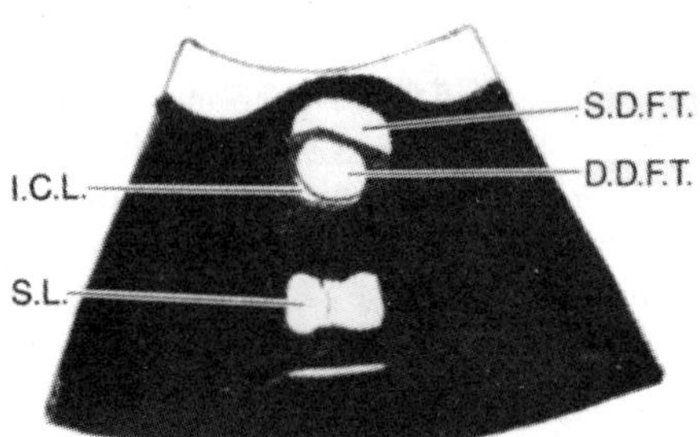

In the proximal part of Zone 2B the I.C.L. starts to merge with the D.D.F.T. This process is completed by the distal part of Zone 2B. In the distal part of this zone the S.L. starts to become bi-lobed in shape in preparation for division into medial and lateral branches in Zone 3A.

Zone 3A

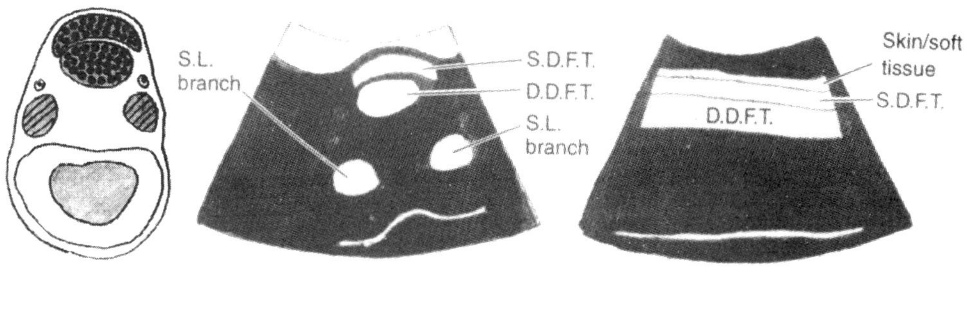

Horizontal view   Longitudinal view

The S.D.F.T. has become markedly more flattened. The I.C.L. is no longer present. The S.L. has bifurcated into two circular medial and lateral branches of approximately 0.8 cm in diameter.

Zone 3B

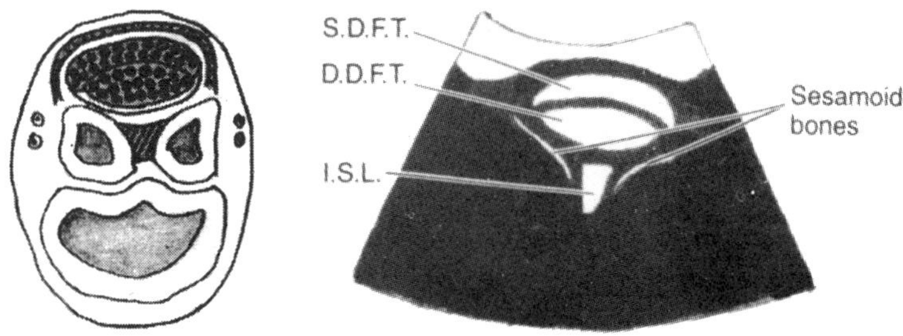

The S.D.F.T. has become very closely associated with the D.D.F.T. At the junction of Zones 3A and 3B it forms a ring through which the D.D.F.T. passes. However, this ring is not usually visible on ultrasound as it is only 1–2 mm in thickness. The S.D.F.T. has become crescent-shaped, conforming to the D.D.F.T. which has become more ovoid in shape. The synovial sheath around the flexor tendons is rarely visible unless thickened or distended due to damage. The annular ligament also is not visible unless thickened due to damage. The medial and lateral branches of the S.L. disappear in the distal part of Zone 3B as they insert on the abaxial surface of the sesamoid bones. The sesamoid bones form a characteristic 'gull-wing' appearance distally in this zone, with the intersesamoidian ligaments (I.S.L.) traversing between. The S.L. branches are best imaged from their respective medial or lateral aspects and can be imaged either in a horizontal plane or in a vertical plane ('Ski jump' view). In the horizontal view, from the medial or lateral aspect, the S.L. branches become almost triangular just before inserting on to the abaxial surface of the sesamoid bone. In the longitudinal view, from the medial or lateral aspect, the insertion of the suspensory ligament onto the abaxial surface of the sesamoid bones can be examined in detail.

The pastern

The structures which are commonly imaged are the straight and oblique sesamoidian ligaments (S.S.L. and O.S.L.), the S.D.F.T and its branches, and the D.D.F.T. Schematic diagrams of the normal anatomy of the pastern are shown in Figs 9.3 and 9.4. The ergot of the fetlock unfortunately interrupts the continuity of the scanned image extending from Zone 3B into the pastern. Distal to the ergot, the pastern can be divided into four sections (see Fig. 9.1). The pastern is a less accessible region to image, due to its angulation and closeness to the ground. By positioning the limb to be examined posteriorly, the fetlock and pastern will become more upright, thus facilitating the procedure. A 10 cm wooden block under the hoof to raise the leg off the ground can also improve the access. It is important, however, to scan the pastern with the leg bearing weight. It is often difficult to visualize the different structures of the pastern simultaneously due to off-normal incidence artifacts (see p. 220) and therefore it is advisable to scan one structure at a time, being careful to move the probe through a range of angles to ensure that the probe is at 90° to the structure being imaged. Normal sonograms appear in Fig. 9.5.

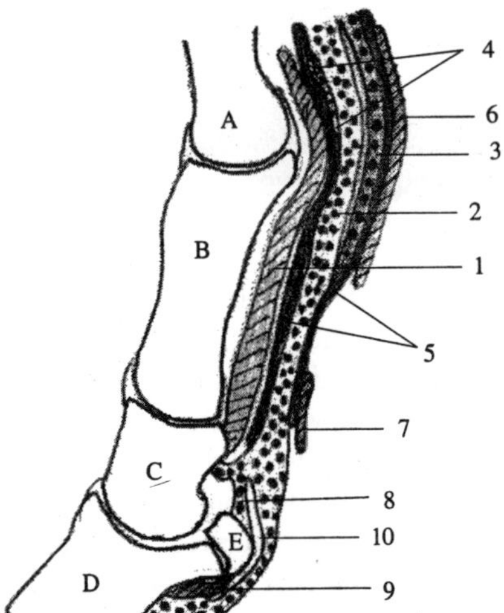

Fig. 9.4. Sagittal section of the digit and distal metacarpus. **1** = straight sesamoidian ligament, **2** = deep digital flexor tendon, **3** = superficial digital flexor tendon, **4** = ring formed by S.D.F.T., **5** = digital flexor tendon sheath, **6** = proximal annular ligament, **7** = distal annular ligament, **8** = collateral sesamoidian ligament, **9** = impar ligament, **10** = navicular bursa; **A** = third metacarpus, **B** = first phalange, **C** = second phalange, **D** = third phalange, **E** = navicular bone.

Zone P1A

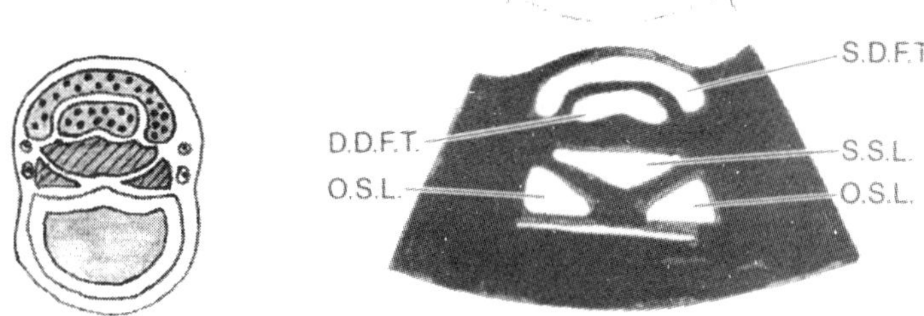

The S.D.F.T. forms a crescent-shaped structure wrapping around the palmar aspect of the bi-lobed D.D.F.T. The S.S.L. forms an inverted triangular structure in the midline, posterior to the palmar border of the first phalange with the medial and lateral O.S.L.s forming small wedge-shaped structures either side.

Zone P1B

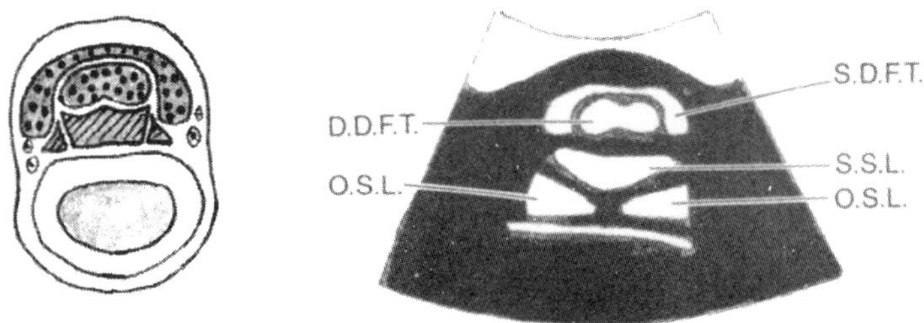

The S.D.F.T. becomes narrow in its midline (approximately 3 mm) but enlarged in its medial and lateral margins to form a bi-lobed structure. The D.D.F.T. remains similar in shape and size, as do the sesamoidian ligaments.

Zone P1C

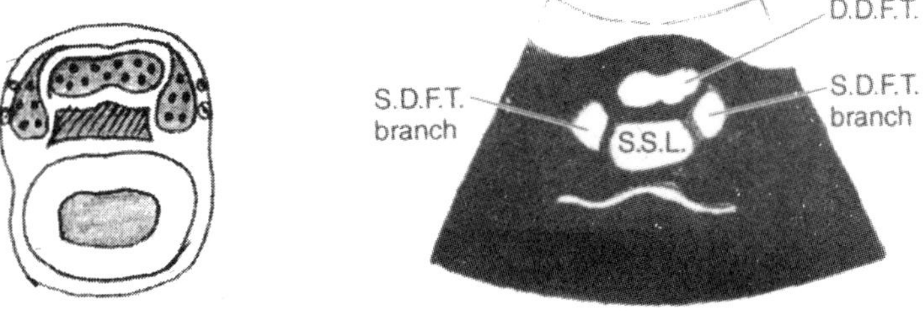

The S.D.F.T. has divided into two branches either side of the D.D.F.T. and extends distally to insert on the distal extremity of the first phalanx and the emi-

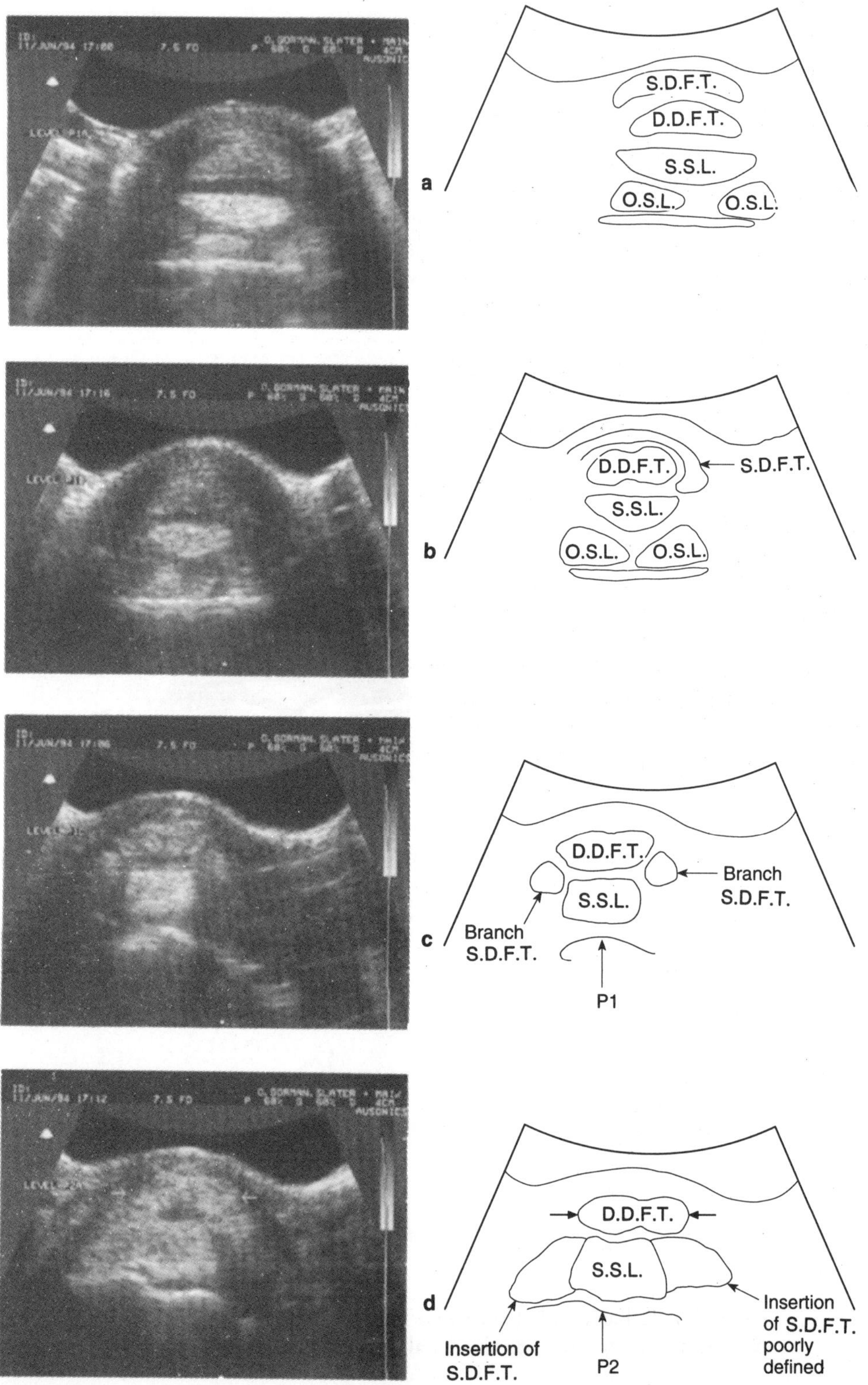
a
S.D.F.T.
D.D.F.T.
S.S.L.
O.S.L.
O.S.L.
b
D.D.F.T.
S.D.F.T.
S.S.L.
O.S.L.
O.S.L.
c
D.D.F.T.
Branch
S.D.F.T.
S.S.L.
Branch
S.D.F.T.
P1
d
D.D.F.T.
S.S.L.
Insertion of
S.D.F.T.
P2
Insertion
of S.D.F.T.
poorly
defined

nences of the proximal extremity of the second phalanx. The S.S.L. has become
more rectangular and the O.S.L.s have disappeared, having inserted on the palmar
surface of the first phalanx approximately at the junction between Zones P1B and
P1C. At the distal end of Zone P1C the insertions of the S.D.F.T. and the S.S.L.
become closely associated, forming a trapezeus-shaped structure which continues into Zone P2A.

Zone P2A

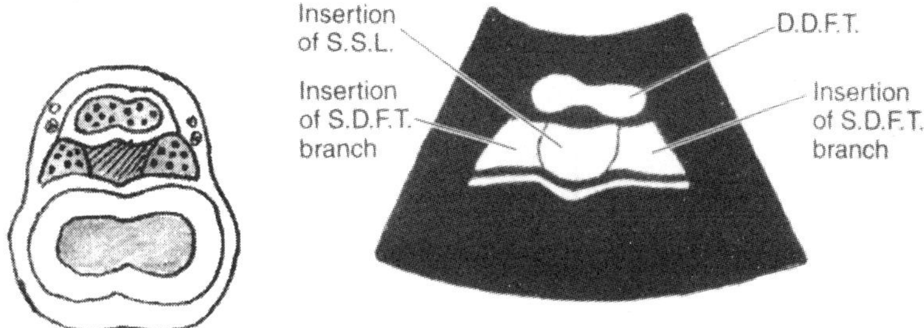

Only a short length of the second phalange (P2) is able to be examined ultrasonically before it disappears below the bulbs of the heel. The insertions of the
S.S.L. and S.D.F.T. form dense echogenic trapezeus-shaped structures palmar to
P2 which end abruptly approximately 10 mm distal to the proximal P2, merging
with the bony prominence on the palmar proximal aspect of P2. The D.D.F.T.
remains bi-lobed and disappears as it continues distally into the hoof.

The carpal canal

The main structures to be imaged in the carpal canal are the S.D.F.T. and
D.D.F.T. and their associated common tendon sheath. The tendon sheath may
only be visible if thickened and/or distended by synovial fluid. The S.D.F.T. in
the carpal canal is more rounded than when seen posterior to the metacarpus. The
carpal canal can be imaged by placing the probe on the palmar medial aspect of the
carpus where the tendons run between the accessory carpal bone and the medial
carpus.

The extensor tendons of the carpus

The tendons which can be imaged are located on the anterior lateral aspect of the
carpus and consist of the long (common) digital extensor tendon (L.D.E.T.), the
lateral digital extensor tendon (Lt.D.E.T.) and the extensor carpi radialis (E.C.R.)

Fig. 9.5. Sonograms of the normal pastern. The scans also demonstrate off-normal incidence (ONI)
artifact in the pastern region. **(a)** Level P1A. The S.D.F.T. is partly hidden due to ONI artifact. **(b)** Level
P1B. The S.D.F.T. is partly hidden due to ONI artifact. **(c)** Level P1C. **(d)** Level P2A.

and their associated tendon sheaths. The probe is placed on the identified tendon and, if the structure is normal, a uniformly echoic round to oval structure is visible with thin anechoic and echoic lines surrounding it, representing fluid within the sheath and the sheath itself. It is useful to use the normal, contralateral leg for comparison when imaging a suspected damaged tendon sheath.

The hock

Schematic diagrams of the normal anatomy of the hock are shown in Figs 9.6 and 9.7.

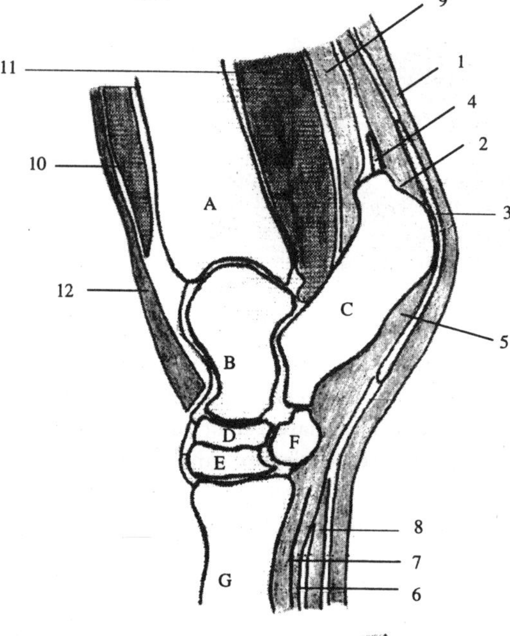

Fig. 9.6. Sagittal section of the hock, cut through lateral aspect. **1** = superficial digital flexor tendon, **2** = gastrocnemius tendon, **3** = gastrocnemius bursa, **4** = calcaneal bursa, **5** = plantar ligament, **6** = inferior check ligament, **7** = suspensory ligament, **8** = deep digital flexor tendon, **9** = tarsal tendon of biceps femoris, **10** = tibialis cranialis muscle, **11** = deep digital flexor muscle, **12** = peroneus tertius; **A** = tibia, **B** = talus, **C** = calcaneal tuber, **D** = central tarsal bone, **E** = third tarsal bone, **F** = fourth tarsal bone, **G** = third metatarsal bone.

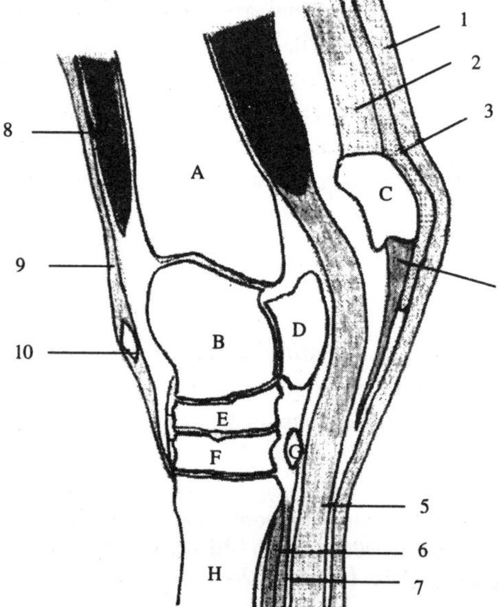

Fig. 9.7. Sagittal section of the hock, cut through middle of groove of trochlear. **1** = superficial digital flexor tendon, **2** = gastrocnemius tendon, **3** = calcaneal bursa, **4** = plantar ligament, **5** = deep digital flexor tendon, **6** = suspensory ligament, **7** = inferior check ligament, **8** = tibialis cranialis muscle, **9** = peroneus tertius, **10** = medial tendon of tibialis cranialis; **A** = tibia, **B** = talus, **C** = calcaneal tuber, **D** = sustentaculum, **E** = central tarsal bone, **F** = third tarsal bone, **G** = fourth tarsal bone, **H** = third metatarsal bone.

Proximal to the tuber calcis

The main structures to be imaged proximal to the tuber calcis are the gastrocnemius tendon and the S.D.F.T. The gastrocnemius tendon forms as the common tendon to the medial and lateral heads of the gastrocnemius muscle. It forms approximately half way between the stifle and the tuber calcis, and initially lies plantar to the S.D.F.T. In its mid-portion, however, it spirals around the S.D.F.T. and comes to lie deep to it. The S.D.F.T. lies under the gastrocnemius tendon proximally. It is a dense, oval echoic structure which becomes more flattened and crescent-shaped as it spirals around the gastrocnemius tendon and runs distally to insert on the tuber calcis. A large bursa (the calcanean bursa) lies between the two tendons from the twist distally to the middle of the hock, terminating around the level of the fourth tarsal bone. When imaged, the calcanean bursa is seen as a thin anechoic line between the S.D.F.T. and gastrocnemius tendon. A small bursa (the gastrocnemius bursa) lies dorsal to the insertion of the gastrocnemius tendon above the tuber calcis. This also appears as a thin anechoic line between the tendon and the tuber calcis. A small subcutaneous bursa may exist over the insertion of the S.D.F.T. on the tuber calcis. This is commonly enlarged and known as a capped hock which, when imaged, is seen as an anechogenic area of variable size, depending on the degree of damage/distension.

Distal to the tuber calcis

The main structures to be imaged distal to the tuber calcis are the S.D.F.T., the plantar ligament and the D.D.F.T. The S.D.F.T. runs distally on the plantar aspect of the hock continuing into the metatarsus. When imaged proximally it appears as a dense, echoic, flattened oval structure which becomes less flattened as it runs distally towards the metatarsus. The plantar ligament arises from the lateral aspect of the plantar surface of the tuber calcis and inserts on to the fourth tarsal bone and proximal fourth metatarsal bone. When imaged, it appears as a dense, echoic, oval structure extending from just below the point of the hock and disappearing at the proximal metatarsus. Approximately half way along its length the D.D.F.T. appears on its medial aspect. The D.D.F.T., when imaged, appears as a dense, echoic structure which is seen from mid-tarsus and continues into the metatarsus.

The metatarsus

The metatarsus appears very similarly to the metacarpus when imaged using ultrasound. The main difference is the greater length of the metatarsus. Therefore the metatarsus is divided into eight zones (1A–4B). The I.C.L. is a much less developed structure in the metatarsus than in the metacarpus, being of less width and depth.

The peroneus tertius

The peroneus tertius (P.T.) forms part of the horse's passive stay apparatus. It lies on the anterior lateral aspect of the tibia, originating from the distal lateral aspect of the femur (extensor fossa), and inserts at the distal tibia dividing into two branches: the cranial branch inserting on the proximal third metatarsal bone and third tarsal bone, and the lateral branch inserting onto the calcaneus and fourth tarsal bone. It is entirely tendinous throughout its length. To image the P.T., place the probe on the anterior lateral aspect of the tibia, just below the stifle joint between the long digital extensor and the lateral digital extensor. The P.T. is a dense, echoic, flask-shaped structure lying between the less echoic muscle bellies of the long digital extensor and the cranialis tibialis.

Artifacts

The formation of artifacts can be a source of misdiagnosis, especially in the hands of an inexperienced operator. A basic understanding of why artifacts occur, and a good knowledge of where the most common artifacts occur is essential. To differentiate an artifact from a potential lesion it is necessary to move the probe up and down, changing the angle of the probe relative to the suspected lesion to check whether it is repeatable and, if possible, to demonstrate the suspected lesion in both the horizontal and vertical planes.

Refraction artifact

When an ultrasound beam travels through a round interface such as the side wall of a blood vessel, the beam becomes slightly diverted producing a shadow deep to the curved interface. This is most commonly seen in the metacarpal region. Figure 9.8 shows a refraction artifact produced by the metacarpal blood vessels giving the illusion of an anechoic area in the suspensory ligament. A schematic illustration of refraction artifact is shown in Fig. 9.9.

Off-normal incidence

Large specular reflectors such as the D.D.F.T. and the S.D.F.T. need to be scanned at 90°. This is easily accomplished when the tendons are running parallel to each other. However, in the region of the pastern the tendons are not parallel and off-normal incidence artifacts are common (Figs 9.8 and 9.9).

Acoustic shadowing

When an ultrasound beam reaches an interface where there is a large difference in acoustic impedence (i.e. soft tissue–bone or soft tissue–air) then a large amount of the beam will be reflected, leaving little to travel deep to the next interface. Hence the structures deep to the interface will be hidden as most of the ultrasound beam will have been attenuated.

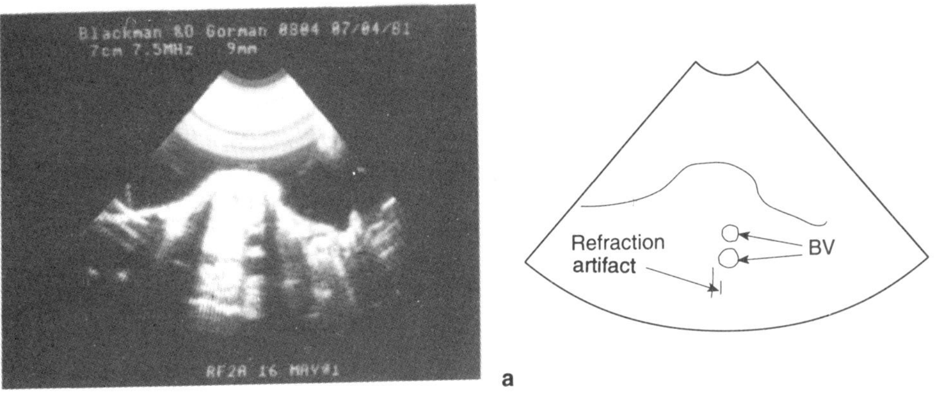

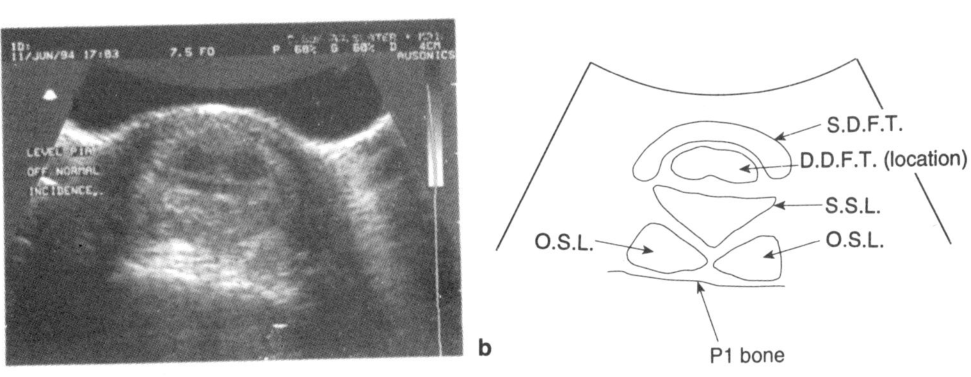

Fig. 9.8. (a) Grade 2 core lesion in the S.D.F.T. with refraction artifact in suspensory ligament from blood vessels (BV). **(b)** Pastern, level P1A. The D.D.F.T. is not visible, due to an off-normal incidence artifact.

Acoustic enhancement

When an ultrasound beam travels through tissue of low acoustic impedence (i.e. with few interfaces) such as fluid, then little attenuation of the ultrasound beam will occur and hence the interfaces deeper to the fluid may appear more echoic. This may be seen when imaging structures such as synovial sheaths, especially if they are distended by excess fluid.

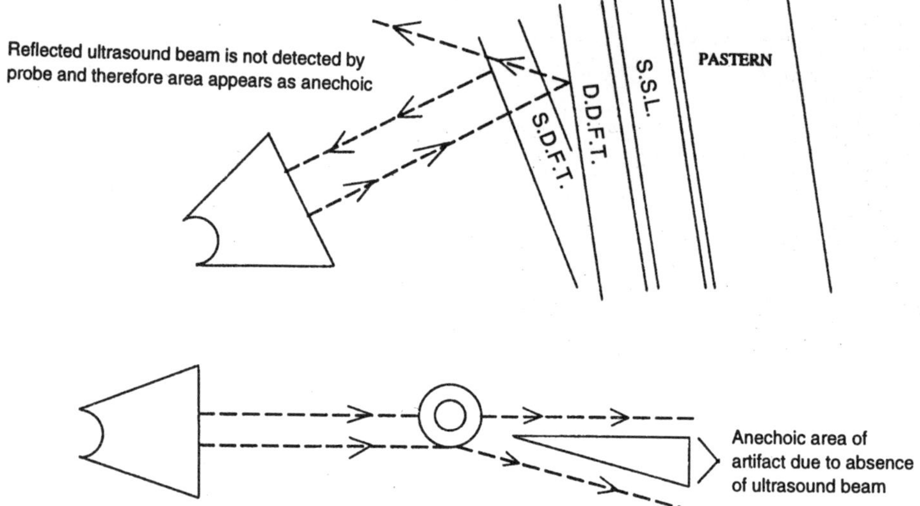

Fig. 9.9. Off-normal incidence artifact (top); refraction artifact (bottom).

Histopathology of Tendon Damage and Healing

Histological examinations of areas of acute tendon damage have demonstrated varying degrees of disruption of collagen fibres in endotendon and peritendon, infiltration by migrating polymorphonuclear and macrophage cells interspersed with haemorrhage, fibrin deposition, and inflammatory exudate containing collagenases and proteases from damaged cells. This initial phase of acute injury is followed by a second phase in which granulation tissue predominates, with the proliferation of endotendon and peritendon (up to approximately two months post-injury), followed by a third phase in which fibroplasia predominates, with increased numbers of fibroblasts and tenocytes and the formation of immature collagen fibres. From six months onwards, a fourth phase consisting of reorganization and maturation of tendon healing occurs, with a reduction in the number of fibroblasts, realignment of the collagen fibres, and an increase in intramolecular and intermolecular linkages. A good correlation between these histopathological changes during tendon healing and ultrasound appearance can be demonstrated (Table 9.1). Re-examination by ultrasound at three, six and twelve months post-injury allows careful monitoring of the macroscopic healing process.

Table 9.1. Comparative histopathological and ultrasound appearance during tendon healing. Time refers to weeks after tendon damage.

Stage of healing	Histopathology	Horizontal ultrasound appearance	Longitudinal ultrasound appearance
Stage 1 (0–1 week): Acute injury	Disruption of collagen fibres/ endotendon/peritendon. Infiltration of polymorphs and macrophages. Haemorrhage, fibrin deposition, inflammatory exudate containing collagenases and proteases	Hypoechoic, hypoechoic/ anechoic mixed, or anechoic (Disrupted collagen fibres can act as non-specular reflectors)	Hypoechoic, hypoechoic/ anechoic mixed, or anechoic reduction in linear echoes. Irregular pattern
Stage II (1–8 weeks): Resorption, granulation	Infiltration of granulation tissue. Proliferation of endotendon and peritendon	Hypoechoic, hypoechoic/ anechoic mixed, or anechoic	Hypoechoic, hypoechoic/ anechoic mixed or anechoic. Reduction in linear echoes. Irregular pattern
Stage III (6–26 weeks): Fibroplasia	Infiltration of fibroblasts. Increased size and number of tenocytes. Formation of immature collagen fibres. Some acute areas of haemorrhage due to stress on immature fibrous tissue	Increasing echogenicity compared to Stage II but still hypoechoic	Increasing echogenicity compared to Stage II but still hypoechoic. Increased numbers of short linear echoes but still irregular pattern
Stage IV (26 weeks onwards): Reorganization	Reduction in number of cells – fibroblasts and tenocytes. Increased collagen fibres. Increased inter- and intra-molecular linkages. Some active areas of haemorrhage (as above)	Increasing echogenicity with lesion starting to blend with surrounding tendon (Realigned collagen fibres act as specular reflectors)	Increasing echogenicity with lesion starting to blend with surrounding tendon. Increased number of long linear fibres and more regular pattern

Ultrasonic Appearance of Common Pathological Lesions

Superficial digital flexor tendon

Peritendinous oedema

This can occur as the result of minor external trauma to the subcutaneous tissues and the paratendon. The most common causes are bandage pinch or a minor blow. The S.D.F.T. will appear normal on ultrasound examination but the paratendon will be separated from the skin by an enlarged anechoic area representing oedematous fluid. The palmar/plantar edges of the paratendon may appear hyperechoic, due to acoustic enhancement as the ultrasound beam travels through the oedematous fluid which forms a fluid–soft tissue interface.

Peritendinous haemorrhage

This is usually seen in association with significant damage to the paratendon and or the S.D.F.T. Haemorrhagic fluid appears as a hypoechoic area between the paratendon and the skin (Fig. 9.10). In severe cases this hypoechoic area may

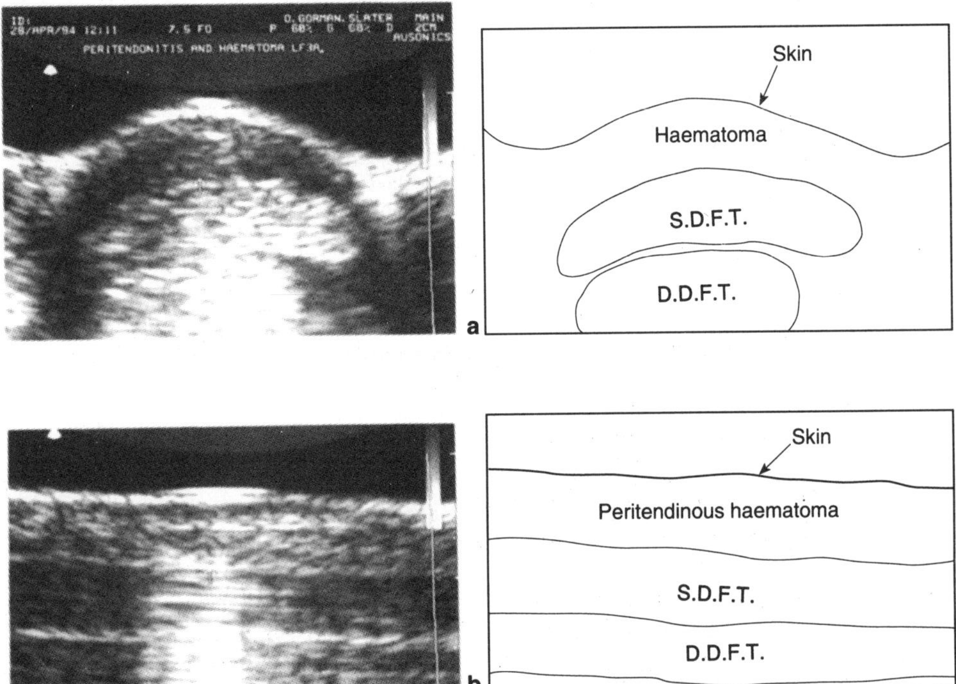

Fig. 9.10. Peritendinous damage. **(a)** Horizontal scan, peritendinous haematoma. **(b)** Longitudinal scan, peritendinous haematoma.

extend around the medial and lateral margins of the S.D.F.T., encroaching on the D.D.F.T., the metacarpal/tarsal blood vessels and the I.C.L. Such extensive haemorrhage may result in later adhesions.

Core lesions

The most common pathological damage to the S.D.F.T. is disruption of tendon fibres within a localized area, forming a damaged core within the tendon. On ultrasound examination in the horizontal plane this core will appear as an area of decreased echogenicity within the normally echoic tendon. The core lesion can be graded I to IV according to the ultrasound appearance in the horizontal plane (Fig. 9.11) and 0 to IV according to the ultrasound appearance in the longitudinal

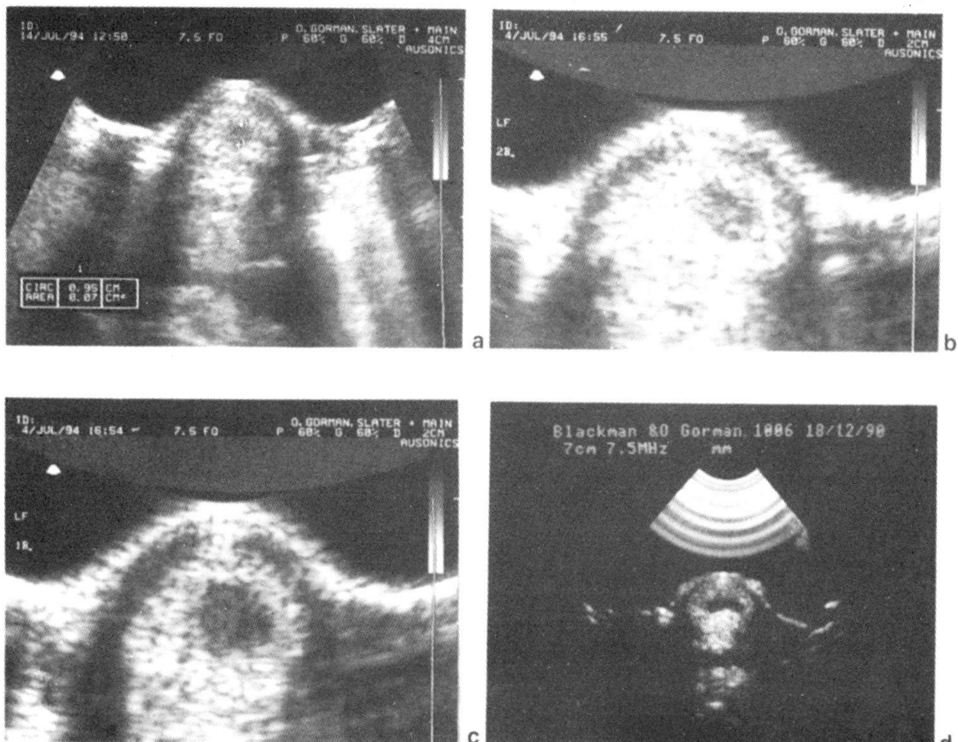

Fig. 9.11. Core lesions of increasing severity in the S.D.F.T. (horizontal view). **(a)** Grade I. **(b)** Grade II. **(c)** Grade III. **(d)** Grade IV.

plane (Fig. 9.12; Table 9.2). The length, width and depth of the core lesion should be measured. If the scanner has the capability, then measurement of the cross-sectional areas of the core lesion, the damaged tendon and the contralateral tendon at the same level should also be made. A simple calculation using these

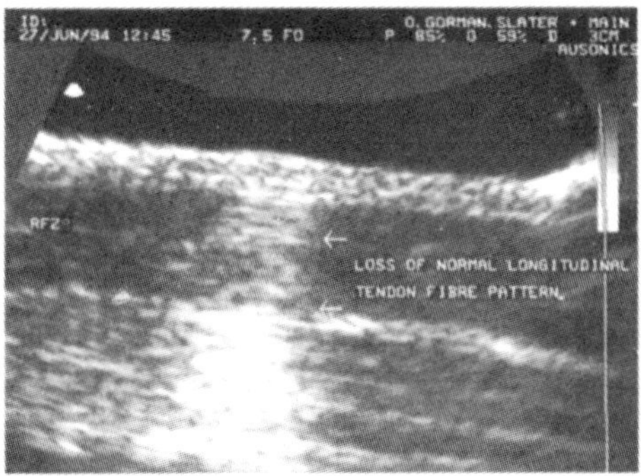

Fig. 9.12. Grade I S.D.F.T. injury (longitudinal view).

measurements allows the area of the damaged core to be expressed as a percentage of the normal tendon area:

$$\% \text{ of tendon damage} = 100 \times (A - (B - C))\,/A$$

where A = cross-sectional area of the normal contralateral tendon at the same level as the damaged tendon, B = area of the damaged tendon, and C = area of the core lesion.

Table 9.2. Classification of core lesions.

	Grade	Description	Severity	
Horizontal plane	I	More echoic than anechoic	Moderate	
	II	Equally echoic and anechoic		
	III	More anechoic than echoic		
	IV	Anechoic	Severe	↓
Longitudinal plane	0	Normal parallel linear echoes	Normal	
	I	Numerous irregular long linear echoes	Moderate	
	II	Few irregular long linear echoes		
	III	Short irregular linear echoes		
	IV	No linear echoes	Severe	↓

Rupture of the S.D.F.T.

If total rupture of the S.D.F.T. has occured then usually clinical signs are sufficient to confirm the diagnosis. More commonly, ultrasound is used to quantify the degree of partial rupture of the S.D.F.T. When examined using ultrasound, the area between the ruptured ends appears irregularly hypoechoic/anechoic in the horizontal and longitudinal planes. In the longitudinal plane there will be no linear echoes within the damaged area. It should be noted that the area of damage can be surprisingly echoic (Fig. 9.13).

Fibrosis and adhesions of the S.D.F.T.

Chronic fibrosis of the S.D.F.T. may occur during the healing phase following tendon injury. On ultrasound examination the tendon appears hypoechoic with irregular hyperechoic foci interspersed. On a longitudinal scan short linear hyperechoic echoes are interspersed. The paratendon may appear hyperechoic and thickened and there may be a lack of differentiation between the D.D.F.T. and S.D.F.T., representing adhesions. It may be helpful to have the leg non-weight-bearing and to gently flex/extend it while scanning in order to identify adhesions.

Deep digital flexor tendon

Remarkably little primary pathological damage occurs to the D.D.F.T. Core lesions within the D.D.F.T. are rare and predominately in the lower third/quarter of the metacarpus/metatarsus. Adhesions around the D.D.F.T. usually involve the S.D.F.T. and/or the I.C.L. The D.D.F.T. may be involved in the annular ligament syndrome involving the digital sheath.

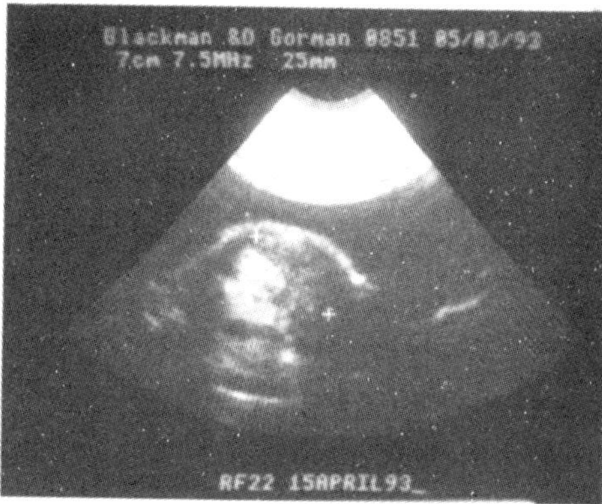

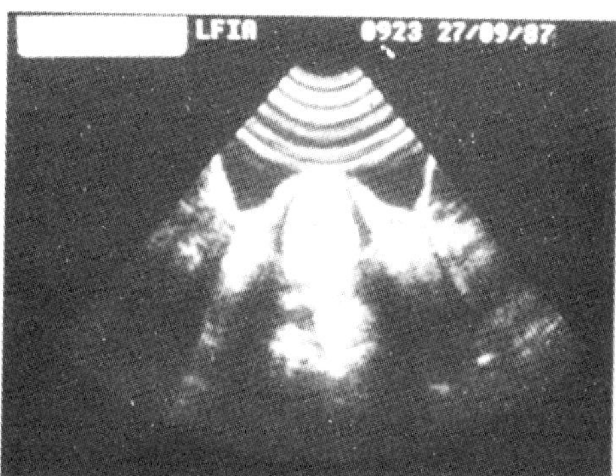

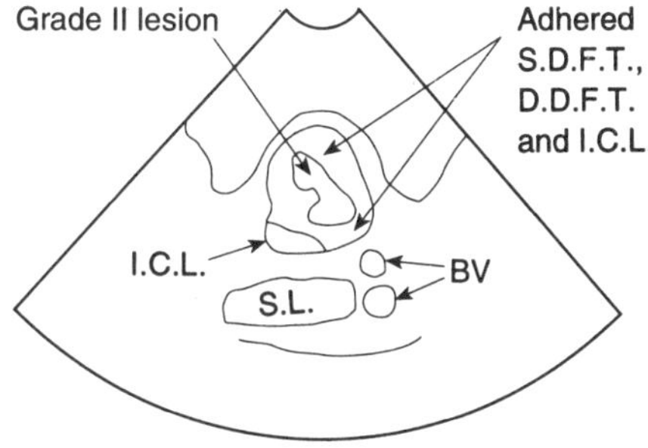

Fig. 9.13. (a) Ruptured S.D.F.T. Diffuse hypoechoic area where S.D.F.T. should be, representing an organizing haematoma. **(b)** Chronic adhesions between S.D.F.T., D.D.F.T. and I.C.L. and a Grade II lesion. BV = blood vessels.

Inferior check ligament

Desmitis of the I.C.L. is seen most commonly in jumping animals and ponies. Ultrasound findings can be variable, but some of the ultrasound features of I.C.L. desmitis are listed below and illustrated in Fig. 9.14.

- Generalized thickening of the I.C.L. with narrowing of the space between the I.C.L. and the S.L.
- An irregular 'ragged' appearance to the outline of the I.C.L.
- A hypoechoic or anechoic core within the I.C.L., or more commonly, a generalized diffuse hypoechoic pattern seen within a large area of the I.C.L.
- Loss of differentiation between the I.C.L., the D.D.F.T. and the S.D.F.T. due to a hypoechoic area between the I.C.L., the D.D.F.T. and the dorsal margins of the S.D.F.T. This hypoechoic area represents adhesions between the I.C.L., D.D.F.T. and S.D.F.T. and may involve the digital blood vessels, which may be enlarged.
- Irregular hyperechoic/hypoechoic and anechoic areas forming a mottled irregular pattern. This irregular pattern is seen particulary in chronic cases where injuries have recurred due to poor healing. The hyperechoic areas represent chronic fibrosis.

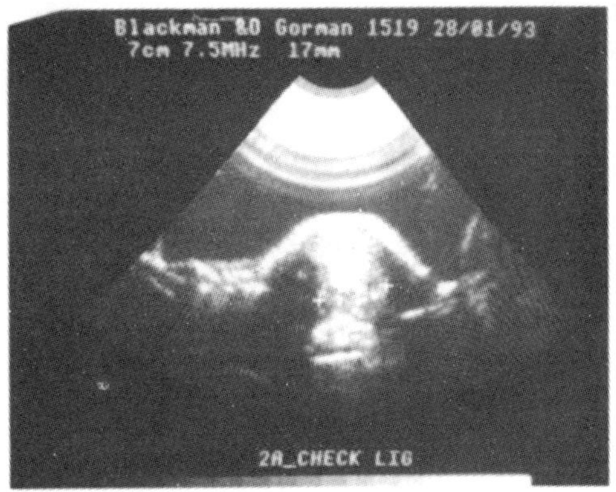

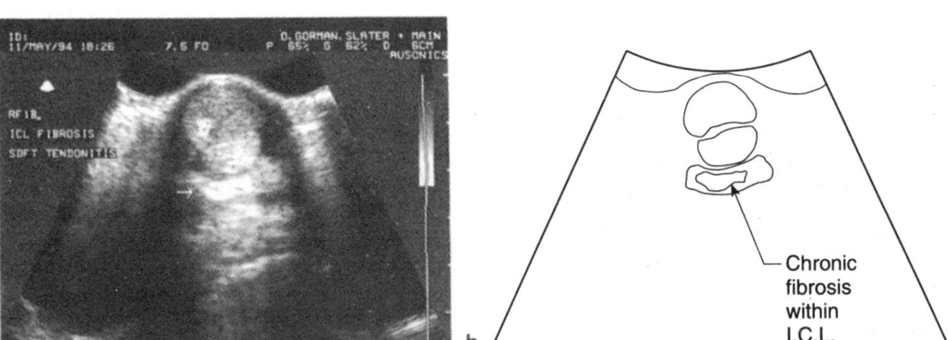

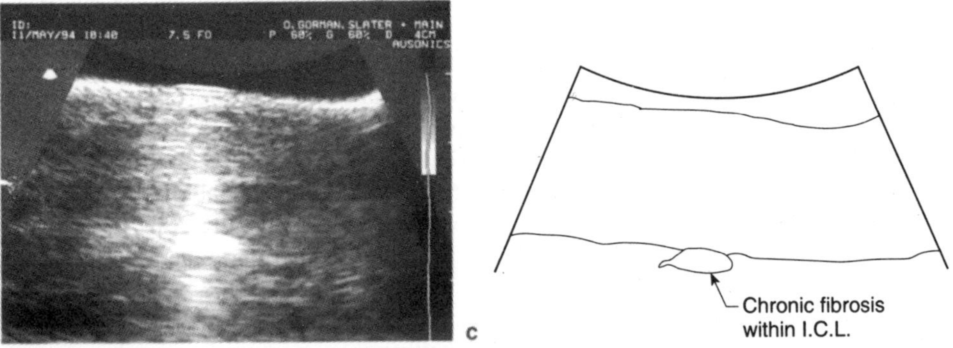

Fig. 9.14. (a) Chronic I.C.L. desmitis between crosses. **(b)**Irregular hypo- and hyperechoic pattern (arrow). **(c)** Hyperechoic lesions within the I.C.L. representing chronic fibrosis (longitudinal section).

Suspensory ligament

The normal appearance of the suspensory ligament is shown in Fig. 9.15. Desmitis of the suspensory ligament can be divided into three main regions: the origin and the proximal third, the middle third to the bifurcation, and the branches, with their insertion onto the sesamoid bones.

The two heads of origin of the suspensory ligament appear as two circular, echoic structures at level 1A. On ultrasound examination these two heads may often appear as a single structure with a central hypoechoic area. It is easy to confuse this hypoechoic area with a significant hypoechoic lesion and it is most important to compare the contralateral leg before diagnosing a pathological lesion in this area. The most common pathological lesion in this area appears as a well-circumscribed anechoic core within the S.L. on ultrasound examination.

Injury to the middle zone of the S.L. is usually associated with a large degree of thickening. Ultrasound evaluation of the thickening often reveals a diffuse hypoechoic area with an obvious increase in width and thickening of the S.L. (Fig. 9.16).

The S.L. branches are easiest to view ultrasonically on their respective medial and lateral surfaces in the horizontal and longitudinal planes (ski jump view). The ski jump view is particularly useful for assessment of the insertion of the S.L. branches and for checking the integrity of the bony surface of the abaxial sesamoid bone. Areas of bony avulsion from the abaxial surface appear on ultrasound as focal hyperechoic areas around the abaxial surface, with acoustic shadowing below if the avulsed bone is of reasonable size (Fig. 9.16). Small hyperechoic areas may be seen up to 4 cm proximal to the insertion of the S.L. branch. This represents small areas of calcification within the S.L. Ultrasound examination of a thickened branch most frequently reveals a hypoechoic core lesion within the branch. However, occasionally the branch appears to be normal on ultrasound examination, and the thickening is due to haemorrhage surrounding the branch. This hypoechoic area may extend to the other branch and the area between the branches. This haemorrhage usually originates from acute damage around the bifurcation of the suspensory ligament.

Annular ligament

The annular ligament (A.L.) forms a canal with the sesamoid bones and intercarpal ligaments through which the S.D.F.T., the D.D.F.T. and their tendon sheaths travel. Any restrictions of movement characterized by lameness, pain, distension of the tendon sheath and a characteristic notch above the annular ligament are collectively known as the annular ligament syndrome. Ultrasound examination has allowed the syndrome to be divided into four categories. It should be noted that the annular ligament is not normally visible unless thickened. The annular ligament of an average Thoroughbred is normally 1-2 mm in thickness, while a thickened annular ligament can measure up to 6 mm. Comparison with the contralateral leg is very useful (Fig. 9.17).

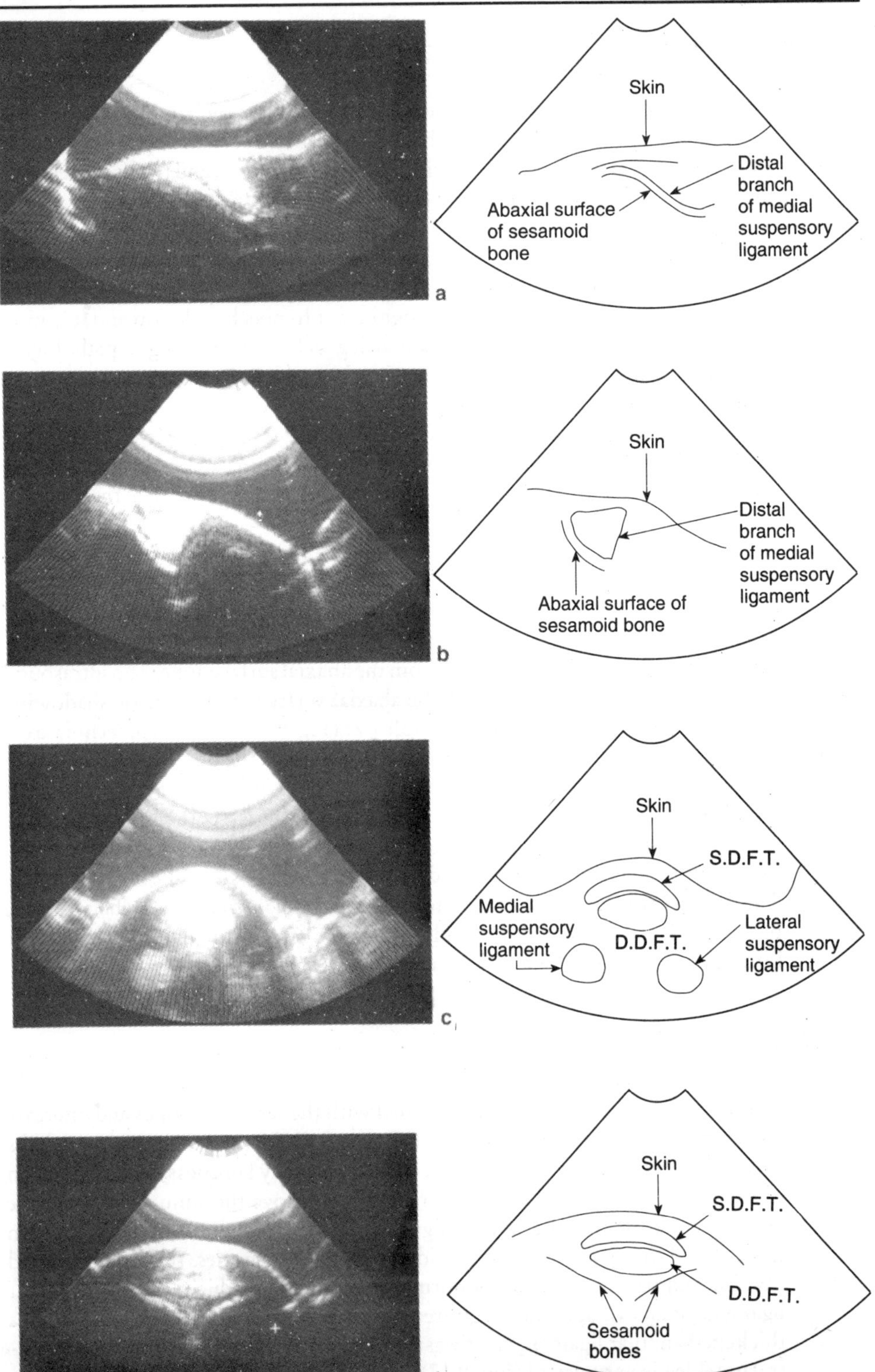

Fig. 9.15. Views of the normal suspensory ligament. **(a)** Longitudinal view of the distal branch of the medial suspensory ligament, taken from medial aspect. **(b)** Horizontal view of the distal branch of the medial suspensory ligament. **(c)** Horizontal view, level 3A. **(d)** 'Gull-wing' view. Horizontal view, level 3B.

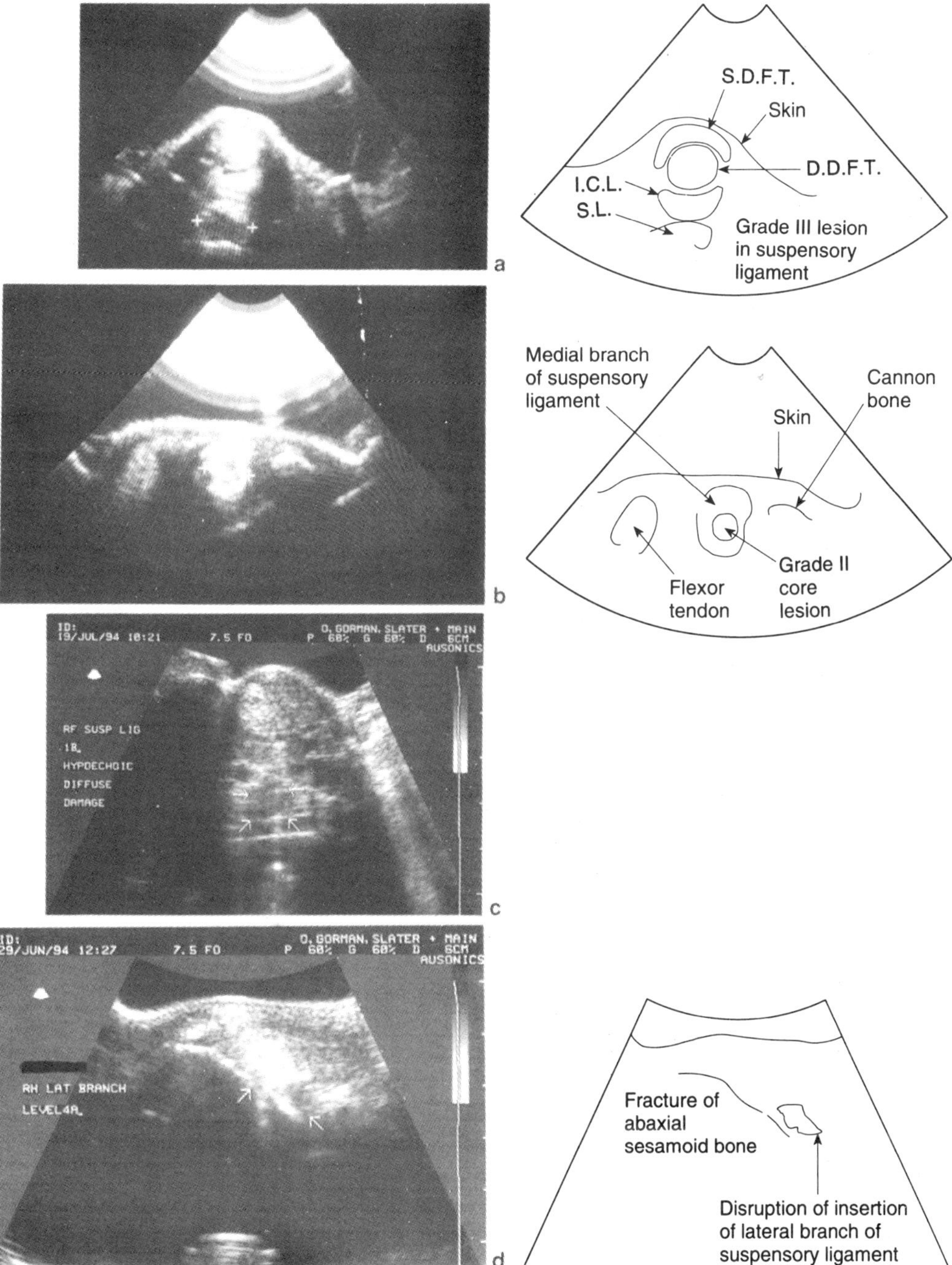

Fig. 9.16. Suspensory ligament lesions. **(a)** Grade III hypoechoic lesion within the body of the suspensory ligament. Horizontal view, level 2A. **(b)** Grade II core lesion within the medial branch of the suspensory ligament. Horizontal view from medial aspect. **(c)** Grade II diffuse hypoechoic lesion (arrows) within the suspensory ligament. Level 1B. **(d)** Longitudinal view of the lateral branch of the suspensory ligament from lateral aspect, showing fracture of sesamoid bone (arrows) and disruption of insertion of the lateral branch of the suspensory ligament. Level 4A.

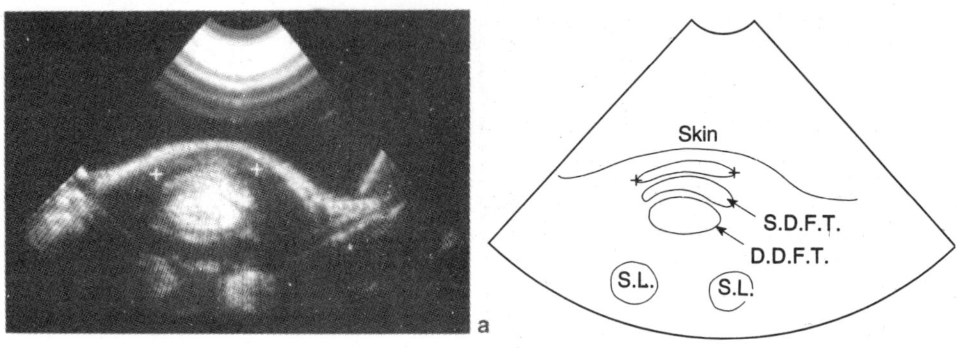

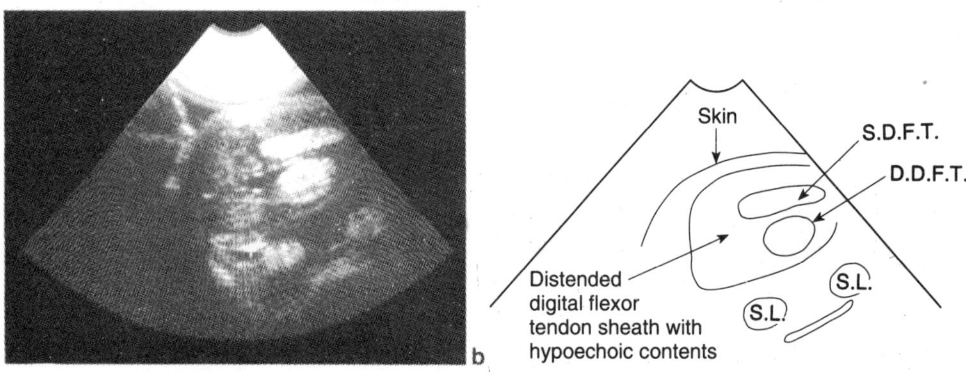

Fig. 9.17. Annular ligament syndrome. **(a)** Type I. Thickened annular ligament between crosses. **(b)** Type II. Distended sheath with hypoechoic inflammatory exudate.

The four categories of annular ligament syndrome are as follows:

Type I   Primary thickening of A.L. with distension of the digital sheath due to constriction. The S.D.F.T. and D.D.F.T. appear normal.

Type II   Distension of the digital sheath with no thickening of the annual ligament. The S.D.F.T. and D.D.F.T. appear normal. A primary synovitis.

Type III   Thickening of the S.D.F.T. usually associated with a hypoechoic core lesion at level 3A/3B. Thickening of the annular ligament, distension of the digital sheath.

Type IV   Thickening of the subcutaneous tissue palmar/plantar to the annular ligament. Distension of the synovial sheath. Normal annular ligament, S.D.F.T and D.D.F.T.

10 Real-time Diagnostic Ultrasound in Bovine Reproduction

J.S. Boyd
*Department of Veterinary Anatomy, University of Glasgow,
Veterinary School, Bearsden Road, Glasgow G61 1QH, UK*

Introduction

The use of real-time, B-mode diagnostic ultrasound has been increasing as an imaging modality in bovine reproduction, as it becomes more apparent that its use can produce solutions to a number of hitherto unanswered questions in dealing with the bovine reproductive cycle and its concurrent disorders. The purpose of this chapter is to attempt to describe the types of equipment necessary for carrying out effective ultrasonographic examinations and to describe the technique involved, as well as taking note of the misinterpretations that can arise due to artifacts. This will be followed by an indication of the applications for use, with illustrations, using ultrasonography to demonstrate the relevant structures of the bovine reproductive tract.

Equipment

Ultrasound scanners fall broadly into two formats, linear and sector, with both being applicable to use in reproductive studies. Linear scanners produce a rectangular image which is easier to interpret with no image distortion in the upper area of the scan picture. They tend to be more robust, as the transducer has no moving parts which can be distorted or wear out, and generally cost less. The transducer face has a larger footprint and therefore requires a larger window for application to the surface to be scanned, although this is not usually a problem with intrarectal reproductive scanning. The majority of linear transducers have a straight linear array (and thus this disadvantage of footprint size), and the scanning face is placed to the side, so that they look laterally when orientated with the longitudinal axis of the body. More recent developments have seen the introduction of microconvex linear transducers which have the array of crystals arranged so that the footprint size is greatly reduced without distortion of the image. Such transducers are now available for reproductive scanning, particularly in transvaginal use. The scanning face can be placed at an angle eccentric to the longitudinal axis, and in some cases this angle can be varied without movement of the transducer.

Sector scanners produce an arc-shaped segmental image, which causes some distortion at the edges, and also a lack of definition in the upper section of the picture. The sector transducers which are generally available in the veterinary field are mechanically driven. They tend to be more expensive than linear transducers, as well as more vulnerable (due to moving parts), and have a shorter working life. Their footprint size of transducer face is much smaller, but this is of reduced value in reproductive scanning. They tend to have their scanning face looking forward in relation to the longitudinal axis, which is less advantageous in transrectal reproductive scanning, although some manufacturers produce eccentrically angled sector transducers.

Phased array transducers, both annular and linear, are used in reproductive scanning in humans but systems of this type tend to be too expensive to be realistically utilized in the veterinary field.

The choice of frequency of transducer is an important issue in obtaining the best scanning results. The lower the frequency of the transducer, the greater the depth at which useful signals can be obtained, but this is counteracted by a loss of resolution. Conversely, a high-frequency transducer will greatly improve resolution but lack penetration. The broad rule, when working intrarectally, is to use 7.5 MHz for ovarian and early pregnancy studies, 5 MHz for routine pregnancy work over 40 days, and 3.5 MHz for late pregnancy or immediately post-partum. Late pregnancy diagnosis can also be attempted transcutaneously using a 3.5 MHz transducer applied in an inguinal position dorsal to the udder.

Most scanning units will provide freeze-frame facilities, text annotation, zoom magnification and a built-in calliper measurement system with the possibility of a programmable computerized gestational age calculation package. The ability to make good hard copy is vital, and most scanners nowadays will have a video outlet to which a video recorder and/or a video thermal copier can be connected. The latter can produce high-quality reproductions at relatively low cost.

Techniques

For transrectal scanning in cattle, it is not normally necessary to administer any sedation or epidural anaesthesia, as the system is well tolerated and non-invasive. The animal for examination should be adequately restrained and the scanning unit placed at a sensible distance from the cow, on the side opposite to the operator's rectalling arm. The animal's rectum should be evacuated of all faeces prior to introduction of the transducer and it is advantageous to carry out a preliminary manual exploration of the topography of the reproductive tract before commencing the ultrasonographic examination. The transducer face is lubricated with a suitable coupling medium and is usually covered by a lubricated plastic sleeve and inserted in a cupped, lubricated hand through the anal opening, before progressing cranially along the rectal floor to overlie the reproductive tract. The transducer face must be pressed firmly against the rectal mucosa in order to effect ultrasound transmission through the rectal wall into the abdominal viscera. Interposition of any contaminating faeces will prevent good transmission and produce poor imaging and artifactual interference. Faeces can be removed, without withdrawing the transducer, by running a finger over the scan face. Abdominal straining can prove an irritation during transrectal scanning, and the transducer must always be protected in the operator's cupped hand to prevent damage as the waves of contraction ride over the transducer. With the transducer proceeding cranially along the rectal floor, the uterus will be imaged as it lies ventral to the rectum with the urinary bladder even more ventral in position. This will appear as an anechoic or echolucent (black) area with the size dependent on the volume of urine retained. With a full bladder, most of the scan field will be occupied by the black image, but with a relatively empty organ the mucosa will be imaged as a corrugated hypoechoic surface at the periphery of the outline of the organ. It is necessary for the operator to be able to identify the bladder and discard its image from the assessment of the reproductive tract. When the pregnancy is in the left horn, the urinary bladder can be used as a landmark to reach the embryo within its vesicle between days 19 and 25 of pregnancy. In these cases the expanded vesicle is located at the top of the loop of the uterine horn, adjacent to the bladder. Between days 30 and 45, detection of the embryo is difficult when the urinary bladder is full, and so stimulation of the perineum may be necessary to induce urination.

As the uterine body, cervix and vagina are midline structures running craniocaudally, they will be imaged in long-axis view as the transducer advances along the rectal floor. With the transducer moving laterally within the rectum, the uterine horns will be imaged in planes varying from cross sectional to oblique. Further lateral movement should permit imaging of the ovaries as the transducer is angled to left and right. It is beneficial to establish a regular examination routine of all of the reproductive tract, as it allows a standard system of reporting. Such a routine could commence with the right ovary, then move to right uterine horn, left ovary, left uterine horn, uterine body, cervix, vagina and vulva as the transducer is gradually withdrawn from the rectum. When trying to identify detail in the conceptus it can be of advantage on occasions to stimulate movement of the fetus by agitating the uterine horn with gentle pressure on the transducer. Between days 80 and 120 of pregnancy the gravid horn becomes more dependent ventrally within the abdominal cavity, and it may be necessary to draw it caudally by manipulating the cervix by means of gentle digital pressure through the rectal wall. Modification of the scanning technique may be required at different stages of the oestrous cycle, as at the time of oestrus the ovaries are drawn into the coiling of the uterine horns so that the transducer has to be moved onto the lateral aspect of the coiled horns to image the ovaries. There will be occasions when the tract or ovaries themselves will require to be manipulated to obtain a more desirable scanning plane, but in general the tract is usually left undisturbed and the transducer does the moving.

The previous description applies to transrectal scanning, which is the technique used for routine scanning of the reproductive tract for examination of the stage of the oestrous cycle, uterine or ovarian pathology, pregnancy diagnosis and fetal sexing. More recently, a technique for transvaginal ultrasonographic examination has been evolved in cattle for the purpose of ova collection by follicular aspiration and sampling of intrauterine fluids. This technique involves a specialized transducer and the administration of epidural anaesthesia, and will be dealt with in a later section.

Interpretation

Interpretation of sonograms of the reproductive tract requires an understanding of the composition of the images and an awareness of the possible artifacts which can occur and lead to misdiagnosis. For example, acoustic enhancement will appear as an hyperechoic region deep to the fluid (anechoic) area. This can often be seen deep to a large follicle (see later, Fig. 10.22). At the other extreme, gas and bone will totally reflect the sound waves and produce the strongest of echo signals, leading to an image which appears on the screen as near-white. So complete is the return of echoes in some cases, that sound waves do not penetrate deep to these areas, resulting in a lack of imaging which manifests itself as a black zone and is referred to as acoustic shadowing. This must not be interpreted as the anechoic image of fluid-filled structures. Another artifact found with strongly echogenic structures such as gas-filled viscera or bone is the rebounding of echoes back and forth between the object and the transducer. With each cycle of rebound there is loss of signal strength, and this is imaged on the screen as a series of layered hyperechoic images repeating themselves between the object and the transducer face. This is termed reverberation and is often encountered in transrectal scanning where gas-filled viscera are present.

During its passage, ultrasound will encounter interfaces of differing natures. If the interface is wide and smooth there will be almost total return of echoes where the sound waves impinge at right angles, giving an intensified signal that appears on the screen as a whiter shade of grey. This is referred to as specular reflection, and is often seen in early pregnancy when imaging the embryonic vesicle (see later, Fig. 10.12). In fact, specular reflection can occur at both the superficial and the deep interfaces of a circular vesicle, giving two strong echo patterns and thus two small near-white images at both faces of the structure. With even larger fluid-filled structures, artifacts can occur at their periphery due to reflection or refraction of the sound waves travelling from the transducer and the returning echoes. Scatter reflection can add to the information received: as the ultrasound waves meet multiple small interfaces (such as one would find in a structure made up of a variety of cell types), a heterogeneous echotexture is produced on the screen. This mixture of signals is often characteristic of an individual structure, e.g. a corpus luteum (CL), and assists in the identification of that structure from the surrounding ovarian stroma. Similarly, the typical echotexture of an organ can be identified, and changes in this echotexture indicate a change in the physiological state of the organ due to an alteration in the nature of the cell or tissue type, and thus in the tissue interfaces.

Normal Ultrasonographic Anatomy

Ovary

The stroma of the ovary produces a mixed echotexture of hypo- and hyperechoic signals. Depending on the physiological state of the organ, a variety of structures can be imaged within the stroma. In a small, inactive ovary the outer layers (cortex) can be seen to contain small, anechoic follicles (2–8 mm in diameter) while the inner zone (medulla) appears free of follicular activity. In a larger, active ovary the differentiation into zones is less distinct, and the stroma is imaged as narrow, echogenic bands displayed around the more obvious features of CLs and pre-ovulatory follicles (Fig. 10.1).

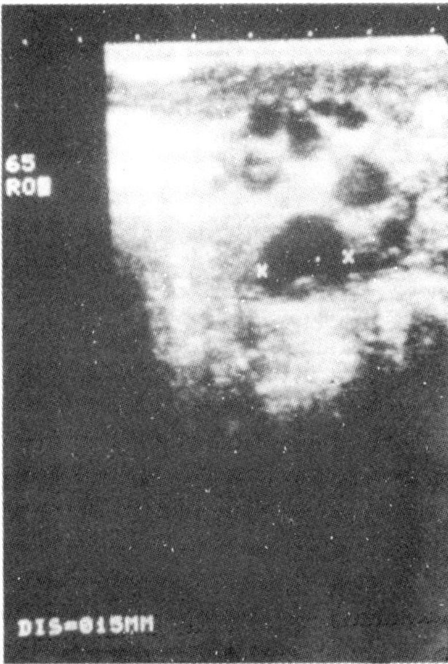

Fig. 10.1. Active ovary from an adult cow. The image of the rectal wall appears longitudinally at the top of the scan field and the ovary is imaged distal to this (7.5 MHz). Anechoic follicles can be seen spread throughout the ovarian stroma. The follicular lumen is indicated by the two cursor crosses which are measuring the overall diameter of the largest follicle.

Corpus luteum (CL)

The cellular components of a mature CL produce an echotexture which is characteristically different from that of the stroma. The echotexture of the image is hypoechoic relative to that of the stroma, and the border is distinct and well-defined. There is intermingling of bright and dark shades within its structure, and the grey shades vary according to the age of the CL, as do its shape, size and position within the ovary. A mature, active CL is large and circular, with a relatively homogeneous echotexture displayed at the periphery of the ovary (Fig. 10.2). The young, newly forming CL (corpus haemorrhagicum) is difficult to discern in its first four days of life, being imaged as an hyperechoic folded structure with a faint dark surrounding line. By six days post-ovulation the CL is well defined in outline and this appearance will persist until 16 days post-ovulation (Fig. 10.3). If pregnancy does not ensue, the CL will regress with a decrease in size

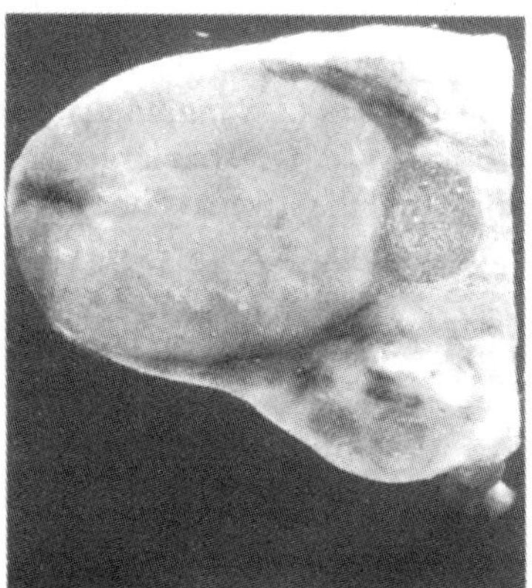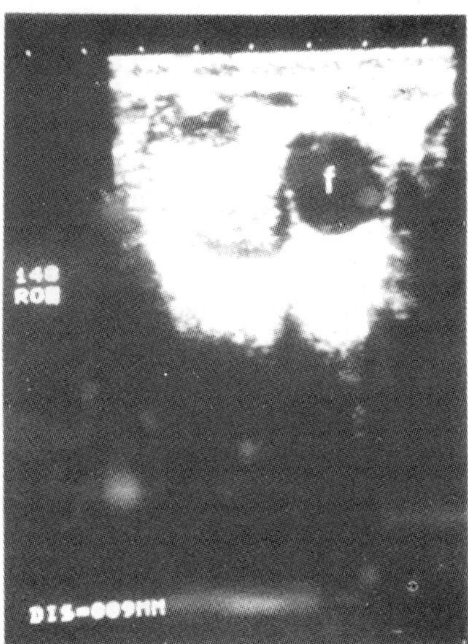

Fig. 10.2. (a) Frozen cross-section of an ovary showing the substance of a corpus luteum (CL) with a follicle placed immediately adjacent to it. Note also the ovarian vessels lying in the top right corner of the ovarian structure. **(b)** Sonogram (7.5 MHz) of an ovary showing the hypoechoic outline of a CL with an anechoic follicle (f) lying adjacent to it. There are small anechoic circular areas in the top right region of the scan image of the ovarian stroma. These are images of ovarian veins. The scan field corresponds to the outline of **a**.

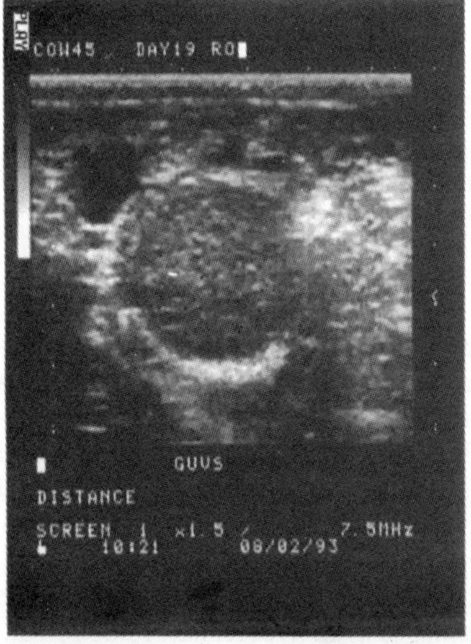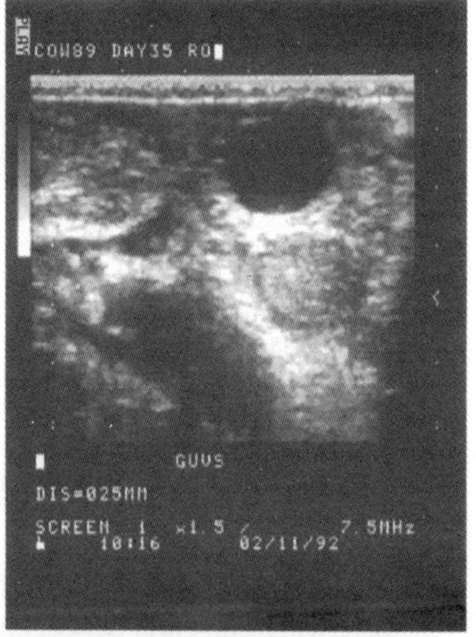

Fig. 10.3. Sonograms (7.5 MHz) of mature active CLs. The CL offers differing acoustic interfaces producing a characteristic degree of scatter with the recognizable outline of its hypoechoic image. The CL in **a** is 19 days post-ovulation. It exhibits a rounded appearance, being placed at the ovarian outer edge, with a good overall even echotexture. In **b**, the ovary lies to the right of the upper scan field. It contains a regressing CL at 5 o'clock, which shows a reduction in size and loss of the homogenous echotexture. There is a new, anechoic dominant follicle apparent at 12 o'clock. A cross-section of uterine horn is imaged at the upper extreme left of the scan.

and a flattening of the outline as the echotexture changes to become increasingly hypoechoic and more heterogeneous. The outline recedes into the stroma and imaging becomes increasingly difficult. By 19 days the appearance has changed considerably and under normal circumstances the next generation of preovulatory follicles will have emerged within the stroma. A CL of pregnancy will retain its shape and consistency beyond 16 days and will continue to be readily imaged within the ovary. A common feature imaged within a CL is the presence of an anechoic centrally placed fluid area (lacuna). Lacunae vary in size in individual cases, but size seems unrelated to the efficacy of the CL, as they are a frequent feature of CLs of pregnancy (Fig. 10.4).

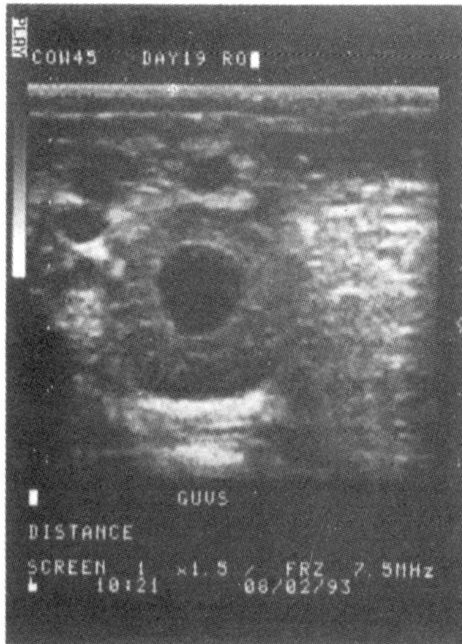

Fig. 10.4. This image (7.5 MHz) is of a CL, centre field, with its hypoechoic echotexture surrounding an anechoic area. The latter represents a fluid-filled lacuna within the CL.

Follicles

In an active ovary, waves of follicles can be followed as they develop and regress during different periods of ovarian cyclicity. Follicles of 2 mm in diameter can be differentiated as individual anechoic structures but their precise outline is not discretely imaged. With increase in size there is increase in definition, and antral follicles are seen as anechoic areas delineated by a sharply imaged follicular wall. Occasional antral follicles are symmetrical and circular (Fig. 10.5) but the more common appearance is asymmetrical, due either to compression by the transducer face or overcrowding within the ovary. The hierarchy of follicular development can be determined and the follicle destined for ovulation can be identified.

The time of ovulation can be predicted by evaluating the structures for a number of factors. The diameter of the follicle will constantly increase as ovulation becomes imminent. Within 12 hours of ovulation, the existing, almost circular, shape changes to a more pear-like shape with pointing of the surface closest to the ovarian perimeter. There is a change in the echogenicity of the follicular wall relative to the ovarian stroma, so that the wall can now be readily differentiated

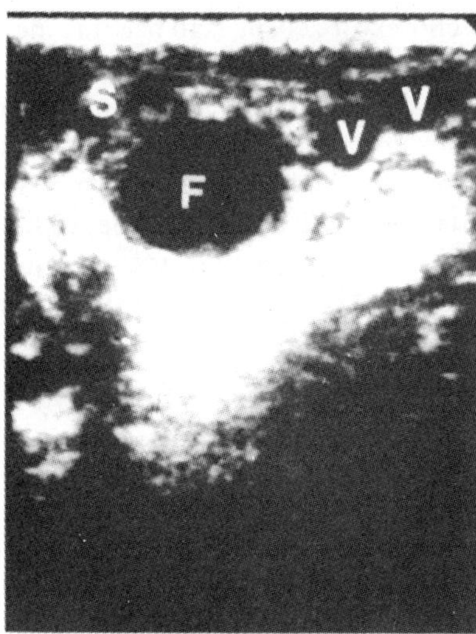

Fig. 10.5. Sonogram (7.5 MHz) of an ovary bearing a follicle (F) within the ovarian stroma. Smaller follicles are to be seen on the left (S) but the anechoic structures on the right are ovarian veins (V). Manipulation of the transducer will maintain the follicle as a circular image, but the veins will become distended longitudinally in shape as the transducer is rotated through 90°.

from its surrounding layers of ovarian tissue (Fig. 10.6), and at this time, when observing in real time, there appears to be undulating movement of the wall surface.

Ovulation has been observed to have occurred by two methods. On occasions there has been abrupt rupture of the follicle with rapid evacuation of

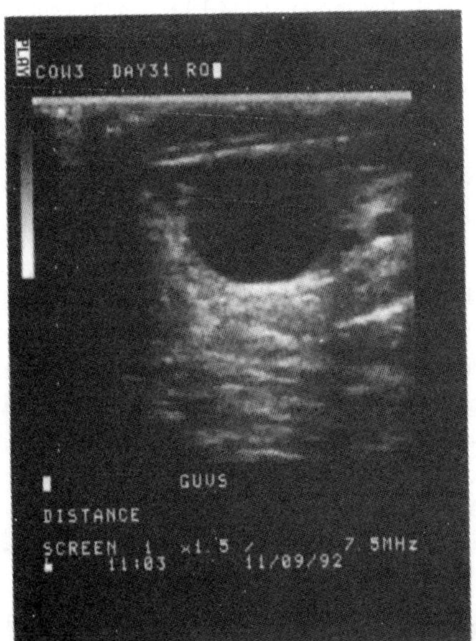

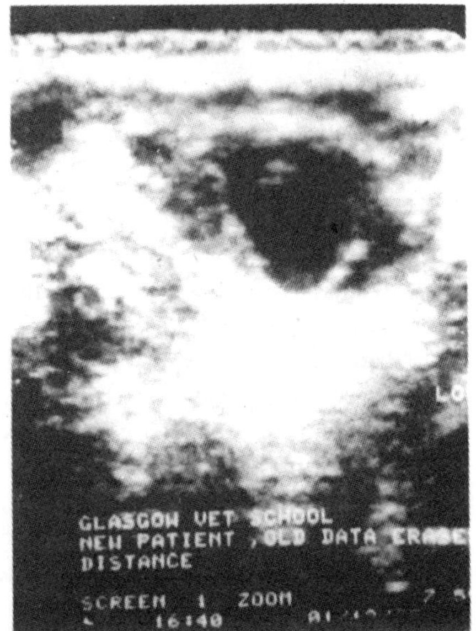

Fig. 10.6. (a) The large, circular, anechoic image of an antral follicle can be seen in centre field with small follicles evident to its right. **(b)** This scan shows an antral follicle imaged immediately prior to ovulation (7.5 MHz). Note the pear-shaped outline with pointing to the ovarian edge, separation of the follicular outline from the ovarian stroma, and the hyperechoic outline of the follicular capsule.

the contents, while at other times of viewing, the follicle has gently decreased in size and liberated its contents over a four-minute period (Fig. 10.7). The different methods could be explained by disruption having occurred to the follicle by transducer pressure in the first instance, while the second may represent a more natural process. Apparent failure to reach ovulation by the predestined follicle has been observed when the follicle loses its tonicity and decreases in size, but on these occasions there usually appears to be a successor follicle which takes over the dominant role and progresses to ovulation.

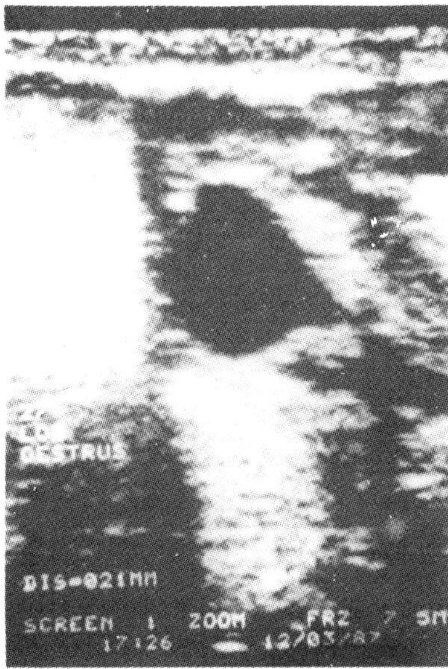

Fig. 10.7. Sonogram (7.5 MHz) of a follicle at time of rupture. Note the point of breakdown at the ovarian edge where the anechoic contents are being liberated.

Ovarian blood vessels

The ultrasonographer should be aware of the presence and appearance of the ovarian vessels to avoid confusion with images of small or medium-sized follicles. Both arteries and veins can be imaged. The veins are seen entering at the caudal pole of the ovary, being imaged as two or three rounded, anechoic structures of 2–5 mm in diameter. By altering the plane of scanning, the images of these structures can be made to change in shape from rounded to elongated, and this helps to differentiate them from follicles, which remain relatively rounded in all scan planes. The arteries appear as a cluster of anechoic rounded areas less than 2 mm in diameter, grouped around the veins. They tend only to be imaged in cross-section and therefore appear rounded in most scanning planes (Fig. 10.5).

Uterine horns

As the uterine horn distal to the interarcuate ligament is spiral in form, the images produced when the transducer passes over the uterine coils will vary. It is customary to describe the appearance of both cross- and longitudinal sections, but variations ranging between these orientations will be seen. The cross-sectional image is of an external hypoechoic layer, outlined by a dark ring, comprising the vascular coat and the longitudinal, circular and oblique layers of the myometrium (Fig. 10.8). This muscular layer is imaged in differing planes and thus produces a signal of varying echogenicity. It is separated by a further dark ring from the

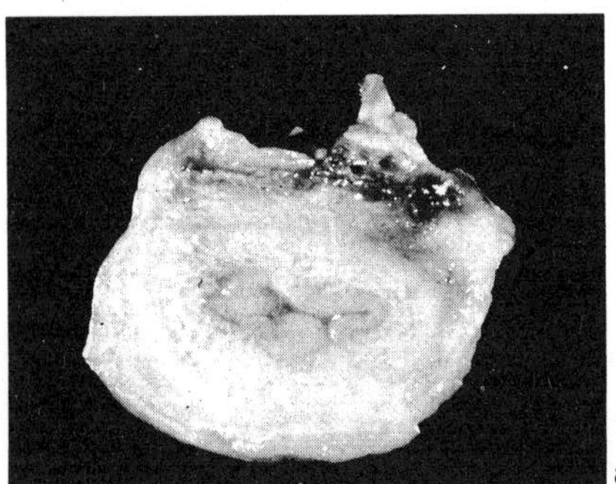
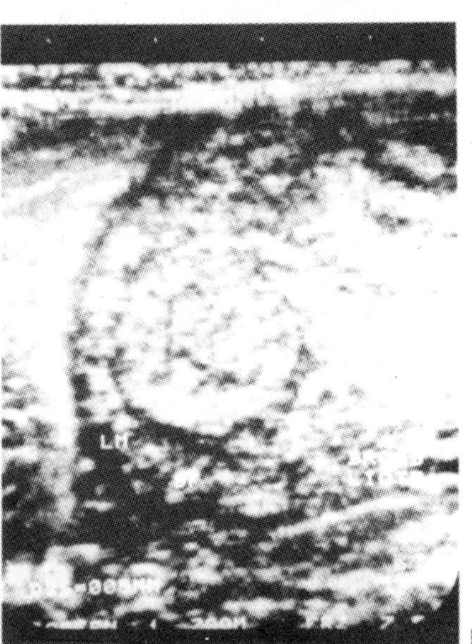

Fig. 10.8. (a) Frozen cross-sectional specimen of a bovine uterine horn. The encircling layers of muscle can be seen surrounding the centrally-placed endometrium with the mucus-filled lumen most central of all. There are uterine blood vessels running in the mesometrium at the top right of the uterine horn. **(b)** Sonogram (7.5 MHz) of a uterine horn in cross-section showing the encircling muscular layers (LM) with the hyperechoic endometrial outline (E) surrounding the anechoic lumen (L) at the centre of the image. The mesometrial structure is imaged approaching from the top right with scattered anechoic areas within it, indicating the presence of uterine vessels. The scan field corresponds to the outline of **a**.

hyperechoic endometrium, which forms a wide concentric layer around the inner anechoic uterine lumen. The latter is always uneven in appearance in adult cows due to the presence of caruncles on the endometrial surface. The identical layers are imaged on longitudinal section but they run parallel with the transducer face, and the lumen is seen as an anechoic central line running between the strongly echogenic endometrial bands (Fig. 10.9). Variations in the ultrasonographic appearance of the uterine horns will occur depending on the state of the reproductive cycle, as the tissue interfaces alter with the oedematous nature of the uterine wall seen at impending oestrus.

Uterine body

The uterine body is usually imaged in long-axis view with the transducer placed cranial to the cervix. By rotating the transducer both clockwise and anticlockwise at the level of divergence of the horns, the continuation of the body with the

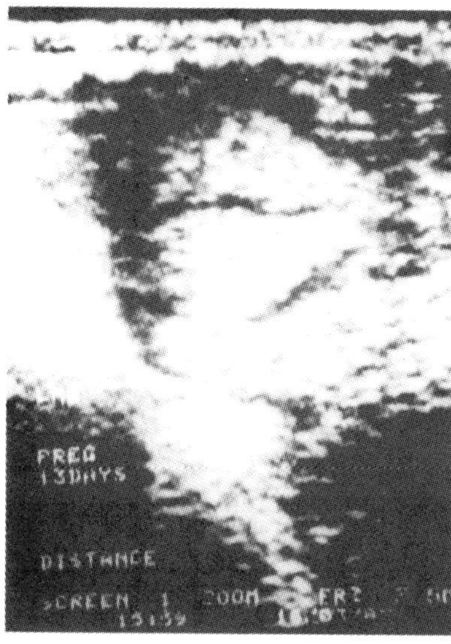

Fig. 10.9. Longitudinal scan (7.5 MHz) of the uterine horn showing an anechoic streak representing the uterine lumen running transversely, being paralleled by the images of the endometrium and the muscle layers.

horns can be imaged. The ultrasonographic appearance is similar to that of the horns but the concentric muscle layers are not as well differentiated.

Cervix

The cervix produces a hyperechoic image and its density can be such as to produce a degree of acoustic shadowing deep to it when viewed in long-axis. However, it is common to observe the bones of the pelvic floor and the urinary bladder deep to the main cervical image. The zigzag course of the cervical canal can be discerned by rotating the transducer, with identification of the external os and portio vaginalis being possible within the cranial portion of the vagina.

Vagina

The cranial portion of the vagina is normally observed as a hyperechoic line close to the transducer face, but when it is fluid-filled, it is seen to have an ovoid, anechoic lumen with enclosing hyperechoic lines.

Urinary bladder

The overall image of the bladder is anechoic but the appearance of the wall will vary according to the degree of distension. An empty bladder has a wall which produces a scatter of echoes from its mucosa, but with distension this layer thins out and the production of echoes decreases. The sonographer should become familiar with the totally anechoic appearance of the bladder at an early stage, and not confuse it with fetal fluids of pregnancy, which will usually contain some echogenic structures on searching in different planes, or with the mixed echogenicity of the uterine lumen in a pyometra.

Applications

Pregnancy diagnosis

Early pregnancy diagnosis is possible using a 7.5 MHz intrarectal transducer and can be performed as early as 17–19 days post-mating. At this stage, the ovaries are observed for the presence of an active, well-formed CL, and the ipsilateral horn is then imaged in cross section. With careful searching over the uterine horn, the lumen will appear anechoic with moderate distension as it contains the conceptus (Fig. 10.10). This fluid can also be seen in longitudinal scans. The fluid distension

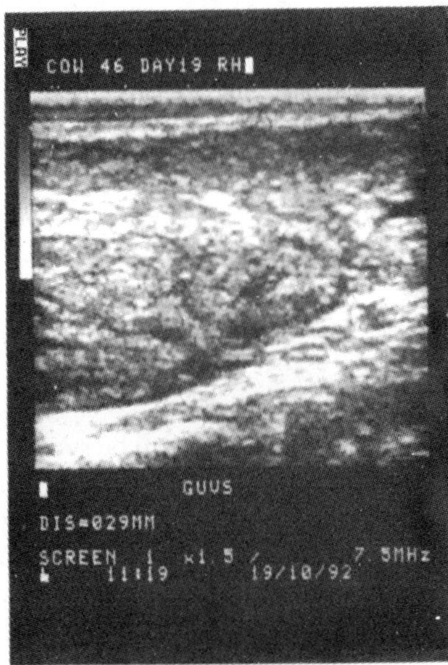

Fig. 10.10. Cross-sectional image of the uterine horn of a 19 day pregnant cow (7.5 MHz). The outline of the uterus can be viewed in the centre of the scan field with the hyperechoic endometrium surrounding the anechoic lumen which has increased in overall diameter as a result of the presence of the conceptus. Taken in conjunction with the presence of an active CL this scan would indicate a positive diagnosis of early pregnancy.

can be followed into the contralateral horn by 17 days post-mating, and by 19 days the amniotic sac greatly expands making imaging of the conceptus more readily detectable in the ipsilateral horn (Fig. 10.11). With a transducer of high frequency, the embryo may be detected as an echogenic streak within the anechoic lumen, but it is not until 22–24 days that the conceptus becomes more consistently imaged, as it now has a detectable heart-beat to assist in its identification (Figs 10.12 and 10.13). Positive diagnosis at this stage still requires considerable expertise, but by 30 days the collection of fluid has so increased that detection is readily made, as is imaging of the viable conceptus (Fig. 10.14). To avoid a false positive diagnosis when embryonic death has already occurred, a positive diagnosis of pregnancy should only be given at this stage if an echogenic embryo with a heart-beat is imaged. By now, the membranes surrounding the fetus will be readily imaged, with specular reflection a commonly observed artifact. From 35 days the uterine caruncles are evident sonographically, further assisting in diag-

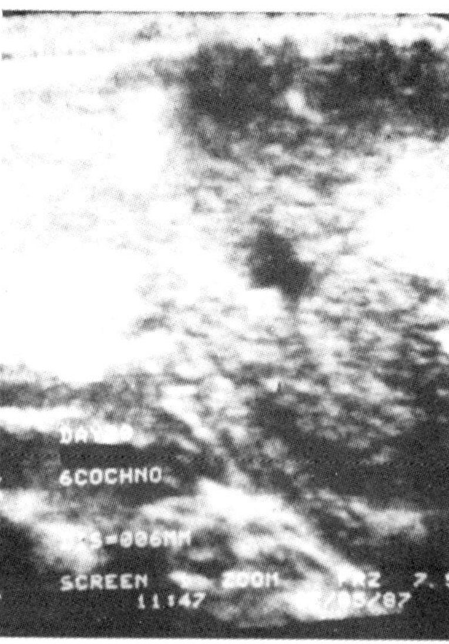

Fig. 10.11. Cross-sectional image of an uterine horn 20 days after artificial insemination (AI) (7.5 MHz). There is a significant collection of fluid within the uterine lumen as seen by the centrally placed anechoic space within the echoic outline of the uterine wall. The amniotic sac has increased in size, producing a more readily detected sonographic image.

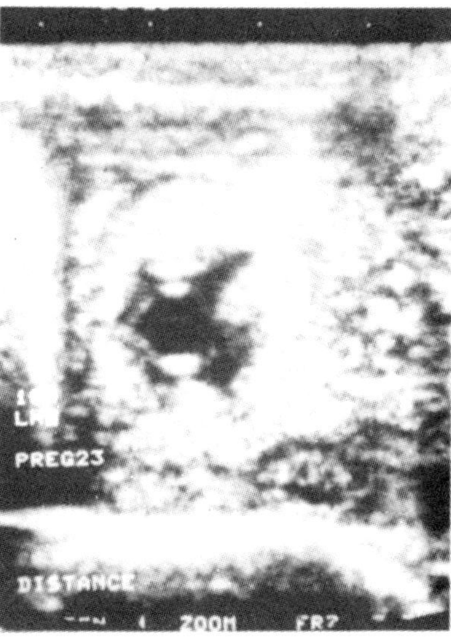

Fig. 10.12. Sonogram of a cross-sectional gravid uterine horn 23 days after AI (7.5 MHz). There has been expansion of the fetal membranes with an increase in fluid content thus producing echoic layers within the anechoic luminal centre. There is specular reflection present as a result of the presence of the fluid-filled sacs, seen as hyperechoic, highlighted spots on the membrane outline.

nosis, and the fetus has such a recognizable image outline that the process of measurement of various body parameters can commence (Figs 10.15 and 10.16).

The most commonly used measurement is the crown–rump length, which can be made using the integral measurement devices commonly fitted into veterinary scanners (Fig. 10.17). Another useful measurement is the biparietal diameter of the skull, where the head region is imaged as symmetrically as possible in a dorso-ventral view, and the distance between the outer line of the parietal bones of each side is recorded (Fig. 10.18). Transabdominal measurements, either circumference or diameter, are taken from cross-sectional images at the level of the

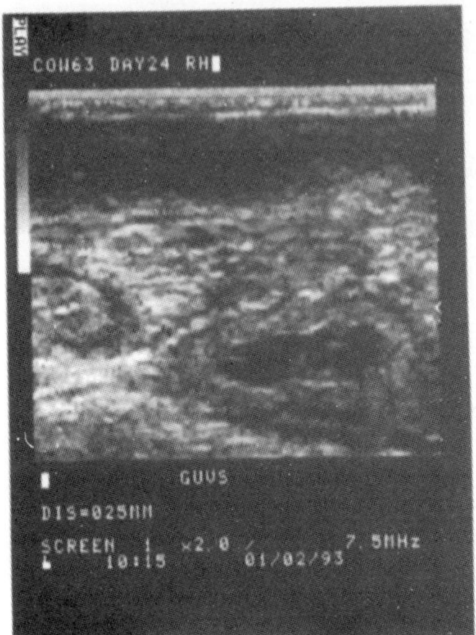 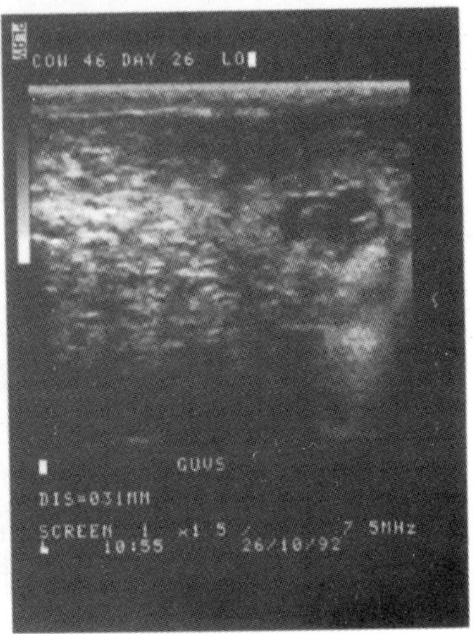

Fig. 10.13. (a) The fluid-filled, anechoic luminal centre is now readily observed in this gravid uterine horn 24 days after AI (7.5 MHz). The anechoic, oval area contains an echoic structure which represents the embryo. By this stage, a fetal heart-beat can be seen in real time within this echoic streak. (b) By 26 days the anechoic luminal centre (mid-field, right) contains echoic membranes enveloping the conceptus from which a heart-beat will be seen in real-time.

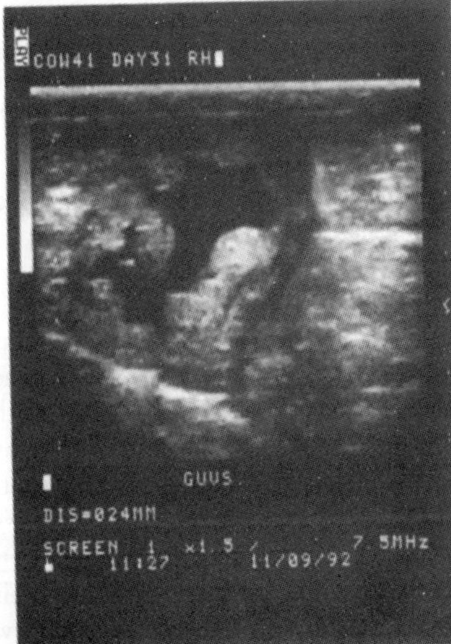

Fig. 10.14. The echoic embryo (day 31) is imaged (7.5 MHz) lying at 10 o'clock within the anechoic luminal centre of the echoic uterine cross-sectional image. The small hypoechoic dot within the embryo's image is the region of the embryonic heart and in real time would be exhibiting a rhythmic beating motion. The embryo has implanted and is attached to the endometrial wall with caruncles beginning to develop, being imaged as raised echoic discs.

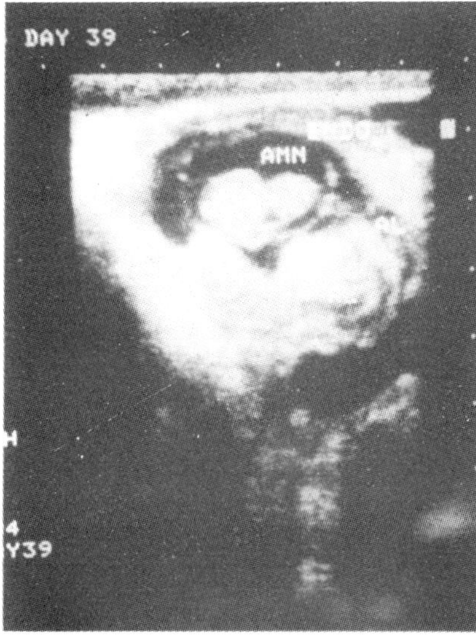

Fig. 10.15. By now, 39 days after AI, the embryo is readily imaged as a hyperechoic structure surrounded by the echoic lines of the placental membranes (AMN) within the anechoic area of the fetal fluid which is situated intraluminally (7.5 MHz).

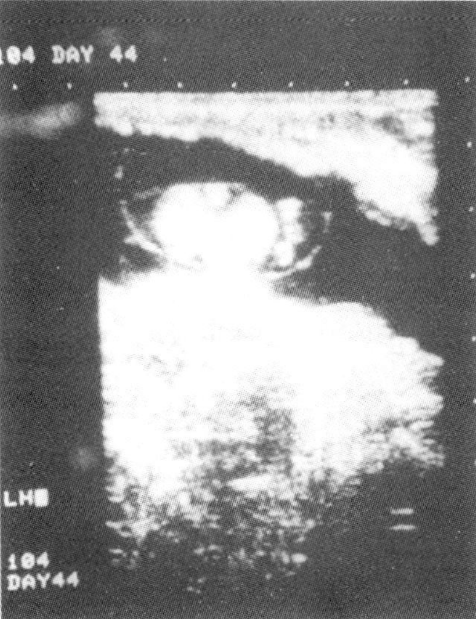

Fig. 10.16. The fetus is recognizable as having identifiable features by day 44 post-AI (7.5 MHz). The head lies to the left with the pectoral limb buds seen adjacent to the thoracic and abdominal outline. The two pelvic limb buds are seen to the right with the image of the tail lying between them. The fetus is surrounded by the echoic line of the fetal membranes.

umbilical attachment (Fig. 10.19), while the transthoracic diameter is recorded with an image showing the rib cage symmetrically displayed on either side of the anechoic outline of the cardiac chambers. Many modern scanning units carry calibrated charts in the computer memories which can indicate predicted days of gestation from a given set of measurements. The development of the fetus and its membranes can be followed sonographically with little difficulty until about 110 days, by which time the pregnant uterus becomes dependent within the abdomen and procuring images of the fetus is increasingly problematic. In late pregnancy, the fetus makes a return into transducer range, but the detection of individual structures at this stage is confusing due to fetal size and reverberation from fetal

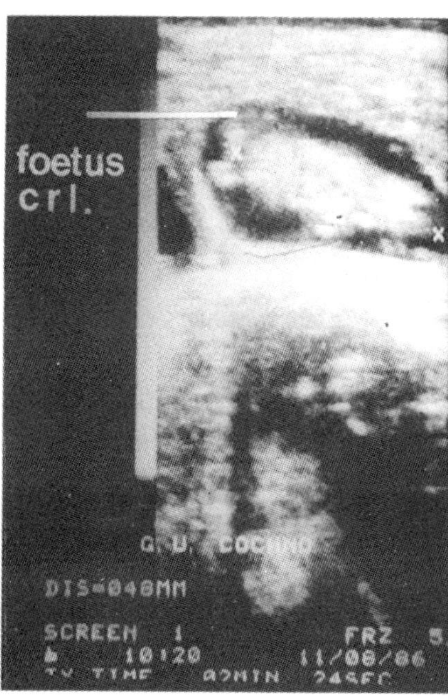

Fig. 10.17. Fetus imaged (5 MHz) at 57 days post-AI. The cranial and caudal extremities can be discerned and are indicated by the measurement cursors, cranial to the right. The distance measured between these points represents the crown–rump length and can be used as a parameter for calculating gestational age. The anechoic line of the developing neural canal can be seen running between the crosses.

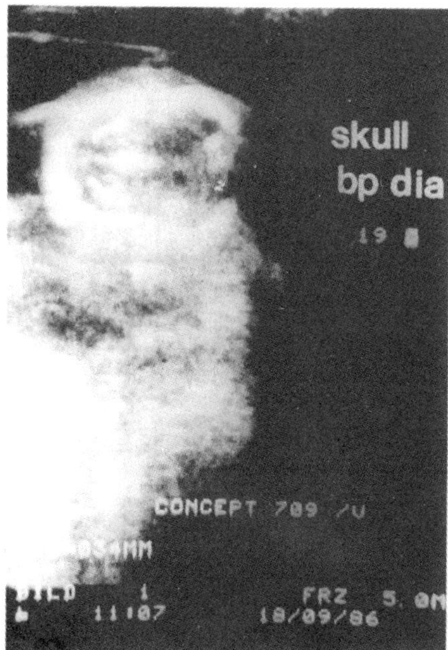

Fig. 10.18. Sonogram (5 MHz) of a fetal skull at 95 days post-AI. The skull is imaged (at the top of the frame) in a coronal plane with the rostral structures lying to the left. Obtaining bilateral symmetry of the developing bones of the skull is essential before a biparietal diameter measurement is taken across the maximum width of the skull image, i.e. from 12 o'clock to 6 o'clock.

skeletal elements. It is possible to scan transcutaneously through the lower right flank with a 3.5 MHz transducer but the detail obtained is generally poor compared with that using the transrectal route.

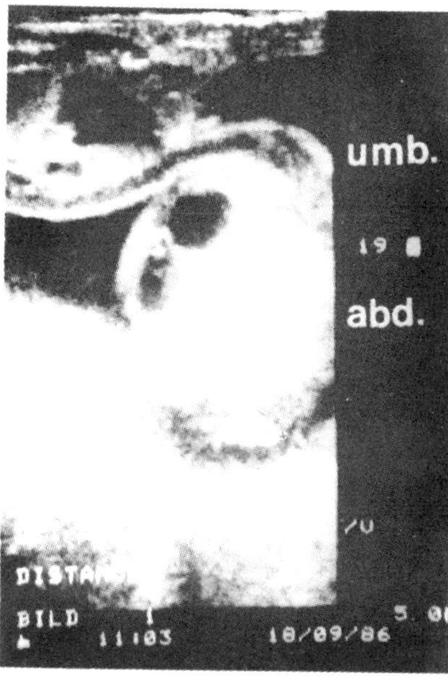

Fig. 10.19. Cross-sectional sonogram (5 MHz) of a fetal abdomen, 95 days post-AI, taken at the level of the umbilicus (umb.) as it enters the abdomen. The vascular contents of the umbilical stalk appear as an anechoic central line within the hyperechoic walls of the umbilicus. This is a site for measuring transabdominal diameter or circumference to calculate gestational age.

Oestrus detection and timing of ovulation

Impending standing oestrus, can be predicted by evaluating a number of criteria in the images of the uterus (e.g. oedema, wall thickness and intrauterine fluid collection) and of the ovary (e.g. follicular shape, position and dimensions).

Ultrasonographic monitoring of the uterus during the time of impending oestrus reveals an increase in endometrial folding accompanied by a disruption in the imaging of distinct layers of the uterine wall due to oedematous swelling (Fig. 10.20). This swelling is at a maximum on the day of standing oestrus, while the endometrial folding starts to recede two days post-ovulation. There is an increase in the anechoic fluid centre to the lumen (Fig. 10.21), which continues up to the day of standing oestrus, when the intrauterine fluid is released per vagina, with a reduction in the diameter of the anechoic lumen. The changes occurring in the ovary and the resultant CL formation are described in the section on normal ultrasonographic anatomy.

Abnormal changes

Failure of follicles to rupture can be detected and followed sonographically with varying results. On occasions the anechoic follicular vesicle develops a degree of echogenicity centrally and this spreads through the follicular structure. Such follicles have been followed to *post mortem* examination when they appeared to contain extensive haemorrhage into the follicular centre. Other follicles appear to develop an enveloping rim of echogenic material which forms a surrounding border, imaging in a manner similar to the echogenicity of a CL. In a number of cases

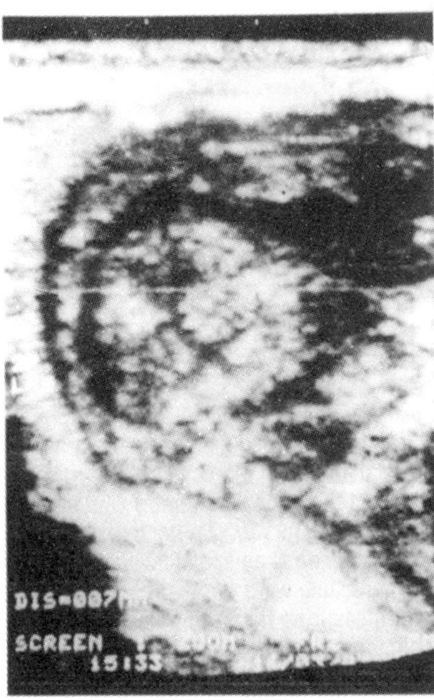

Fig. 10.20. Cross-sectional sonogram of a uterine horn imaged (7.5 MHz) two days prior to standing oestrus. There is evidence of the oedematous infiltration of the myometrial layers which shows as mixed hypo- and hyperechoic areas. The endometrium at the centre of the field exhibits exaggerated folding which will only decline after standing oestrus has occurred.

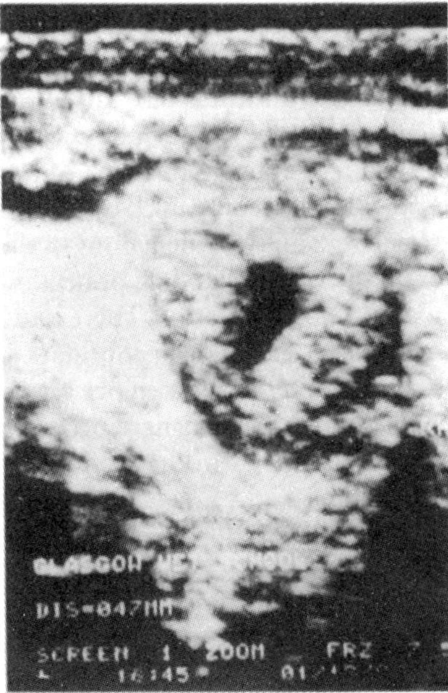

Fig. 10.21. Cross-sectional image (7.5 MHz) of a uterine horn immediately prior to standing oestrus. There is a distended anechoic lumen in centre field due to the accumulation of intrauterine fluid.

these structures, assumed to be cystic follicles, developed fine echogenic strands appearing to extend across the anechoic follicular centre (Fig. 10.22).

Intrauterine pathology (e.g. fetal death and abortion, macerated fetus and

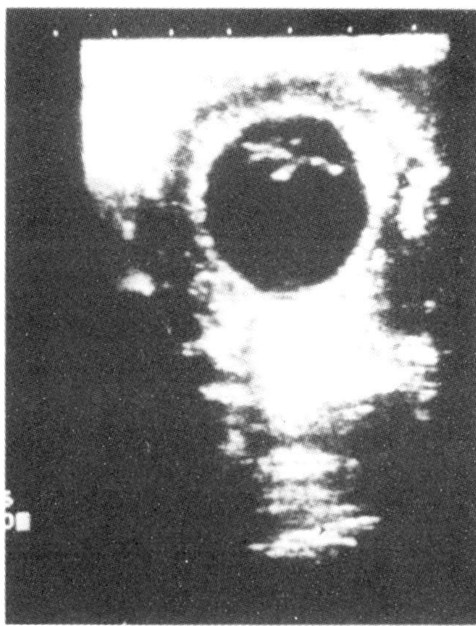

Fig. 10.22. The anechoic central structure represents the fluid retained within a follicle which has failed to rupture and is now being luteinized. This is imaged as a hyperechoic layer, surrounding the anechoic centre, and from which echoic strands run through the centre of the structure. Note the acoustic enhancement deep to the fluid-filled follicle giving the false impression of a hyperechoic layer in this deep position.

pyometra) can be discerned sonographically. Pyometra usually appears as a distension of the uterine lumen with an image of mixed echogenicity, containing hypoechoic material intermingled with some hyperechoic signals, often producing a swirling effect in real-time. With a mummified or macerated fetus, irregular hyperechoic images are randomly detected within what may be either an anechoic or hypoechoic background, although usually these strong signals are without a regular anatomical outline. Fetal death is initially detected by an absence of heart-beat and this is accompanied by detachment of the fetal membranes from the endometrial layer. The membranes lose their tense appearance and begin to image as if floating within the anechoic uterine lumen. The conceptus, with membranes, will traverse through the uterine body, cervix and vagina, and may be imaged in any of these areas accompanied by anechoic fluid. Even after the conceptus is expelled, the CL will maintain good size and echogenicity for a number of days post-abortion, and thus it is of importance when giving a positive pregnancy diagnosis from 24 days onwards that the operator should seek out the fetus and confirm viability with a heart-beat, and not just rely on imaging a distended anechoic uterine lumen and a large CL.

Early sexing of the fetus

Sexing of the fetus is a possibility at the 49- to 52-day phase of gestation but requires considerable skill and experience for a high degree of accuracy. The fetus is imaged transrectally using a 7.5 MHz transducer, which has to be manipulated to try to achieve both cross-sectional and dorsal plane (section parallel with the dorsum of the fetus) images of the conceptus.

At this stage of gestation the target structure for imaging is the genital tubercle from which the penile structure or clitoris is formed, depending on the sex of the fetus. At 42 days of gestation, in the male, this structure commences to migrate from its perineal position close to the developing anus, and arrives in a position closely approximated to the umbilical stalk where this attaches to the midline, ventral abdominal wall. In the female, migration does not occur and so a hyperechoic structure can be imaged at 49–52 days, in a position immediately caudal to the pelvic limbs and cranial to the tail. Conversely, on ultrasonographic investigation of this area at this time in the male, there is a lack of a structure in this location, but by investigating the region of the abdominal umbilical attachment a hyperechoic structure can be discerned caudal to the umbilical stalk. The former imaging is best conducted in a cross-sectional plane, while the latter is carried out in a dorsal plane.

Later scanning of the fetus, between 75 and 110 days, can also be used to differentiate sex, but here the structures to be imaged are the scrotal swellings and the mammary glands. In the male, a recognizable scrotal outline can be detected in the inguinal region from 75 days and the gonad descends into the sac between days 90 and 130. The female has an image of the mammary glands in the same location during the same period of scanning. The later the date of scanning, the more difficult it is to reach the fetus consistently, as the uterus is becoming increasingly dependent within the abdominal cavity.

Transvaginal Ultrasonography

This new approach to reproductive ultrasonography offers an exciting potential for extending the uses of real-time imaging of the ovary and uterus in cattle. The technique requires more expensive equipment and better preparation of the cow prior to examination, and so its uses will be more restricted to research purposes and specialized activities such as ova collection.

The type of scanning unit used by this author is a linear machine equipped with a 6.5 MHz microconvex linear transducer designed for human transvaginal investigations. The transducer face is mounted at the end of an extended rod, and the scan plane is angled and covers a field of 65°. The unit incorporates a biopsy guide through which a needle can be inserted so that aspiration from the ovary or uterus can be achieved under real-time ultrasound guidance (Fig. 10.23). Cow preparation is important, with sedation required and accompanying epidural anaesthesia.

Aspiration of ova direct from ovarian follicles

This technique requires two operators, one to carry out the scanning and manipulate the transducer and the other to perform the needle insertion and aspiration. The first operator evacuates the faeces from the rectum of a prepared cow and palpates the ovary through the rectal wall. The transducer is then inserted through the cleaned vulva and pushed cranially to image through the vaginal wall in the vicinity of the external os of the cervix. By grasping the ovary through the rectal wall the gonad can be lifted to lie adjacent to the vaginal wall and thus within the scanning field (Fig. 10.24a). Ovarian structures can be imaged

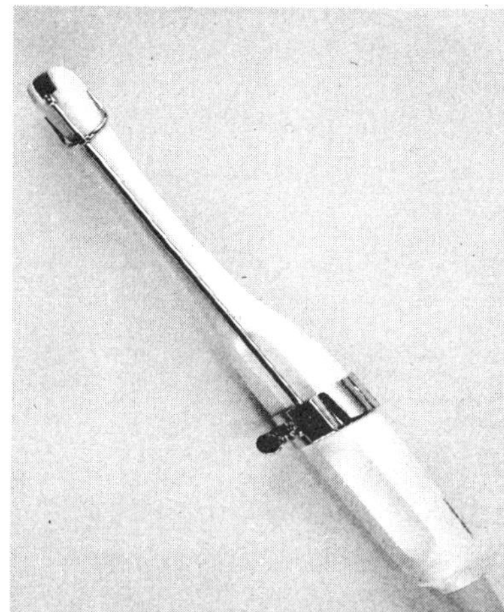

Fig. 10.23. Transvaginal transducer (Toshiba, 6.5 MHz) with biopsy guide attached. The grey area at the tip of the transducer is the region from which the beam is emitted in a wedge-shaped fashion, giving a scanning arc of 65°. The biopsy needle, when fed down the guide channel, emerges at the tip and appears within the left-hand field of the scanning arc, along a predetermined line.

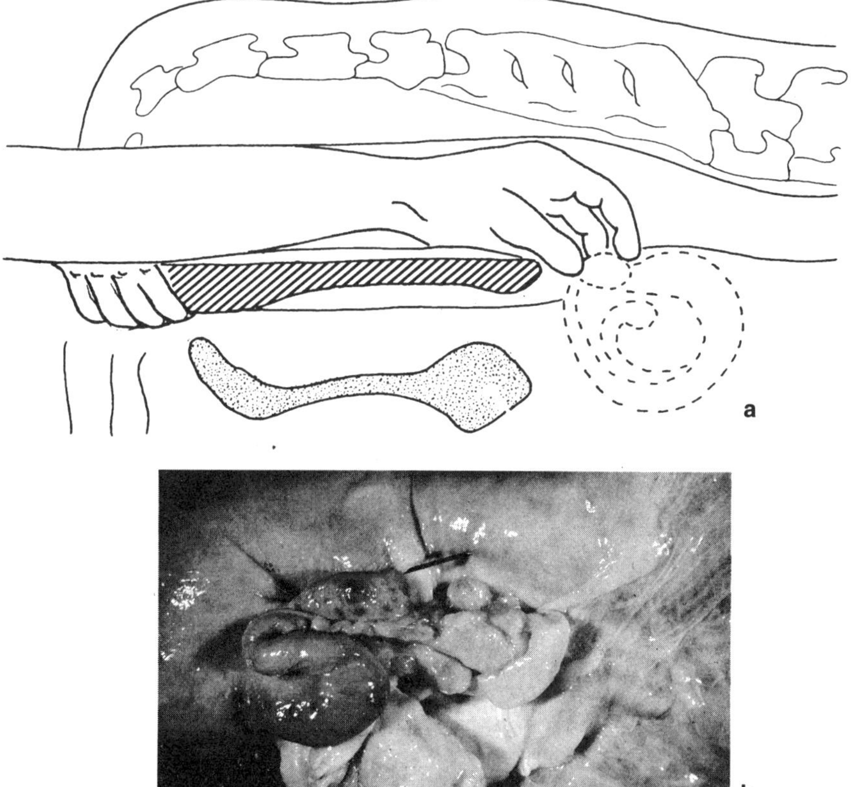

Fig. 10.24. (a) Line diagram of the transvaginal transducer in place with the operator's hand intrarectally guiding the ovary to the external vaginal wall to allow transvaginal imaging. **(b)** Demonstration of the position of the aspiration needle, having perforated the vaginal wall from the vaginal lumen, as it comes to lie adjacent to the manipulated ovary.

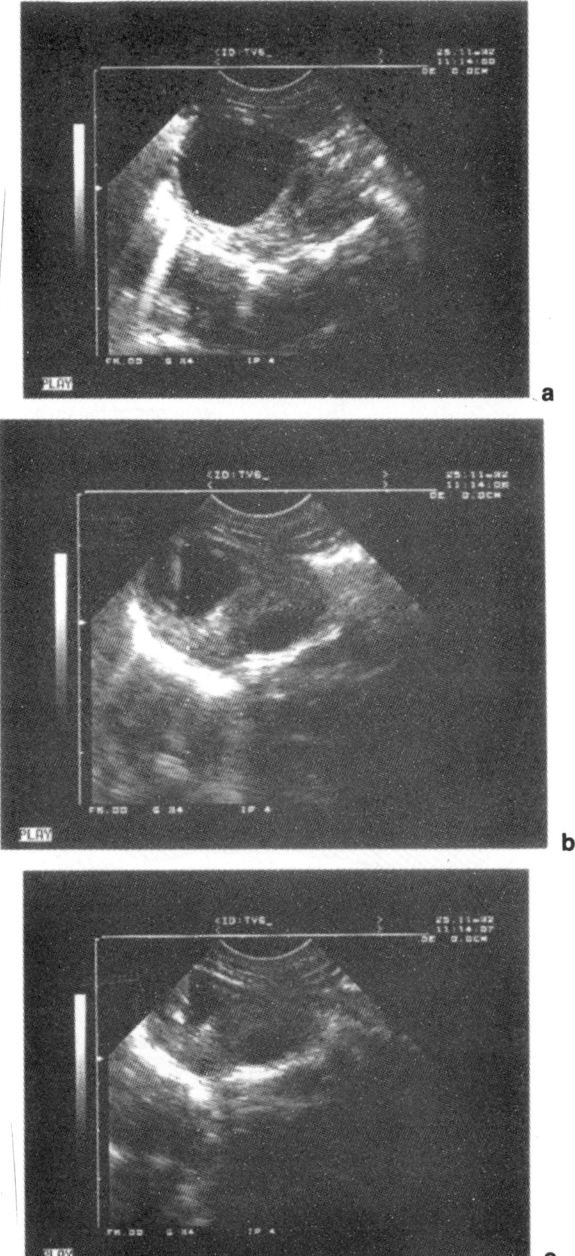

Fig. 10.25. (a) Transvaginal sonogram (6.5 MHz) of an ovary with a large anechoic preovulatory follicle in the centre of the field. The biopsy guide line can be seen as a dotted white line running from the top left corner through the anechoic follicular structure. The needle tip is just entering the scan field at the extreme top left of the guide line. **(b)** The needle has been advanced along the guide line so that it is now imaged as an hyperechoic vertical bar lying within the anechoic follicle. Penetration of the follicle has occurred and aspiration can commence. **(c)** The needle is still imaged within the follicle at the top left of the frame but there has been collapse of the follicle as a result of the aspiration, with subsequent decrease in size.

in considerable detail and the ovary can be manipulated as desired so that follicles can be brought to the area of the scan field where a biopsy cursor line is displayed. A long, fine needle is introduced into the needle biopsy guide which runs along the surface of the transducer handle and is progressed cranially until it pierces the vaginal wall (Fig. 10.24b). The echogenic needle tip will now appear on the scanner screen as a hyperechoic area producing some reverberation. By pushing the needle further through the vaginal wall, an image of the tip can be seen to proceed down the cursor line and, if the alignment of the ovary is correct, it will perforate the ovarian stroma and any intervening follicle which it encounters. On entering a follicle, negative pressure can be applied through the needle and the follicular contents aspirated into a collection receptacle (Fig. 10.25). Multiple collections can be achieved and both ovaries explored by this technique. This method can also be used to obtain fluid samples from early pregnancies, as the uterus can be gently manipulated per rectum into the scanning field.

Acknowledgements

The author wishes to thank the following who assisted in providing sonograms for this chapter: Dr S.N. Omran, Iraq, R. de Moura, Brazil, and C. Paterson, Scotland. Thanks also go to A. May for his assistance and expertise in the production of the photographs.

Further reading

Boyd, J.S. and Omran, S.N. (1991) Diagnostic ultrasonography of the bovine female reproductive tract. *In Practice*, 13, 109–118.

Taverne, M.A.M. and Willemse, A.H. (1989) *Diagnostic Ultrasound and Animal Reproduction*. Kluwer Academic Publishers, Dordrecht, The Netherlands.

11 Small Ruminant Reproductive Ultrasonography

A.J.F. Russel[1] and P.J. Goddard[2]

[1] *The Macaulay Land Use Research Institute, Hartwood Research Station, Hartwood, Shotts, Lanarkshire ML7 4JY, UK*

[2] *The Macaulay Land Use Research Institute, Craigiebuckler, Aberdeen AB9 2QJ, UK*

Ultrasonography is widely used in many aspects of small ruminant reproduction. Its first major application was in the diagnosis of pregnancy and determination of fetal numbers in sheep. This remains numerically the most important use of the technique, with approximately ten million ewes, or half of the flock in the UK, being scanned each year. Ultrasonography is used for the same purposes in goats and to diagnose pregnancy and estimate fetal age in farmed red deer and in the South American camelids which, for present purposes, are considered as being small ruminants. The camelids, unlike, sheep, goats and deer, are induced ovulators and do not have regular oestrous cycles, and ultrasonography has also been used in camelids to study ovarian activity and chart the development of ovarian follicles.

Ultrasonography also has a role in male reproduction and is used in work on testicular structure and function in rams and bucks.

The Need for Pregnancy Diagnosis and Fetal Number Determination

Results from research on the nutrition of the pregnant ewe have shown clearly that lamb birth weight, and consequently lamb survival, can be influenced to a significant extent by the feeding of the ewe during the final six to eight weeks of gestation. Nutrition over this critical period also has an important effect on the ewe's body reserves at parturition which, in turn, affects lactation performance and levels of disease and mortality. There is thus a clear need for, and economic advantage to be gained from, a technique which can be used to provide immediate, accurate and rapid determinations of fetal numbers prior to 90–100 days of gestation and to do so without hazard to the health of operator or animal.

Non-ultrasonic Techniques

Clinical examination by rectal palpation, as used to diagnose pregnancy in cattle, is, for reasons of physical size, not possible in sheep, goats or deer and is difficult in even the largest camelids.

Concentrations of circulating hormones, such as progesterone, and metabolites, such as non-esterified fatty acids and 3-hydroxybutyrate, could theoretically serve as indices of fetal numbers but in practice are affected by too many other factors to be used with confidence for this purpose. The time taken for their determination also precludes the possibility of obtaining an immediate diagnosis.

Radiographic techniques, including equipment specifically developed for the rapid examination of ewes, are capable of providing high levels of accuracy of both pregnancy diagnosis and determination of fetal numbers. Such equipment is, however, expensive and its use potentially hazardous, and it can be employed successfully only after about 80 days of gestation thus limiting its application to ewes mated within a period of about 20 days.

Other non-ultrasonic techniques such as abdominal palpation, ballottement and measurement of various characteristics of cervical or vaginal mucus have proved to be unsatisfactory. Only ultrasonic techniques fulfil all the criteria of safety, accuracy, speed of operation and the provision of an immediate diagnosis.

Ultrasonic Instruments for Pregnancy Diagnosis and Fetal Number Determination

Doppler shift and A-mode instruments

The Doppler shift principle, whereby movement is measured by a change in sonic frequency, has been used to detect fetal heart-beats and the flow of blood in uterine and fetal vessels. Early work showed that this approach could be used with a single-crystal probe applied externally to the sheep's abdomen to diagnose pregnancy with an accuracy approaching 100% when used in the second half of gestation. The lightweight nature of some versions of the equipment and its requirement for only battery power are significant advantages in field situations.

Later work demonstrated that this approach could be used successfully at earlier stages of pregnancy by incorporating the crystal in a slim rectal probe. This enabled the transducer to be placed in closer proximity to the uterus than was possible in early gestation with an externally applied probe. Although there are numerous reports of high rates of success in accurately diagnosing pregnancy by the use of intra-rectal Doppler probes, there is a considerable potential for causing serious damage to the animal, and the technique is not to be recommended.

When used by skilled operators, Doppler shift instruments with external probes can provide acceptable levels of accuracy of pregnancy diagnosis in small ruminants and other species. The principle has not, however, been used successfully to determine fetal numbers or estimate fetal age.

The problems of determining fetal numbers with simple Doppler instruments are two-fold. Firstly, the ultrasound emitted from the single stationary crystal will, in most cases, be reflected from only one moving target, and hence convey information from only a very limited area. Secondly, the returning signal is generally transformed to sound in the audible range so that the operator 'hears' the fetal heart-beat or blood flow. If twin fetuses were present and the operator was able, by altering the angle of the transducer, to 'switch' from one fetus to the other, it would still be extremely difficult to distinguish between the two returning signals. To be certain that these signals were from different fetuses and not from two parts of the same fetus it would be necessary to measure the rates of the pulses and to assume that the two fetal hearts were beating at detectably different rates. It would be technically possible to separate and display two such signals received simultaneously from a wide-beam Doppler instrument, but the sophistication required would outweigh the advantages of simplicity and inexpensiveness which the Doppler equipment marketed for pregnancy diagnosis offers.

A-mode scanners have also been used to diagnose pregnancy in small ruminants and other species. As with most Doppler instruments, they use a single piezoelectric crystal to transmit ultrasound through the body and to receive echoes from tissue interfaces. The returning signals are displayed in such a way that the depths of the interfaces beneath the skin surface are represented as one-dimensional distances on the screen. Most of the trials with this type of instrument have been carried out on sheep with the transducer placed on the abdomen lateral to the udder, and the presence of a strong signal indicating an interface at a depth of about 90 mm or greater has been regarded as a positive sign of pregnancy. The information obtained from such an approach is clearly very limited and many of the shortcomings of the Doppler technique apply equally to A-mode instruments. Not surprisingly, the results from the use of such instruments have been disappointing.

Real-time instruments

Whereas A-mode scanners have only a single and stationary crystal and provide information regarding the depth of tissue interfaces in only one dimension, real-time instruments have either a row of crystals (linear array scanners), or a single or small number of moving crystals (sector scanners), and portray the returning signals as two-dimensional images on a cathode ray tube or screen (see Chapter 1 for a fuller description). By moving the probe across the skin surface, or merely by altering the angle at which the probe is held, the operator can readily build a mental three-dimensional model from a series of two-dimensional images. The movement of fetal limbs and the beating of fetal hearts is very easily recognized in the live, real-time images provided by these instruments.

Linear array instruments typically have a row of 60–80 crystals arranged in a line generally about 60–100 mm in length. Groups of crystals, or elements, are energized sequentially and the display consists of a series of close parallel scanning lines giving a rectangular image of up to about 200 mm in depth. This gives a field of view between 120 and 200 cm^2, depending on the instrument and the settings selected. In practice it can be difficult to maintain contact with the animal's skin over the entire length of a 100 mm linear array probe.

Sector instruments generally have either a single oscillating crystal or two to four rotating crystals. The area of skin contact required is much less than with linear array instruments and the image afforded by the moving crystals is that of an arc. In the only instrument known to the writers to have been developed specifically for work on farm livestock (the Oviscan 3, or its variant the Vetscan 2, BCF Technology Ltd, Livingston, Scotland) the angle of the arc is 170°. (This can be reduced to 85° to give improved resolution of features of particular interest.) Depth of field can be varied from 50 to 400 mm, although it would be unusual to operate at more than 250 mm. At that depth the area of the 170° image is more than 900 cm² or about five to seven times greater than that offered by most linear array instruments. Scanning is generally undertaken at 3.5 MHz to optimize tissue penetration.

Scanning Techniques

Linear array instruments

Linear array instruments can be used for pregnancy diagnosis and fetal number determination in all small ruminant species, although in some cases they would not be the equipment of first choice. In scanning sheep with linear array instruments the ewe is normally turned on her back and restrained either horizontally or in a semi-recumbent position. The area over which the transducer has to be moved extends across the width of the abdomen, passing from one side of the udder, across in front of the udder, to the other. To achieve accurate results it is advisable to shear the wool from an area some 150–200 mm anterior to the udder.

The transducer is generally held at right angles to the longitudinal axis of the ewe and moved in a systematic W-shaped searching pattern from one side of the abdomen to the other, always ensuring that good contact is maintained with the skin throughout the course of the scan. During the movement across the abdomen, the angle of the transducer against the skin surface is continually altered so that the path of the ultrasound beam sweeps or scans in the longitudinal axis of the ewe and covers all areas of potential interest.

It is, of course, possible to image a fetus from more than one position of the transducer and the mistake most commonly made by inexperienced operators using linear array instruments is to count a single fetus twice. This type of error can be avoided if the operator can build a mental three-dimensional model of the uterus and its contents from the series of two-dimensional images displayed on the screen.

The technique outlined for scanning sheep does not work particularly well with goats. Goats generally have a more prominent spine than sheep and are not easily restrained on their backs. They also resist such restraint strongly and vocally! They can either be held in a semi-recumbent position or placed on their side on a table or a rectangular straw bale. The same systematic pattern of scanning as outlined for sheep should be adopted with goats. It is seldom necessary to clip hair from the abdomen.

As indicated above, transrectal probes are not recommended for routine use on sheep or goats; the risk of causing damage is high, and in any case, these animals are relatively easily restrained for transabdominal scanning. With red deer and camelids, scanning rectally with a small linear array transducer is less hazardous to both animal and operator. Because these animals are larger there is less likelihood of damaging the rectum with the probe, although care must always be exercised. Also, it is much easier, and safer for the operator, to scan these species transrectally when they are restrained in a normal standing position than to apply a probe to the abdomen, regardless of the method of restraint.

The technique of transrectal scanning in red deer and camelids is simple. The probe must be introduced very carefully into the rectum, using a suitable lubricant to facilitate entry. As the probe is moved slowly forward, gentle pressure should be applied to maintain contact between the face of the probe and the ventral wall of the rectum.

In many cases the first recognizable feature to be imaged is the bladder, which appears as a smooth-walled, fluid-filled structure which generally contains no echogenic material save a little echogenic sediment. As the probe is slowly moved forwards, the uterus will come into the field of view. If the animal is pregnant this will be recognized as another fluid-filled structure, but the wall is less sharply defined than that of the bladder, and some echogenic material will be observed within the fluid-filled area. The volume of the uterus and the size of the fetus and placental structures will obviously depend on the stage of pregnancy (see below), but the imaging of the fluid-filled uterus is itself usually a sufficient basis on which to make a positive diagnosis of pregnancy.

When the uterus has been located, the entire area of interest can be imaged by rotating the probe through a small angle (no more than 15-20°) to either side of the vertical plane.

The placentation in red deer and camelids takes the form of a thickening of discrete areas of the uterine wall, unlike the development of cotyledons (placentomes) in sheep and goats. These denser and, therefore, more highly echogenic areas of tissue may, on occasion, make it difficult to image the fetus. This, however, is of little practical importance unless the objective of scanning is to estimate fetal age. Twinning in these species is virtually unknown and thus the need to determine fetal numbers does not arise.

Sector instruments

The size and configuration of sector scanner transducers or probes are generally such that they cannot be used transrectally in small ruminants. Examinations are therefore made externally, usually with the probe placed on the wall of the abdomen in the groin and lateral to the udder.

Sector instruments have several advantages over linear array equipment for work on small ruminants. First, animals can be scanned in the standing position as opposed to being turned on their backs. This causes less stress to the animals and saves the physical effort of manually turning the ewes or does on their backs, or of using the elaborate handling equipment which enables this to be done semi-automatically.

Scanning ewes in the standing position also allows the use of simple systems of restraint and higher rates of throughput than are generally possible with linear array equipment.

The second main advantage of sector instruments for pregnancy diagnosis and fetal number determination in small ruminants is the greater area visualized on the screen at any time. This, and the fact that the probe does not require to be moved from one side of the abdomen to the other, means that there is a greater likelihood of viewing multiple fetuses in the one image and a lesser risk of viewing the same fetus from more than one position. These factors make for greater accuracy.

Finally, there is also some evidence that the problems of gas in the rumen and intestines and its adverse effect on image quality are less with ewes scanned in the standing position than when they are turned over for linear array scanning.

The technique generally adopted for scanning sheep or goats with a sector instrument is for the operator to sit parallel to the animal, on its left side and beside its back legs. The probe is then placed in the groin area, between the udder and the right leg on the naturally bare area of skin. The probe is first pointed posteriorly, towards the root of the tail. The bladder is sometimes, but not always, visualized at this stage. The probe is then gradually turned in a clockwise direction until it is pointing anteriorly without necessarily moving it from the original point of contact. During this turning movement the ultrasound beam will have traversed the length of uterus and all its contents will have been viewed.

In the operation as described above, the plane of the ultrasound beam remains approximately vertical. To examine areas of particular interest the probe may be turned through 90° so that the beam is more nearly horizontal. This allows the operator to alter the image from, say, a transverse section of a fetus to a longitudinal section, or vice versa, and aids fetal identification.

For ewes in the later stages of pregnancy, when the uterus has become very large, or where there are multiple fetuses, it may be useful to move the probe anteriorly on the abdomen for a distance of approximately 100 mm.

Left-handed operators find it more convenient to work from the ewe's right and to place the probe on the left side of the abdomen.

Red deer and camelids can also be scanned transabdominally with sector instruments. The method is essentially the same as that described for sheep, the main difference being in the handling equipment used. With deer the difficulty is to prevent the animal kicking with its hind legs, to the risk of both the operator and the probe. A modified drop-floor crush which permits access from the side has been found to be effective. The same approach can be used with camelids although many llamas and alpacas are sufficiently docile to be restrained with only a halter during the scanning operation.

Stage of Pregnancy

The size of sheep fetuses at different gestational ages can be judged from Fig. 11.1. These give an indication of the period over which pregnant ewes can be scanned.

In most sheep and goats it is possible by careful examination to detect the presence of a significant quantity of fluid in the uterus between 20 and 25 days

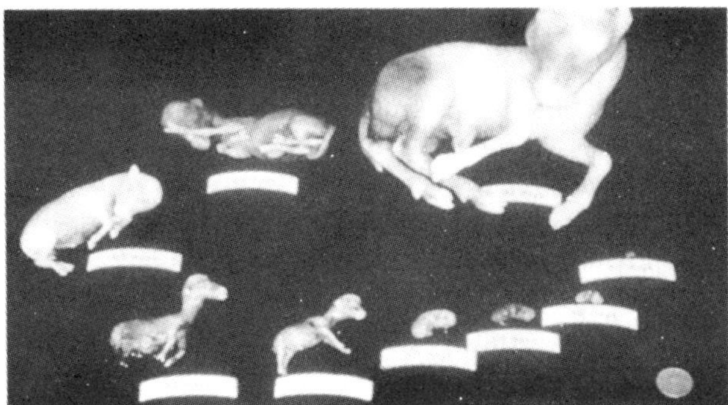

Fig. 11.1. Development of the ovine fetus. From right, clockwise: 20, 30, 35, 40, 50, 55, 65, 75 and 90 days after mating.

of gestation. This is generally assumed to constitute evidence of pregnancy, although embryos are not always imaged at this stage. Individual fetuses can generally be distinguished from about 30 days but at that stage they are still extremely small and it can be difficult to determine numbers accurately, particularly when scanning large flocks or herds. At the high rates of throughput practised by commercial sheep scanning operators, individual fetuses can be confidently identified and accurately counted from about 45–50 days of age.

By about 100 days of gestation, sheep and goat fetuses are of a size such that their images can more than fill the screen of most linear array instruments; only parts of fetuses can be viewed. By this stage the fetal skeleton is calcified and large bony structures, such as the skull and scapulae, cast shadows. It can then be extremely difficult to see beyond the fetus lying nearest the transducer to one or more other fetuses which may also be present.

Scanning to determine fetal numbers in sheep and goats should therefore be restricted to the period from about 50 to 100 days of gestation. In practice, however, the spread of gestational age within any flock or herd and the commercial pressure to scan for as long a season as possible are such that many operators attempt to extend this period by five to ten days at either end. Experience indicates that the interval over which sheep flocks can be scanned with a high degree of accuracy is some five to seven days earlier for operators with sector instruments than for those with linear array equipment.

Where operators are required to identify ewes with triplets or quadruplets, as distinct from merely distinguishing between singles and multiples, this is more readily done at earlier rather than later stages of gestation. It should also be remembered that the different nutritional regimes for single- and multiple-bearing ewes should be applied from no later than 100 days if they are to be fully effective.

The diagnosis of pregnancy, as distinct from the determination of fetal numbers, can, of course, be made from the earliest stages indicated above until the date of parturition. Thus, in red deer and camelids, where twinning is virtually unknown, scanning can be carried out at any time after about 30 days.

Estimation of Fetal Age

Most scanning instruments incorporate features whereby the image can be 'frozen' and measurements of structures of particular interest made, using callipers which move over the screen in response to a joystick manipulated by the operator. This enables measurements of the size of fetal parts to be made and from these it is possible to obtain an estimate of fetal age and hence to predict the likely date of parturition.

Equations for estimating fetal age from measurements of the biparietal head diameter and diameter across the widest part of the thorax in sheep, goats, red deer and camelids are presented in Table 11.1. As pregnancy progresses, breed differences which result in size differences at birth will cause a small departure from the estimate, particularly for goats.

Some of the scanning instruments developed specifically for animal use incorporate look-up tables relating fetal size and age and have the facility to display an estimated age on the screen when a measurement has been made. It is important to ensure that the fetus is viewed in the optimum orientation and callipers are used accurately if results are to be reliable.

Image Interpretation

The image portrayed on the real-time scanning instrument screen can be thought of as a two-dimensional section through the tissues of the animal in the area immediately beyond the transducer. The operator can imagine that the animal has been cut across in the plane of the beam and that they are looking at a portion of

Table 11.1. Estimation of fetal age from size.

Species	Stage of gestation (days)	Prediction equation
Sheep	50–110	A = 36.6 + 0.88 TD A = 17.3 + 1.58 HD (Russel, 1989)
Goat	40–100	A = 26.0 + 1.78 HD (Haibel, 1988)
Red deer	35–170	A = 26.8 + 1.64 TD A = 28.9 + 1.83 HD (White *et al.*, 1989)
Camelid	66–235	A = 18.8 + 3.79 HD (Haibel and Fung, 1991)
	50–170	A = 44.2 + 1.97 TD (Iason *et al.*, 1993)

A = age (days)
TD = trunk diameter (mm)
HD = head (biparietal) diameter (mm)

the cut surface. If the instrument used has a linear array transducer, the area of the cut surface viewed will be a rectangle probably measuring 60–100 mm wide and 200 mm deep, with the skin of the animal at the top of the screen. With sector instruments the area viewed will most probably be pie-slice shaped (170°), with the point where the probe is in contact with the skin being the origin of the radial scanning lines.

The relationship between the size of the image and the actual area represented on the screen will vary according to the particular instrument and its depth settings, but in most cases the image is approximately half actual size.

The areas of black, white and grey on the screen represent different tissues and their interfaces. Fluid-filled structures are non-echogenic and appear on the screen as black areas (Fig. 11.2). If the bladder is at least partly full it can be imaged and will appear as an almost spherical black area with well-defined smooth margins and lying in the midline position. The fluid-filled uterus of a pregnant animal also appears as a black area but is readily distinguished from the bladder. In the early stages of pregnancy before the fetus and cotyledons or other forms of placentation develop to a significant extent, the uterus is convoluted and appears as several apparently discrete sacs (Fig. 11.3) which, by altering the angle of the transducer, can be shown to be parts of one structure.

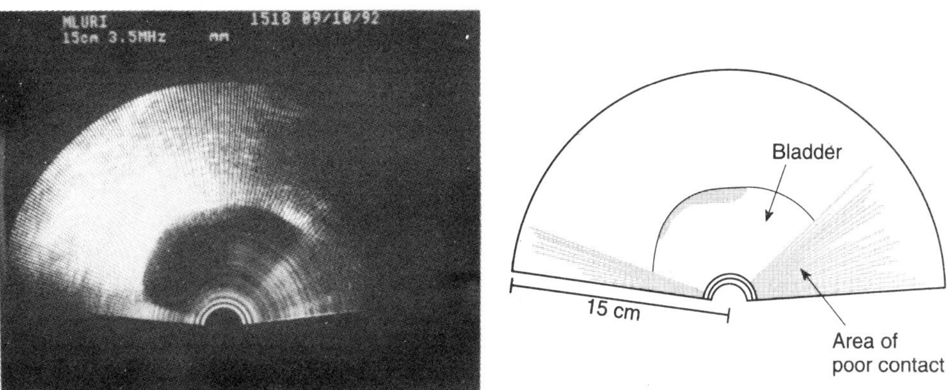

Fig. 11.2. Visualization of the non-echogenic bladder in a ewe.

As pregnancy advances, the volume of fluid in the uterus increases very rapidly and the convoluted appearance of the structure is lost, but it is unlikely to be confused with the bladder. The latter is always wholly non-echogenic while the uterus, by the time it is of a volume similar to a full bladder, will contain echogenic fetal material and cotyledons or areas of placentation.

In sheep and goats cotyledons can be distinguished from about 40 days as echogenic (white) structures with hollow centres which appear and disappear as the angle of the transducer is altered (Fig. 11.4). Cotyledons continue to grow in size until about day 90 and their size can be used by experienced operators as a guide to the stage of pregnancy. Points of placental attachment in red deer and

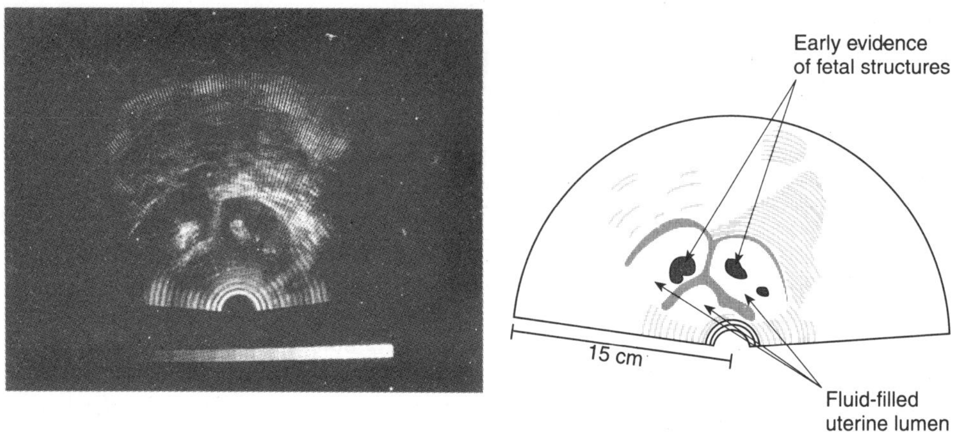

Fig. 11.3. Appearance of the reproductive tract of a ewe in early pregnancy, *circa* day 35.

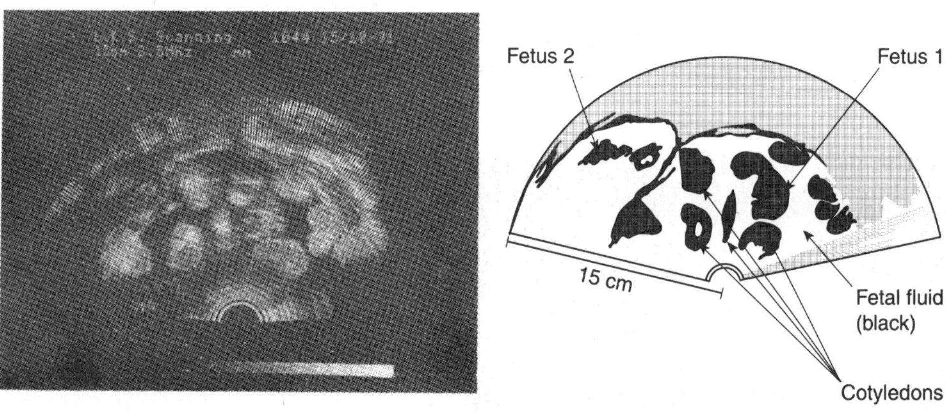

Fig. 11.4. Appearance of cotyledons.

camelids are more diffuse and appear as more highly echogenic (whiter) areas on the uterine wall.

Fetuses can be identified before individual cotyledons are distinguishable. They appear as almost circular highly echogenic structures, which seem to be freely floating in the uterine fluid, although implantation is in fact complete by this stage. The fetuses grow rapidly, as illustrated in Fig. 11.1, and by 45–50 days they can be observed to move independently of the surrounding tissues. At this stage the head is about half the size of the trunk, limb buds are evident and the crown–rump length is about 40 mm.

Fetal bones appear as highly echogenic, white images from about 70 days. As ultrasound cannot pass through the calcified skeleton, strong black shadows appear beyond well-formed bony structures such as the skull and scapulae. Images of the ribcage have a very characteristic striated appearance, with black shadows beyond each rib alternating with white lines where the ultrasound passes through the intercostal spaces (Fig. 11.5).

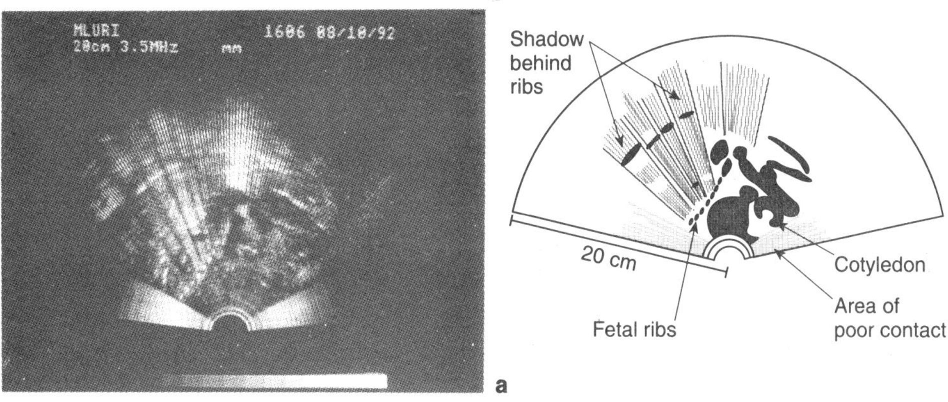

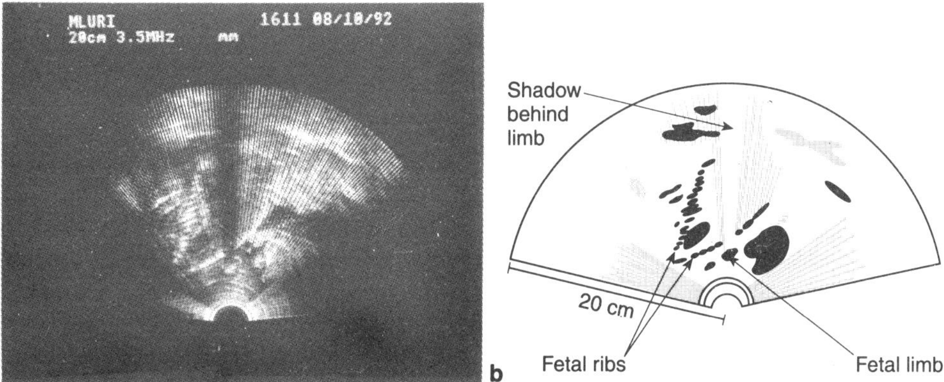

Fig. 11.5. Characteristic shadowing caused by calcified fetal structures: **(a)** ribs, **(b)** limb.

The beating of fetal hearts can be readily observed in scanning images. This, the often very rapid movement of fetal limbs, and the presence of shadowing all help to draw attention to the location of a fetus which, particularly if lying towards the periphery of an image, might otherwise be difficult to detect. These movements, which are an important aid to image interpretation, are, of course, lost when the image is frozen. The interpretation of frozen images or photographs are therefore much more difficult than in the case of 'live' real-time images.

The umbilicus is another structure which is readily recognized and can be an aid in locating a fetus. It appears either as an empty white circle, if imaged transversely, or as a longer tube-like structure if seen in longitudinal section (Fig. 11.6). This can be followed to the abdomen by a very slight alteration in the angle of the transducer.

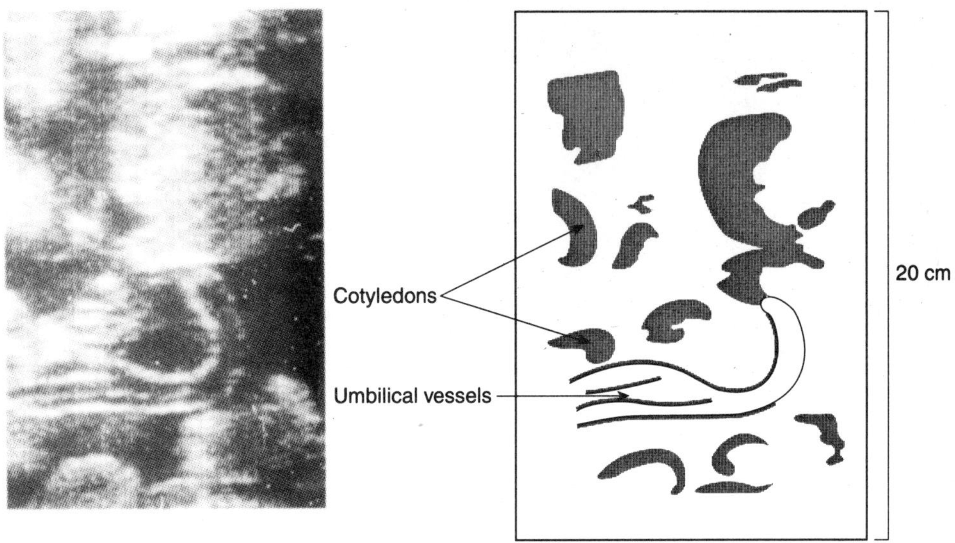

Fig. 11.6. Umbilical vessels. Longitudinal section seen on a linear array image.

The accurate counting of fetal numbers is more difficult than the diagnosis of pregnancy. One clue to the possible presence of a multiple pregnancy is the imaging of what is sometimes referred to as a 'septum' dividing the uterus into two compartments (Fig. 11.7). This is, in fact, the walls of the two uterine horns, and is seen only where both horns are fluid filled and are lying one against the other so that the two walls appear as a single structure. The imaging of this 'septum' is strongly indicative of a multiple pregnancy with one or more fetuses lying in each uterine horn. It is not, however, conclusive proof of the presence of two or more fetuses, as it is possible for the membranes and fluids associated with a single fetus to extend from one horn to the other.

Where two fetuses lie in the one horn, this clear division is not seen. In such instances the amniotic membranes surrounding and effectively separating the two fetuses appear as extremely fine echogenic lines which may only be seen in very high quality images.

A condition which occurs infrequently in goats, but which appears to be unknown in other small ruminants, is hydrometra, pseudopregnancy or false pregnancy. It is known as 'cloudburst' by goatkeepers. In this condition, does develop all the symptoms of pregnancy without the presence of a fetus. The uterus fills with fluid and some membrane-like structures may be imaged within the uterine lumen (Fig. 11.8). There are, however, no cotyledons nor, of course, any fetal structures.

In cases where the fetus has recently been aborted some placental contents, including cotyledons, may still be present although generally most fluid will have been lost too. If a fetus dies it may become mummified, possibly alongside a normally developing twin. In these cases disparity of size and absence of a heart-

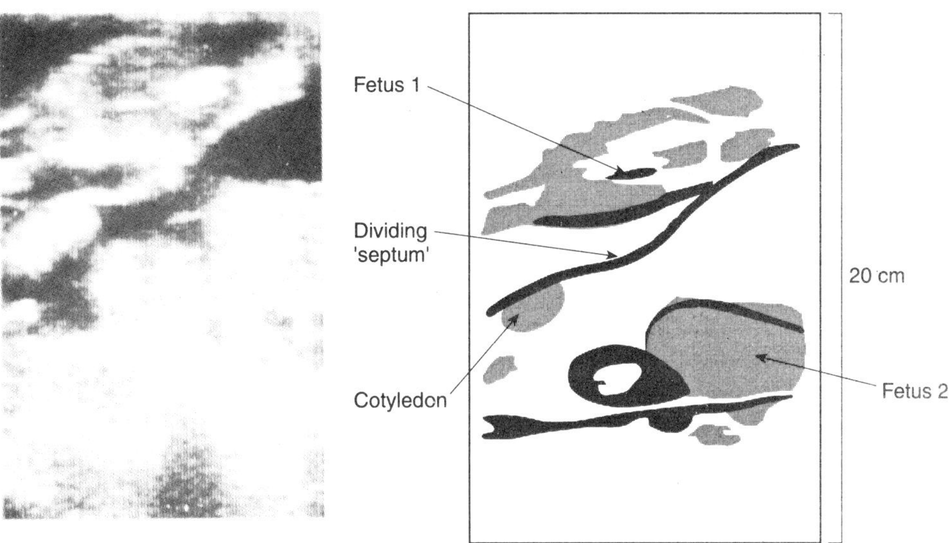

Fig. 11.7. Prominent demarcation between twin fetuses.

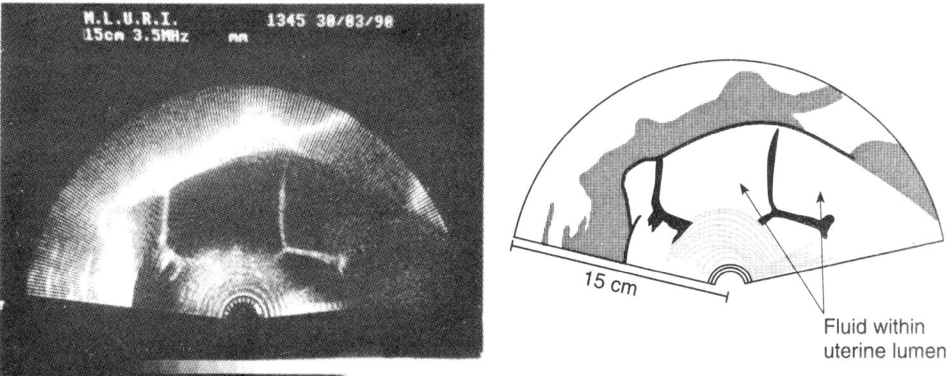

Fig. 11.8. Hydrometra in a goat. The uterus is grossly distended by fluid but no fetal structures can be seen.

beat are useful diagnostic signs. Uterine infection may result in pyometra, in which case floccular material can be seen within the uterine lumen.

Other Applications

Assessment of ovarian activity

Ovarian activity in small ruminants can be monitored by ultrasonography. The examination has to be carried out transrectally, as it is virtually impossible to obtain a clear path unimpeded by loops of bowel from any external placement of the transducer. As far as we are aware, this application of ultrasonography has been used only in the llama; it is theoretically possibly to examine the ovaries of other small ruminants by this technique, but the smaller physical size of sheep and goats demands the use of a very slim probe and extreme care on the part of the operator to avoid damage to the subject.

The technique is especially useful in camelids as these are induced ovulators and do not exhibit regular oestrous cycles as do sheep and goats during the breeding season. Ultrasonography has been used in llamas (Fig. 11.9) to evaluate ovarian status and, particularly, to follow the development of waves of follicles (which can be clearly seen around the edge of the ovary) and corpora lutea, so allowing strategic mating. Similarly the technique can be used to monitor ovarian responses to exogenous hormones. Studies on uterine morphology and early pregnancy diagnosis are possible, although there are insufficient reports to state the earliest stage at which a single examination will allow a reliable diagnosis of pregnancy to be made. To date, all recorded single pregnancies have been found in the left uterine horn. It is a technique destined to become more widely practised in the reproductive management of these animals.

Use in the male

Ultrasonography is finding an increased use in the investigation of male fertility in small ruminants, and may in a short time come to be considered as a routine part of pre-breeding examination as an adjunct to palpation and other techniques. The testes and epididymides are principally studied (Fig. 11.10). As with all ultrasound investigations, it is important for the sonographer to be familiar with the normal appearance of the tissues concerned and to adopt a standard technique. Once this familiarity is achieved, the study of abnormal structures and echotexture will allow identification of testicular and epididymal changes. Insufficient data are currently available to permit correlation of such changes with pathological conditions which may affect fertility.

Practical Considerations

Attention to some simple practical points is important if good results are to be achieved in practice. The quality of ultrasonic images is affected by a number of factors, including the acoustic coupling medium used and presence of gas in the intestines.

Two principal types of coupling agents are used. Vegetable oil can give a good contact on the often greasy skin areas on the abdomen and is readily absorbed by hair and wool. It is, however, difficult to wash off the animal after scanning and, where large numbers of sheep are being scanned at a time, the area around the operator inevitably becomes covered in oil and is physically hazardous. Oil can also interact with the plastic covering of the cabling connecting the transducer to the instrument, making it brittle and liable to split. Proprietary cellulose gels are more widely used and are generally to be preferred. They are water-based and easily washed off both the subject and the operator's hands. It is

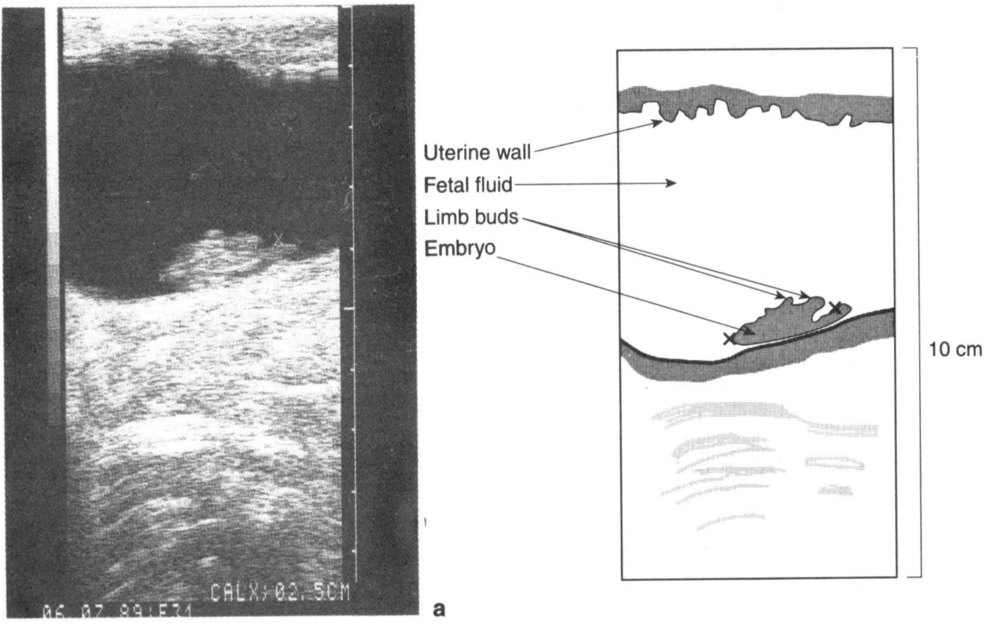

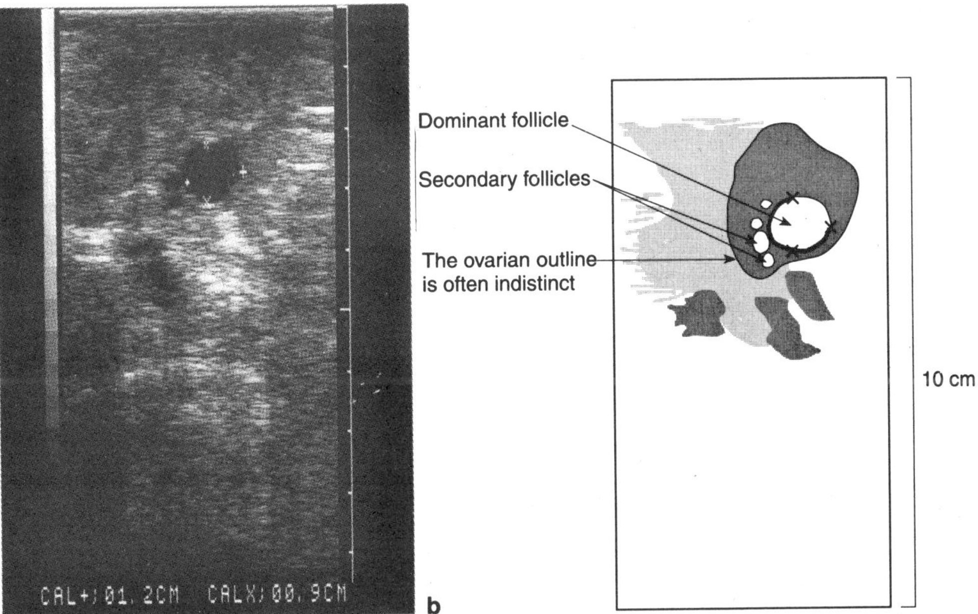

Fig. 11.9. Use of transrectal ultrasonography in the llama. **(a)** 30-day old embryo, 2.5 cm long. Note the large volume of fluid. **(b)** One large dominant follicle (12 × 9 mm) and several smaller follicles.

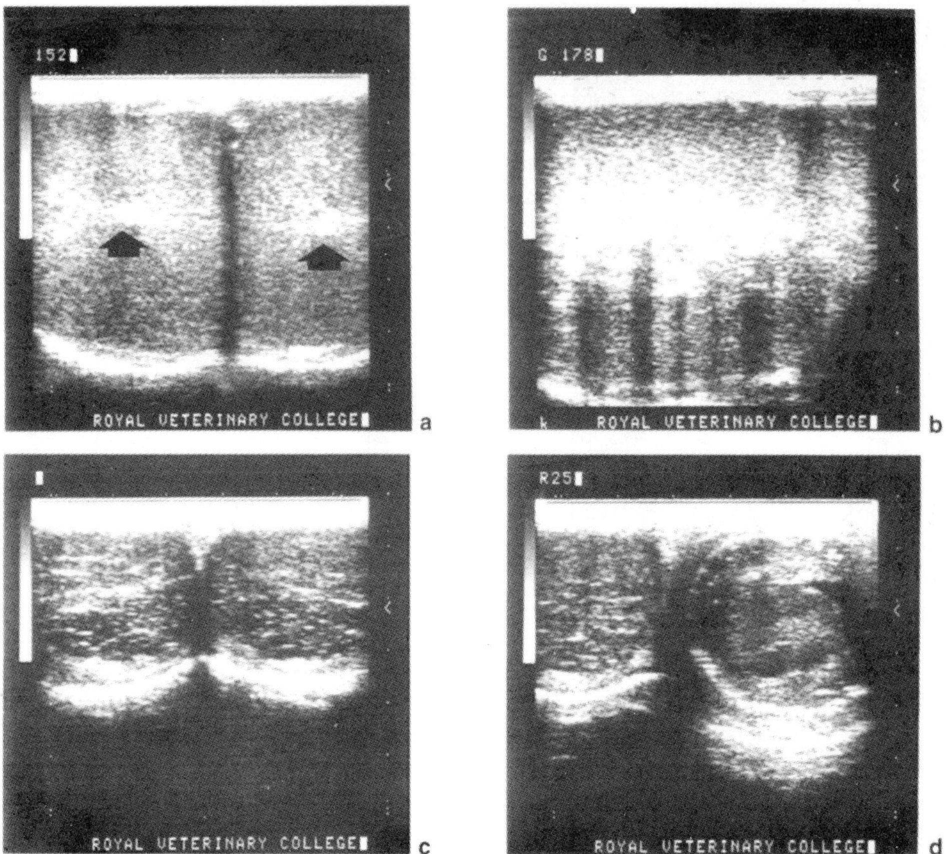

Fig. 11.10. Sonograms of the male reproductive tract. (Taken by Dr N. Ahmad, Royal Veterinary College.) **(a)** Transverse image of the paired testes of a normal ram, showing circular echogenic areas representing the mediastinum testis (arrows). **(b)** Longitudinal image of a testis from an infertile buck with testicular degeneration and mild mineralization represented by echogenic areas with acoustic shadowing. **(c)** Transverse image of the paired epididymal tails of a normal ram. **(d)** Transverse image through the paired epididymal tails of a ram. There are sperm granulomas in the right tail. The left tail is unaffected.

important to use only gels supplied specifically for animal use; similar products manufactured for other purposes may contain additives such as fungicides which could prove harmful both to the subject and the operator.

The presence of excessive gas in the lower part of the alimentary tract can adversely affect image quality. It is not possible to define the circumstances which affect gas production in the bowel, but diet and time since last feeding are clearly important. Practical experience indicates that withholding roughage (hay, silage and straw) for 12–15 hours before scanning is helpful in minimizing this problem. There is no reason to withhold water from the animals prior to scanning, nor is there any apparent disadvantage in scanning animals immediately after grazing.

Consideration should also be given to the physical layout of the scanning instrument and the equipment used for restraining the animal. Scanning should be carried out indoors, both from the point of view of the danger of using electrical equipment under wet conditions and because of the difficulty of viewing the screen in bright light. The instrument should be positioned indoors so that direct light does not appear immediately above the screen and indirect light is not reflected in the screen. Both situations make it difficult to interpret images.

Attention should also be paid to the comfort of the operator! Many commercial sheep scanning operators scan more than one thousand sheep per day and their performance is undoubtedly affected by the physical conditions under which they work; if they are comfortable and warm they are more likely to achieve a high degree of accuracy.

Accuracy

The accuracy achieved in the diagnosis of pregnancy and determination of fetal numbers in sheep and goats is dependent primarily on the skill of the operator. In theory the accuracy of both assessments should be 100%. In practice many experienced operators achieve accuracies close to this figure. Overall reported accuracy may be influenced by the actual pregnancy rate in the flock or herd.

The most common error in the diagnosis of pregnancy is the classification of a pregnant ewe as being not in lamb. This is invariably a consequence of scanning at too early a stage of pregnancy. If there has not been a ram with the ewe flock for at least six weeks, this type of error should not occur. The incidence of this type of error would, with many operators, be less than one per thousand ewes scanned.

Failure to identify one of a number of multiple fetuses is the main error in the determination of fetal numbers. This type of inaccuracy is serious if a twin pregnancy is determined as only a single, but is less serious if triplets or quadruplets are determined as only twins or triplets. The principal cause of this type of error is scanning at a too advanced stage of pregnancy when the volume of the uterus is very large and when extensive shadowing is caused by the fetus nearest the transducer. Despite the difficulties experienced by commercial operators in scanning flocks with a large range of gestational ages, many consistently achieve accuracies in excess of 98% in the determination of fetal numbers.

References and Further Reading

Ahmad, N., Noakes, D.E. and Subandrio, A. (1991) B-mode real time ultrasonographic imaging of the testis and epididymis of sheep and goats. *Veterinary Record*, 128, 491–496.

Bourke, D.A., Adam, C.L. and Kyle, C.E. (1992) Ultrasonography as an aid to controlled breeding in the llama (*Lama glama*). *Veterinary Record*, 130, 424–428.

Haibel, G.K. (1988) Real-time ultrasonic fetal head measurement and gestational age in dairy goats. *Theriogenology*, 30, 1053–1057.

Haibel, G.K. and Fung, E.D. (1991) Real-time ultrasonic biparietal measurement for the prediction of gestation age in llamas. *Theriogenology*, 35, 683–687.

Iason, G.R., Elston, D.A. and Sim, D.A. (1993) Ultrasonic scanning for determination of stage of pregnancy in the llama (*Lama glama*): a critical comparison of calibration techniques. *Journal of Agricultural Science*, 120, 371–377.

Russel, A.J.F. (1989) The application of real-time ultrasonic scanning in commercial sheep, goat and cattle production enterprises. In: Taverne, M.M., and Willemse, A.H. (eds) *Diagnostic Ultrasound and Animal Production*. Kluwer Academic Publishers, Dordrecht, The Netherlands, pp. 73–87.

White, I.R. and Russel, A.J.F. (1991) Determination of fetal numbers in sheep by real-time ultrasonic scanning. In: Boden, E. (ed.) *Sheep and Goat Practice*. Baillière Tindall, London, pp. 40–50.

White, I.R., McKelvey, W.A.C., Busby, S., Sneddon, A. and Hamilton, W.J. (1989) Diagnosis of pregnancy and prediction of fetal age in red deer by real-time ultrasonic scanning. *Veterinary Record*, 124, 395–397.

12 Porcine Reproductive Ultrasonography

M.J. Meredith and S.J. Maddock
Department of Clinical Veterinary Medicine, University of Cambridge, Madingley Road, Cambridge CB3 0ES, UK

Current Usage of Ultrasonography in Pigs

Doppler and A-mode ultrasound instruments are used extensively on commercial farms, all over the world, for pregnancy diagnosis. Real-time (B-mode) scanning (RTS) is used for reproduction research purposes but is, as yet, little used on commercial farms or even, diagnostically, by veterinary surgeons. However, we expect that, sometime in the future when instruments become cheaper and more portable, RTS will become the method of choice for pregnancy diagnosis on farms. Some specialist breeders have used A-mode or B-mode scanners for *in vivo* assessment of carcass quality characteristics in genetic improvement programmes. Ultrasonography is rarely used, at present, for diagnosis of genital disorders, but this could increase when real-time scanners become more readily available on pig farms.

Restraint for Scanning

Good restraint is essential for accurate positioning of the transducer and for systematic sweeping of the abdomen with the ultrasound beam. Too much movement of the sow, or of the transducer against the skin, can prevent a clear image being obtained or, in the case of Doppler instruments, produce uncomfortable and confusing artifactual sounds. Ideally, sows are restrained in stalls, tethers, individual feeders or even weighing or farrowing crates. Electronic sow feeders are becoming more common but often have solid sides with poor access for scanning.

Some loose-housed sows can be scanned while feeding. Outdoor pig units often have trailers for holding pigs for artificial insemination. If all else fails, sows can be restrained with a pig catcher or rope snare around the upper jaw, although this may prove too noisy for use of Doppler instruments! Movement of the sow during examination will produce artifactual sounds which decrease the accuracy of the technique. Often examination is carried out after feeding since sows may get restless prior to feeding. Bristles on the sow's skin can interfere with scanning, particularly if the transducer has a large contact area. The less hairy areas of the abdomen, lateral and dorsal to the mammary glands, are generally more suitable.

Rectal probes, for use with Doppler or RTS instruments, do not require a hand in the rectum, but there is a danger of damaging the rectum or colon when these accessories are inserted 'blind'. Transrectal RTS is undertaken with a hand inserted in the rectum to guide and hold the probe. Gilts are usually too small for this and only operators with small hands should undertake transrectal RTS of primiparous or small breed sows.

Pregnancy Diagnosis

Pregnancy testing has become a routine procedure on most commercial pig units in order to monitor the success of breeding management and to monitor boar fertility. Early identification of non-pregnant sows enables rapid re-serving or culling, resulting in a reduction in the number of productive days lost and therefore a substantial improvement in reproductive efficiency (pigs reared per sow per year).

The practical realities of pregnancy testing on commercial pig farms, are, firstly, that it is usually too expensive to employ veterinarians, so testing is mostly done by stockpersons. Secondly, most sows are pregnant at the time of testing, because of the high conception rate in pigs, so there are usually very few non-pregnant animals to detect. This means that, unless there is an infertility problem, the benefit of negatives detected is small compared with the cost of testing all the pigs that have been served (Meredith, 1989). Re-testing of pigs assumed pregnant is even less cost-effective. This severely limits the economic viability of pregnancy testing in herds with good performance. However, pregnancy testing is widespread because pig breeders place a high value on the reassurance value of routine testing. Commercial success is very dependent on being able to reliably predict and control the number of expected farrowings and the consequent availability of progeny to fill marketing contracts.

Strategies for pregnancy testing

What is the optimum time for pregnancy testing? Theoretically it would be beneficial to detect non-pregnant mated sows before their first return to oestrus, but this is not usually possible with ultrasound at present, despite the extravagant claims of some companies selling Doppler and A-mode instruments. Even if testing could be reliably done, diagnosed pregnancies could fail during subsequent days because embryo losses are common in the first month of pregnancy. Most sows which return to service do so at 21 ± 3 days after the initial service, but there is a second peak of returns between 24 and 30 days after service. These delayed returns are mainly due to embryo losses and commonly account for 20–30% of all sows that do not hold to service (Meredith, 1995).

Ultrasonic pregnancy testing seems to be of most value as a confirmatory test on pigs that have not shown return to oestrus by 30 days. At one month after mating, ultrasonic pregnancy testing is highly accurate and the pregnancies diagnosed should be reasonably secure from failure. This is also a time when a reliable confirmation of pregnancy can be very helpful, because sows are often moved away from the service area into housing which is less suitable for detecting oestrus. In situations where pregnancy testing of every mated pig is not cost-effective (in highly fertile herds), testing a proportion of the sows mated may be sufficient for fertility monitoring purposes.

For research, or infertility diagnosis purposes, real-time ultrasound can be highly accurate from 23 days after the first day of mating or insemination. Occasional pregnancies may be apparent a few days earlier than this – the stage of development of embryos can vary. Doppler and A-mode instruments can give some correct positives at 21–28 days of pregnancy, but negatives are unreliable before 28 days (preferably 30 days).

Pregnancy Diagnosis Instruments

Doppler ultrasound

Doppler ultrasound instruments constitute the most widely used special test for pregnancy in UK pig units at the present time (Fig. 12.1). Rectal probes are available, but external hand-held transducers are safer and more convenient. Doppler ultrasound allows the detection of a number of different indicators of pregnancy:

1. increased blood flow in one or more uterine arteries*;
2. fetal heart-beats;
3. umbilical artery* pulsations;
4. fetal movement.

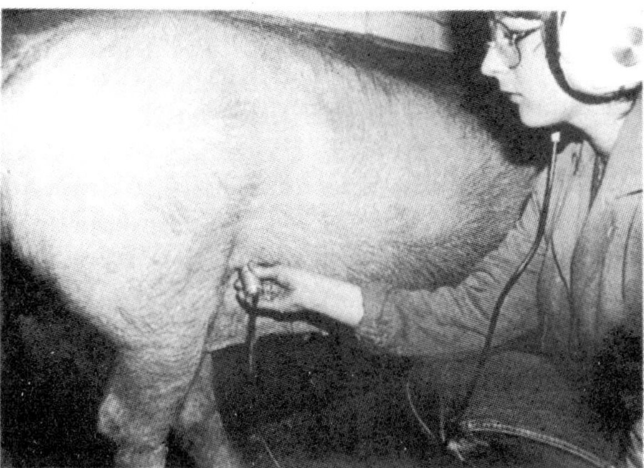

Fig. 12.1. Pregnancy testing of a sow at one month after service by means of a Doppler instrument. The transducer is aimed at a uterine artery. In pregnancy, pulsatile sounds will be heard in the headphones.

---

* Pulsations may also be detected in major branches of these arteries.

Detection of one or more of the above indicates that a gilt or sow is pregnant. Fetal circulation (heart or umbilical arteries) pulsations occur at a much faster rate than the sow's pulse rate, which is about 80 beats per minute at rest. An audiotape of typical sounds is available (Meredith, 1980).

Method

During the first half of pregnancy, sows are examined in the standing position since this facilitates location of the uterus. During late pregnancy, the uterus is more easily located and it may be more convenient to scan a sow in lateral or ventral recumbency.

Positioning of the probe depends on both the stage of pregnancy and the type of sounds required. Uterine artery sounds can be heard by placing the probe just medial to the stifle skin fold, on a horizontal line level with the stifle joint and a vertical line level with the second from last teat. The probe should then be directed dorsally and slightly caudally, aimed approximately one-third down the opposite flank. In the non-pregnant sow, the uterine artery is too small to be heard, except during oestrus when the pulsating of the uterine artery may be sufficient to be detected (Meredith, 1980).

To detect fetal sounds during the first half of pregnancy, the probe should be placed further forward on the abdomen, level with the third from last teat, pointed dorsally but not caudally. Late pregnancy uterine artery sounds may also be heard from here. Fetal sounds during later pregnancy can be heard by placing the probe on the boundary of the mammary tissue, level with the third or fourth from last teats, pointing the probe dorsally.

At all three scanning sites it may be necessary to move the probe around on the skin in order to locate the diagnostic sounds, since the beam is only about 2 cm in diameter and the position of the reflecting structures varies. If no evidence of pregnancy is found on one side of the sow, the other side should be examined.

Accuracy

Doppler ultrasound is unreliable before day 23 post-service and does not achieve good accuracy until four weeks after service (Almond *et al.*, 1985; Almond and Dial, 1986). At this stage, diagnosis is based on detection of uterine artery pulsations and both false negatives and false positives are possible. After six weeks, detection of fetal pulses is possible and both false positives and false negatives are rarer.

Reported accuracies range from 60 to 99% on sows that later prove to be non-pregnant (the *specificity* of the test) and 83 to 100% on sows that subsequently farrowed (the *sensitivity* of the test). The specificity, defined as the number of correct negatives as a proportion of the total test results for truly non-pregnant pigs (Meredith, 1994), is generally high. In contrast, however, the sensitivity of the Doppler instrument (defined as the number of correct positives as a proportion of all results from truly pregnant animals) tends to be lower. This means that, although the test is efficient at detecting non-pregnant animals, the lack of sensitivity will result in a number of pregnant animals being diagnosed as non-pregnant, leading to expensive errors if these supposedly non-pregnant animals are culled (Almond *et al.*, 1985). In practice, farmers rarely act on an initial negative result, but will re-test the sow once or twice, or wait until return to oestrus is detected, before culling a sow.

False negative results can be a problem with Doppler instruments because the operator is attempting to detect small structures in a large abdomen with only a small beam. Background noise from ventilation fans, sows or friction of the transducer on the skin can also be a problem. Operator care and skill is important in minimizing errors. When using a rectal probe, packing of faeces around the probe can decrease accuracy.

There are several causes of wrong positive results. Uterine artery sounds are occasionally present in normal sows as a result of oestrus or endometritis. A further possibility is that an agitated sow may have an elevated pulse rate which is mistaken for a fetal pulse. Finally, mistakes in recording or identifying sows during testing can lead to recording of erroneous diagnoses.

Almond and Dial (1986) compared the accuracy of Doppler ultrasound instruments with abdominal and rectal probes. The overall accuracy was similar for both types. Sows did not react to penetration of the rectum with the Doppler probe and no clinical consequences were detected. In stalls or crates, rectal examination took no longer to perform than abdominal scanning, and the rectal probe eliminated the problem of friction rubs encountered during abdominal scanning. Sows in oestrus or pro-oestrus during rectal scanning were occasionally wrongly identified as pregnant due to the increase in uterine circulation during these stages. To minimize this, sows should be observed for signs of oestrus prior to scanning. Rectal probes do, however, have the important physical limitation in that they cannot be used on gilts or small sows.

A-Mode (pulse–echo/amplitude–depth) ultrasound

This type of instrument differs from Doppler ultrasound in that pulses of sound are emitted and it is the amplitude (as opposed to the frequency) of the reflected sound which is detected. Reflections are displayed as either an audible tone, light-emitting diode(s), or as an oscilloscope trace. These instruments were popular in the 1970s, but are prone to giving false positive results and have now largely been replaced by Doppler instruments. Oscilloscope-type A-mode scanners can also be used for backfat measurement in breeding stock selection.

An audible tone and/or a diode lighting up is the simplest type of display for A-mode instruments. These signals occur when the reflection of ultrasound received by the probe is of sufficient amplitude and depth to be due to the pregnant uterus. Instruments with an oscilloscope display are the most sophisticated, and give detailed information about sound echoes as a series of peaks on an oscilloscope screen. Limitations of oscilloscope instruments are their expense, bulkiness, and fragility, and the more complex interpretation of output required. On the credit side, there is more possibility of discounting reflections from the bladder (Meredith, 1980).

The characteristic reflections of the pregnant uterus are thought to be from fluid/tissue interfaces. The proportions of fetal fluids and fetal tissues change during pregnancy, which limits accurate use of this technique in diagnosing pregnancy to days 30–70 after service.

Method

Restriction of sow movement and a quiet testing environment are less crucial than for Doppler instruments. The pig should be in a natural standing position to facilitate location of the uterus. A suitable contact medium is applied to the probe, which is placed on the hairless skin just cranial to the stifle and midway between the stifle skin fold and the margin of the udder. The probe is manipulated to slowly scan the area between the external angle of the ilium and the last rib, and ventrally to scan the entire depth of the abdomen. It is important to avoid the pre-pelvic area where false positive signals can be obtained from the bladder.

If no positive signal is obtained, the scan should be repeated on the opposite flank of the sow before recording a negative result.

Accuracy

Both false negatives and false positives are problems with this technique, particularly where a simple diode-type of reflection display is used. A-mode ultrasound instruments are only reliable 30 to 70 days after service (Gecele *et al.*, 1982; Inaba *et al.*, 1983; Almond *et al.*, 1985; Taverne *et al.*, 1985; Pyörälä, 1989), with the peak accuracy being reached at approximately 56 days (Gecele *et al.*, 1982).

False negatives are of low incidence with A-mode instruments (high sensitivity), but cause expensive errors when they do occur as they undermine the confidence of the operator when using this technique and may result in the culling of pregnant animals. False negatives can arise from inadequate scanning technique, poor skin contact (some A-mode displays give warning of this), uterus too close to the probe due to distension of the bladder or the gastro-intestinal tract (Taverne *et al.*, 1985), or small litter sizes (Pyörälä, 1989).

In contrast, the specificity of A-mode instruments is low for all types of display (Meredith, 1984; Taverne *et al.*, 1985; Botero *et al.*, 1986; Almond and Dial, 1986), and these false positives have compromised the economic viability of A-mode testing and led to them being largely superseded by Doppler instruments on commercial pig units. Wrong positives are mainly due to detection of the fluid-filled urinary bladder (Almond *et al.*, 1985; Taverne *et al.*, 1985; Almond and Dial, 1986; Glossop and Foulkes, 1988; Pyörälä, 1989; Guerra and Zavala, 1992) which is interpreted as a gravid uterus. These errors can be reduced if sows are scanned shortly after urination. Accumulations of fluid within a non-gravid uterus, such as pyometra or endometrial oedema, can also be misinterpreted as a gravid uterus (Almond *et al.*, 1985; Almond and Dial, 1986; Pyörälä, 1989).

Special merits

Minimal restraint is required for A-mode scanning and the small diode-type instruments are particularly cheap, light, robust and quick and easy to use.

Real-time (B-mode) ultrasound

Both linear array and sector scanners can be used for the porcine reproductive system. Sectors scanners are preferable because of the smaller skin contact area required, but linear array transducers are more suitable for ovary scanning by hand-held intrarectal manipulation.

The lower the frequency of the transducer, the greater the penetration of tissues and depth at which images are obtained, but, conversely, the poorer the resolution of detail in that image (Boyd and Omran, 1991). Thus 3.5 or 5 MHz instruments are most suitable for pregnancy detection (Cartee *et al.*, 1985), while 7.5 MHz is more suitable for ovary scanning.

Method

Sows must be more securely restrained when using real-time ultrasound than when using other ultrasound techniques, because of the inherent weight, bulkiness and fragility of these instruments. Care must also be taken if the scanner has a mains lead that could be chewed.

In the first two months of pregnancy, sows are best scanned in the standing position, to facilitate location of the uterus. The transducer is placed on the skin in the area of the flank medial and slightly ventral to the pre-crural skin fold (Fig. 12.2). The transducer is directed dorsad, towards the genital tract. In the second half of pregnancy, the gravid uterus will extend futher ventrad and craniad. It can be located by scanning from the flank, lateral to the mammary glands, between the first and third from last teats. As with all scanning for pregnancy, the scan should be repeated on the opposite flank if the first side is negative.

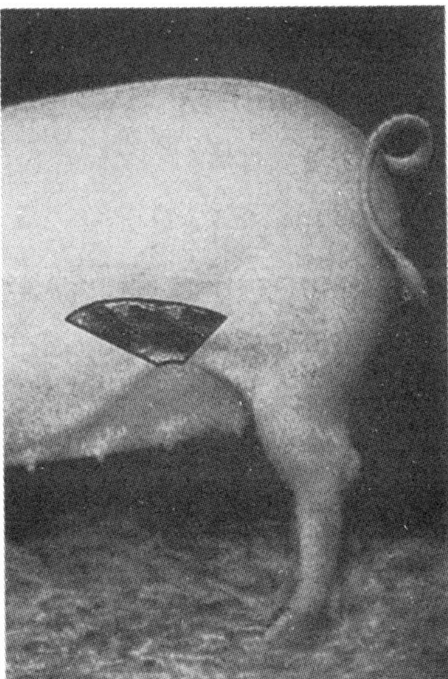

Fig. 12.2. Pregnancy testing of a sow at 25 days after service by means of a real-time sector scanner. The position of the fan-shaped ultrasound beam is illustrated. Detail of the image is shown in Fig. 12.3.

Interpretation of the display

In the non-pregnant gilt or sow, the uterus is difficult to visualize but may present as an indistinct, hypoechoic structure within the caudal abdomen and dorso-cranial to the bladder. The bladder can be identified and clearly distinguished from uterine structures by its location (caudal to the uterus) and appearance (an-echoic area with no echoic content resembling an embryo or fetus). Intestinal contents may appear as floccular masses of no definite structure.

The earliest reported changes in early gestation are enlargement and lobula-tion of the uterus, as early as 10 days post-breeding, with an increase in size but no change in appearance until days 21–22 when anechoic areas begin to appear (Car-tee *et al.*, 1985). These changes were only seen with a 5 MHz transducer and are too subtle and variable to be of use in routine pregnancy diagnosis.

At approximately 18 days, embryonic vesicles begin to appear in the uterine lumen. These are formed by rapid accumulation of amniotic and allantoic fluid in the lumen of the gravid uterus between days 18 (5 to 10 mm diameter) and 23 (15 to 20 mm). They are seen on the display as well-defined, regular, anechoic (black) areas, often surrounded by hyperechoic rings and embedded in the hypoechoic uterus. The presence or absence of these vesicles is the major criterion for diag-nosing early pregnancy. Reliable diagnoses can be made in the period from day 23 until full term (Inaba *et al.*, 1983; Cartee *et al.*, 1985; Botero *et al.*, 1986; Jackson, 1986a, b).

From approximately day 25, embryos become visible inside the embryonic vesicles as hyperechoic masses (Fig. 12.3) which reach 10–20 mm in size by day 30 (Botero *et al.*, 1984; Cartee *et al.*, 1985; Botero *et al.*, 1986; Jackson, 1986a, b; Martinat-Botte *et al.*, 1988; Meredith, 1988). The vesicles themselves are 40–50 mm at day 30. Cartee and colleagues (1985), using a 5 MHz transducer,

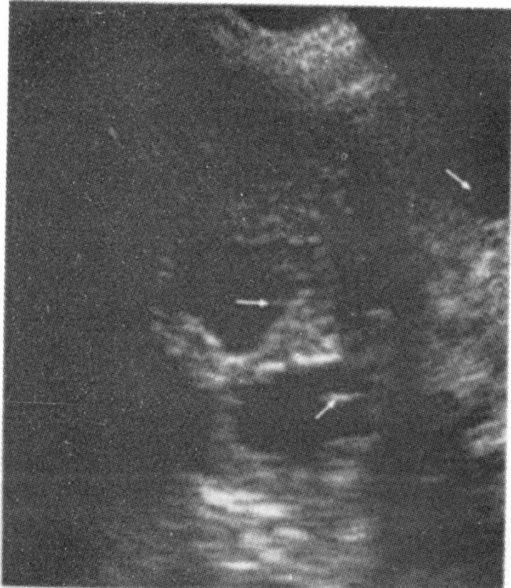

Fig. 12.3. Embryonic vesicles at 25 days of pregnancy (5 MHz sector scanner). Arrows indicate embryos.

reported detecting pulsatile movement within the hyperechoic fetus (representing cardiac activity) from day 25 of pregnancy. This was not detectable with a 3.5 MHz transducer. Embryo movement, represented by movement of a hyperechoic mass within the anechoic vesicle, was detected from 28 days post-service. Other investigators have detected fetal movement (the fetal period begins at 35 days in pigs), but only from 60 days post-service (Inaba *et al.*, 1983; Martinat-Botte *et al.*, 1988).

By 40 days, fetal structures such as the thoracic cavity, skull, liver and limbs have become evident (Fig. 12.4), and by 60 days the fetus may fill as much as half of the screen. Skeletal details, such as vertebrae and ribs, are visible at this time. Details of the placental wall can also be seen if a 5 MHz transducer is used (Fig. 12.5).

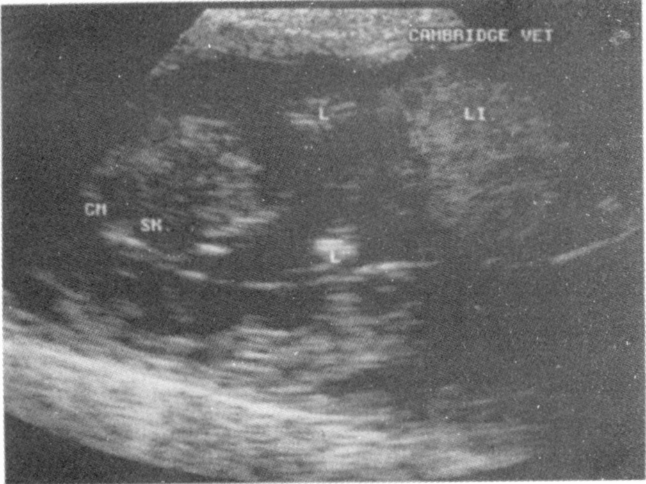

Fig. 12.4. Pig fetus at 42 days (7.5 MHz sector scanner). L = forelimbs, LI. = liver, SK. = skull.

Accuracy

Real-time ultrasonography can be used from 23 days and is close to 100% accurate (in both sensitivity and specificity) by 30 days (Martinat-Botte *et al.*, 1988). Early usage risks errors in predicting farrowing if embryo death occurs after the time of scanning. Other possible sources of false positives are abnormal accumulations of fluid in the uterus – endometritis or endometrial oedema appear similar to the pregnant uterus at three to four weeks after service (Inaba *et al.*, 1983; Jackson, 1986a, b). Ovarian cysts can also appear similar to embryonic vesicles (Jackson, 1986a, b). At 30 days, however, the absence of embryonic hyperechoic tissue in the embryonic vesicles allows the experienced operator to distinguish these pathological conditions from the pregnant uterus (Martinez *et al.*, 1990) – an advantage of B-mode instruments over their A-mode counterparts.

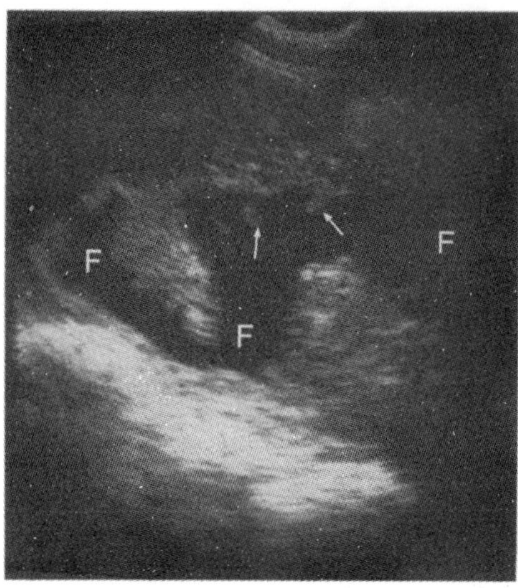

Fig. 12.5. Uterus at 42 days of pregnancy (5 MHz sector scanner). F = allantoic fluid, arrows indicate placental folds.

Another important advantage of the B-mode instrument is the ability to distinguish bladder from gravid uterus.

When false negatives occur, it is usually due to careless or insufficient scanning of the abdominal cavity, especially during early gestation (18 to 25 days post-service) and in sows with litters of fewer than five piglets (Botero *et al.*, 1986).

Problems and limitations

There are two principal limitations preventing the widespread application of B-mode instruments on commercial pig units. The first is the high capital cost of these instruments compared with the economic benefit obtainable on a single farm (Inaba *et al.*, 1983; Jackson, 1986a, b; Martinez *et al.*, 1990). Using an instrument on more than one farm is difficult because pig farmers are very wary of people or equipment that have been on another farm and may be carrying disease. Current instruments are difficult to clean and disinfect efficiently.

The second limitation of B-mode ultrasound is their inconvenience (Taverne *et al.*, 1985; Szenci *et al.*, 1992). Even the 'portable' instruments are heavy, bulky and relatively fragile. Recently, however, Szenci and colleagues (1992) reported that a battery-operated real-time scanner, using a 3.5 MHz sector transducer, was a highly accurate, rapid, on-farm method of pregnancy diagnosis in sows. The battery-operated instrument permitted a single operator to carry the scanner between sows by means of a shoulder case.

Special merits

Because embryos and fetuses are clearly visible, their state of development and health can be assessed (Inaba *et al.*, 1983). Early use of RTS allows some detection of embryo and fetal losses in cases of poor breeding performance (Taverne *et al.*, 1985; Botero *et al.*, 1986; Martinez *et al.*, 1990).

Detection of Pathological Conditions

A number of physio-pathological conditions can be detected by real-time ultrasound instruments.

Dystocia

Detection of retained fetuses during farrowing is possible by means of both real-time and Doppler (if the fetus is alive) instruments, provided that quantities of air have not entered the uterus.

Follicular cysts

In an extensive study, Madec and colleagues (1987) detected the ovaries in 73% of sows scanned and found that the ovaries were easier to detect when sows were in the follicular phase compared with the luteal phase. Cystic follicles were easily demonstrated (100% accuracy) on the ovaries. They were generally bilateral, appeared as an accumulation of anechoic vesicles each with a diameter of 10 to 40 mm, and were well circumscribed by a thin wall (Fig. 12.6). Normal follicles appear as small anechoic spots, 4 to 10 mm diameter, within echoic ovarian tissue.

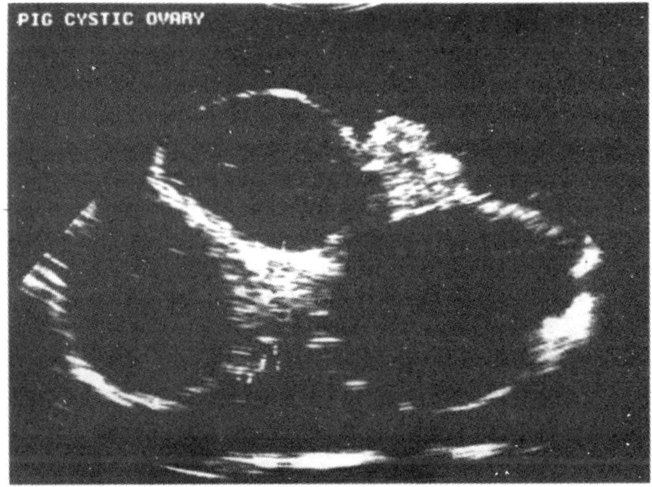

Fig. 12.6. Partially luteinized follicular cysts 30–40 mm diameter (7.5 MHz sector scanner).

Corpora haemorrhagica

Corpora lutea are difficult to visualize because of their low fluid volume. In contrast, corpora haemorrhagica are often seen (55% accuracy), appearing as anechoic zones, rarely greater than 20 mm in diameter, and sharply demarcated by thick walls as compared to cystic follicles (Madec *et al.*, 1987). However, these structures are generally of no pathological significance in pigs.

Endometritis

Endometritis can lead to false positives during pregnancy testing with Doppler, A-mode and B-mode instruments (see above). However, B-mode can discriminate between endometritis and pregnancy (Jackson, 1986a, b; Martinez *et al.*, 1990), since the fetus can be visualized in the gravid uterus after 30 days.

Miscellaneous

An abscess in the broad ligament has been observed by real-time scanning, appearing as a defined oval echogenic mass (Madec *et al.*, 1987). It is also possible that mummified piglets might be revealed by echography because of their morphology and structure (Jackson, 1986b; Madec *et al.*, 1987).

Acknowledgements

The technical help of Dr H. Rudorf and Mr J. Moyle of the University of Cambridge, and of Mr R. McIver of Dynamic Imaging Limited is gratefully acknowledged.

References

Almond, G.W. and Dial, G.D. (1986) Pregnancy diagnosis in swine: a comparison of the accuracies of mechanical and endocrine tests with return to oestrus. *Journal of the American Veterinary Medical Association*, 189, 1567–1571.

Almond, G.W., Bosu, W.T.K. and King, G.J. (1985) Pregnancy diagnosis in swine: a comparison of two ultrasound instruments. *Canadian Veterinary Journal*, 26, 205–208.

Botero, O., Martinat-Botte, F. and Chevalier, F. (1984) Ultrasonic echography for early pregnancy diagnosis in the sow. *Proceedings of the International Pig Veterinary Society*, 306.

Botero, O., Martinat-Botte, F. and Bariteau, F. (1986) Use of ultrasound scanning in swine for detection of pregnancy and some pathological conditions. *Theriogenology*, 26, 267–278.

Boyd, J.S. and Omran, S.N. (1991) Diagnostic ultrasonography of the bovine female reproductive tract. *In Practice*, May, 109–118.

Cartee, R.E., Powe, T.A. and Ayer, R.L. (1985) Ultrasonographic detection of pregnancy in sows. *Modern Veterinary Practice*, 66, 23–26.

Gecele, P., Diaz, I. and Skoknic, A. (1982) Pregnancy diagnosis in pigs. 1. Ultrasonic method (amplitude-depth analysis). *Proceedings of the International Pig Veterinary Society*, 232.

Glossop, C.E. and Foulkes, J.A. (1988) Occurrence of two phases of return to oestrus in sows on commercial units. *Veterinary Record*, 122, 163–164.

Guerra, D.C.G. and Zavala, R.L. (1992) The use of ultrasound, heat reappearance and exfoliative cytology for pregnancy determination. *Proceedings of the International Pig Veterinary Society*, 463.

Inaba, T., Nakazima, Y., Matsui, N. and Imori, T. (1983) Early pregnancy diagnosis in sows by ultrasonic linear electronic scanning. *Theriogenology*, 20, 97–101.

Jackson, G.H. (1986a) Pregnancy diagnosis in the pig using real-time ultrasonic imaging. *Proceedings of the International Pig Veterinary Society*, 9.

Jackson, G.H. (1986b) Pregnancy diagnosis in the sow using real-time ultrasonic scanning. *Veterinary Record*, 119, 90–91.

Madec, F., Martinat-Botte, F., Forgerit, Y., Le Denmat, M. and Vaudelet, J.C. (1987) Utilisation de l'echotomographie en elevage porcin: premiers essais de codification de quelques cas physiopathologiques concernant les organes genito-urinaires des truies. *Journées de la Recherche Porcine en France*, 19, 135–142.

Martinat-Botte, F., Bariteau, F., Lepercq, M., Forgerit, Y. and Terqui, M. (1988) L'Echographie d'ultrasons: outil de diagnostic de gestation chez la truie. *Recueil de Médecine Vétérinaire*, 164, 119–126.

Martinez, E., Vazquez, J.M., Coy, P., Ruiz, S., Carrizosa, J. and Roca, J. (1990) Early pregnancy diagnosis in the sow: comparison of A-mode, Doppler and real-time ultrasonography. *Proceedings of the International Pig Veterinary Society*, 476.

Meredith, M.J. (1980) *The Detection of Pregnancy in Pigs. Part 1: Tests for Pregnancy.* Tape–slide programme. Unit for Veterinary Continuing Education, Royal Veterinary College, London.

Meredith, M.J. (1984) Pitfalls in evaluating the accuracy of pregnancy tests. *Proceedings of the International Pig Veterinary Society*, 377.

Meredith, M.J. (1988) Pregnancy diagnosis in pigs. *In Practice*, January, 3–8.

Meredith, M.J. (1989) Pregnancy diagnosis in higher performance pig herds – is it a waste of resources? *Pig News and Information*, 10, 477–480.

Meredith, M.J. (1995) Pig breeding and infertility. In: Meredith, M.J. (ed.) *Animal Breeding and Infertility*. Longman, Harlow, pp. 278–353.

Pyörälä, S. (1989) Pregnancy diagnosis in swine by palpation and by amplitude-depth ultrasound scanning. *Theriogenology*, 31, 1067–1073.

Szenci, O., Fekete, C. and Merics, I. (1992) Early pregnancy diagnosis with a battery-operated ultrasonic scanner in sows. *Canadian Veterinary Journal*, 33, 340–342.

Taverne, A.M., Oving, L., van Lieshout, M. and Willemse, A.H. (1985) Pregnancy diagnosis in pigs: a field study comparing linear-array real-time ultrasound scanning and amplitude depth analysis. *Veterinary Quarterly*, 7, 271–276.

13 Ultrasonic Examination of Fish

P.J. Goddard
The Macaulay Land Use Research Institute, Craigiebuckler,
Aberdeen AB9 2QJ, UK

Introduction

There are a number of areas where ultrasound may have a valuable role to play, not only in the rapidly developing aquaculture industry but also in the hobby sector. The potential benefits have yet to be quantified but will derive from facilitating management practices, saving feed and improving diagnostic techniques.

This chapter considers some potential applications before discussing techniques so far found to be useful. It concludes with a section on image interpretation.

Applications

Sex determination

Ultrasonography offers a noninvasive method of sex determination in a variety of fish. For fish breeding enterprises it is important to differentiate the sexes for the optimum sex ratio to be maintained. As fish approach sexual maturity significant physiological changes occur, yet external phenotypic differences may never occur or are often not apparent until relatively late. Thus even experienced personnel may have difficulty in selecting male and female breeding stock at the optimum time. These secondary sexual characteristics include changes in body coloration and the appearance of the kype on the lower jaw or the dorsal adipose fin (Naesje *et al.*, 1988). Typically, maturing male salmon may be selected from July and females from August in the northern hemisphere. Absolute age will depend on growth characteristics but generally two sea-winter or possibly three sea-winter fish are involved, making them four or five years old respectively. Trout may be selected a month or two later. Determination of sex hormones from blood samples is possible. However, blood collection is stressful to the fish and, since the result is not available immediately, the fish needs to be permanently identified to allow sorting when results are known. Keeping excessively large numbers of fish to the time when separation can be reliably achieved, or making an earlier, less certain decision both have significant financial implications. In the former case not only are there additional feed costs, but the later rejected fish have a poorer meat quality (as tissue reserves are converted to energy) and hence a lower sale value. There is every indication that the use of ultrasound can aid this decision-making process by differentiating the developing female gonad at a relatively early stage, and thus has the potential to play an extremely valuable role in the management of fish stocks. However, there are currently insufficient data to indicate precisely at what stage differentiation based on scanning becomes reliable, since discrimination between the early developing gonad and the liver is sometimes difficult, and this approach has yet to be economically tested in a commercial environment. Ultrasonography may also have a useful role to play in surveys of wild fish in the same context.

Reproductive organ development

In fish breeding, direct collection of ova (roe) and semen (milt) with subsequent controlled fertilization is necessary to achieve good fertility. By monitoring the development of the ovary and testis the optimum time of collection could be predicted. Gross increase in external size can be used as a guide but this alone may provide insufficient information to allow egg and milt collection at the optimum time. By monitoring the development ultrasonically, a more precise correlation between developmental stage and post-collection fertility could be achieved.

Waves of development of gametes occur at intervals of a few days. By examining fish ultrasonically, repeat collections may be more precisely timed. Ultrasonic techniques allow the physical disturbance and associated stress on the fish to be minimized, and it may even be possible to dispense with the use of anaesthesia in appropriate situations. Reducing the stress fish are subjected to is likely to reduce the level of manifestation of subclinical disease. Current examination methods are also often time consuming. For example, it has been proposed that ultrasonography may have a role to play in the management of Pacific herring (*Clupea harengus pallasi*) (Bonar *et al.*, 1989). Here the technique was reported to be useful in determining the time when roe quality was highest and the maximum ratio of gonad weight to body size had been reached.

Tissue quality

It is possible that optimum harvesting time could be predicted by *in vivo* ultrasonic examination. Tissue elasticity and density are important contributors to the eating quality, and hence value, of the fish and are characteristics which ultrasonography can quantify. As fish approach maturity, fat and protein contents decrease and water content increases, and these and other organoleptic changes contribute to a deterioration in meat quality (Aksnes *et al.*, 1986). The speed of application of the technique would allow a large batch of fish to be examined relatively quickly. The stress to and mortality of the fish which can accompany repeated physical examination could also be reduced. However, it must always be remembered that harvesting is usually dictated by market forces which may override the desire to produce fish with ideal tissue quality. Currently, for example, salmon of 5–6 kg are desired.

The presence of tissue cysts of *Henneguya saminicola* leads to a marketing problem for the affected fish. Parasitism occurs only occasionally in batches of fish, with cysts reaching up to 15 mm in size. The cysts are normally first detected when fish are filleted. They have been detected in Pacific salmon using a 10 MHz device (Boyce, 1985). The ability to make a rapid diagnosis in whole fish would lead to better quality control and allow more rapid instigation of disease control measures. It may also be possible to image the cysts resulting from parasitism by cestodes. Other aspects of quality control could be examined, including monitoring tissue bruising and the efficiency of bone removal.

Diagnostic applications

When small numbers of ornamental fish are kept there is often the need to provide advice on individuals. There are a number of granulomatous diseases, fungal, bacterial and parasitic, which cause large swellings of the kidney, spleen or liver. A number of neoplastic conditions occur sporadically and enlarged organs with abnormal density may be identified. The diagnosis of a number of diseases affecting the internal organs may be facilitated by noninvasive techniques. The corollary of this is also true, since these techniques may also show the normal appearance of organs suspected to be diseased. Foreign bodies may be detected, if of appropriate density, and other abnormalities of internal organs and eyes studied. For farming situations disease may have a significant economic impact.

Anatomical studies

The ability to visualize many structures *in vivo* allows the correct anatomical disposition of tissues to be determined.

Techniques

It is important firstly to consider safety matters. The scanner may be required to work in a relatively humid environment and electrical safety must be assured. In addition to normal practices it is useful to be able to provide additional earthing to the holding tank, which is often metal. Since there will often be splashing it is important to ensure that no water can enter the machine. It is the responsibility of the sonographer to ensure that safety measures are appropriate. It is also important to secure the machine to prevent it being damaged. It may be valuable to provide a transducer with an extended cable. The highest scanning frequency consistent with adequate tissue penetration should be employed. For larger fish 5 MHz will usually be chosen but for smaller animals 7.5 MHz will be more appropriate and provide enhanced detail. There is no consistent benefit of using a linear rather than a sector instrument, although the former may allow easier interpretation of structures for the infrequent user, particularly if these structures are of circular cross-section.

This having been said, ultrasonography is a relatively easy technique to apply in submerged fish because the necessary acoustic coupling is provided by the water itself, through which attenuation of ultrasound is relatively low. Thus no other coupling medium is required. Flat fish in particular can be examined in a partially drained tank with no other restraint, the transducer being held a few centimetres from the target area. Fish generally remain quieter if the transducer is held a short distance from their surface rather than in direct contact. Alternatively, they can be temporarily removed from the water and examined on an appropriate table but the period for which they will remain static is relatively short and this time constraint does not facilitate a thorough study. For these animals their mucus coating provides the necessary coupling agent. In smaller fish particularly, unless a transducer with a very short focal length is used, a stand-off will help to optimize the resolution of the image. Specular reflection from the fish's scales does not generally cause substantial attenuation of the ultrasound beam.

It is most satisfactory if fish can be examined without removal from their environment, but for salmonids this is often not feasible and it will usually be necessary to administer an anaesthetic to facilitate examination. A system has been described in which the fish are encouraged to swim through a conduit below which the transducer is mounted (Reimers *et al.*, 1987). This allows an instantaneous image to be recorded for subsequent study but does not allow an interactive examination to be undertaken.

Whatever method of contact is employed, it is necessary to develop a protocol for systematic examination based on a knowledge of the anatomy of the subject. This is particularly important with reproductive tract development which will displace the viscera, since the pre-ovulatory ovary may well occupy the majority of the abdominal cavity and extend caudally between the muscles to near the anus. Details of anatomy can be found in Harder (1975) and Lagler *et al.* (1977). The structures to be examined may be larger than the width of the transducer and it will be necessary to devise an accurate measurement system.

When examining flat fish it is only generally necessary to scan in one plane, perpendicular to the lateral surface. Angling the transducer will allow alternative views if necessary. Essentially examination of the area behind the operculum and below the midline is required to visualize the body cavity. Skeletal structures occupying a conventional dorso-ventral position may make it difficult to visualize the ventral side when a high scan frequency is selected. When examining salmonids, two planes are available for examination, with the transducer head held either transversely or longitudinally, although it may be sensible (and less confusing) to use consistently either the ventro-dorsal or lateral approach (Fig. 13.1). If a large number of fish are to be examined it is useful to prepare a suitable holding cradle. When flat fish are studied the views are restricted.

It has been suggested that a period of starvation of up to three days may be necessary to enhance the image quality by reducing gut fill in salmon (Reimers *et al.*, 1987), although the author does not practise this.

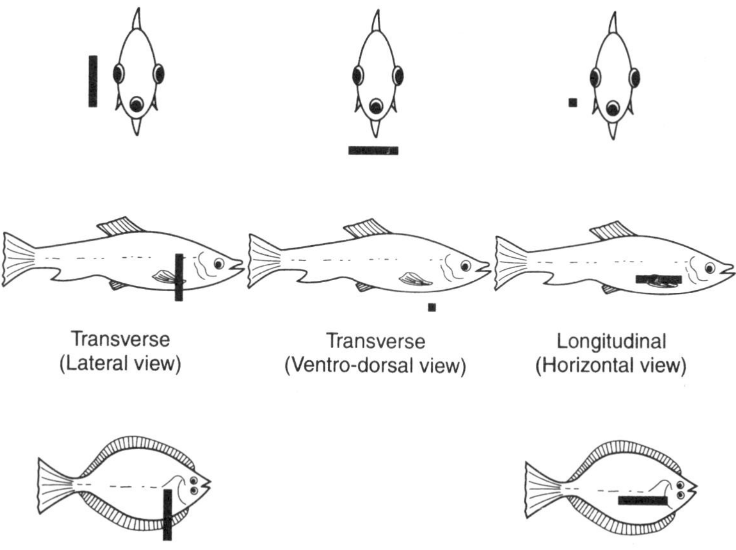

Fig. 13.1. Standard scanning planes for fish.

Storing Images

Conventional methods of image storage can be used, although due regard must be given to the environment in which devices are required to work. Video recorders and video printers must be made safe to work in a hostile damp atmosphere. Polaroid stills can be made but the low temperature often experienced during field work in temperate latitudes leads to problems with development: it is difficult to keep film packs and the processing environment warm enough.

Image Interpretation

Initial experience should be gained with fish that can subsequently be killed and examined. The examination of fish which have been frozen and subsequently thawed is not a helpful exercise, as during these processes water leaves the intracellular spaces leading to a great reduction in ultrasonic contrast. As with any ultrasonic investigation, successful image interpretation requires a knowledge of the area being scanned. Use should be made of standard landmarks, especially if comparative measurements are to be made, and a standard examination procedure should be adopted. Much more value will be derived from an interactive examination than from studying static images such as those presented here, which are included simply for guidance.

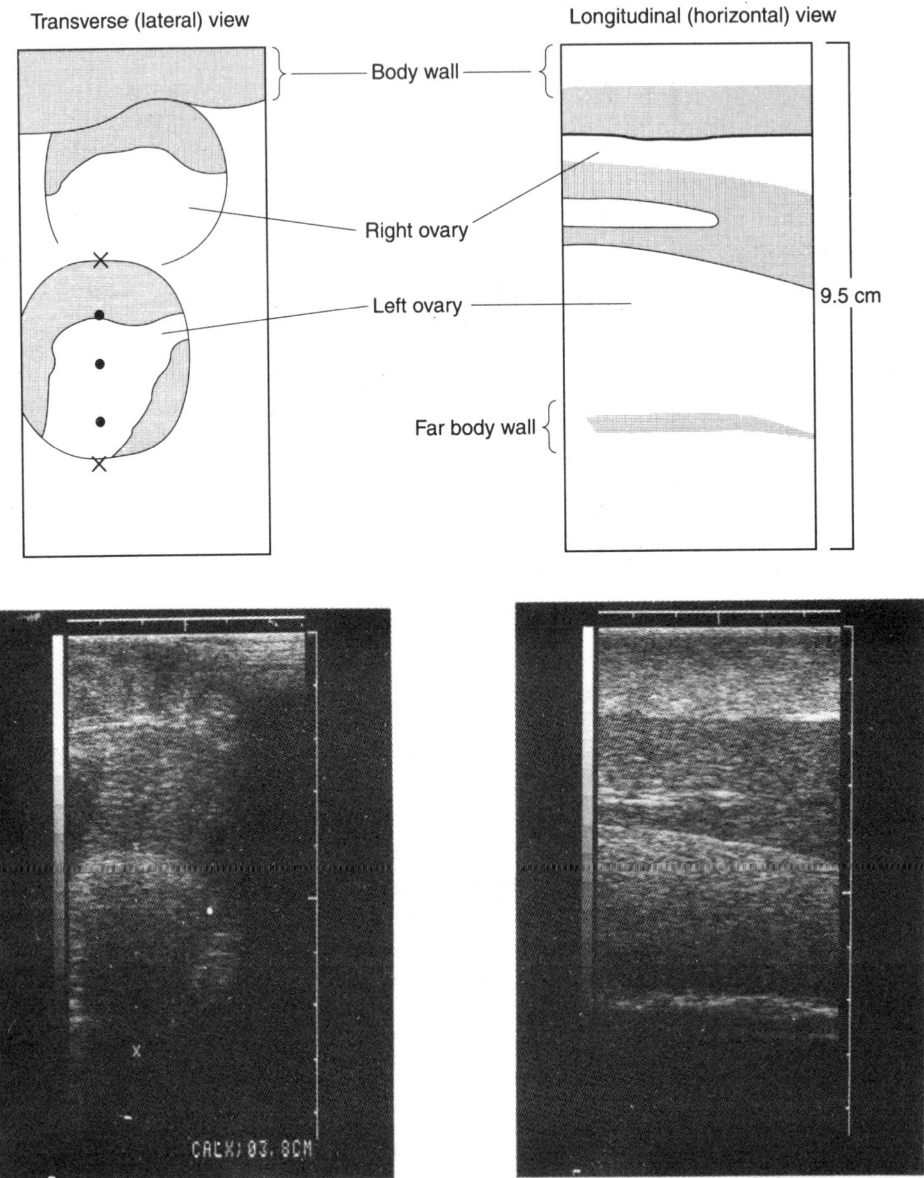

Fig. 13.2. Bipartite ovary in a mature salmon. The two halves of the ovary can be clearly seen. At the level scanned, the left ovary diameter is 3.8 cm. Thus the ovaries occupy most of the body cavity.

Reproductive organs

Sex determination becomes easier as maturity is approached. One important difficulty arises in fish with prominent swim bladders (air bladders) which can cause marked reverberation echoes. The swim bladder lies adjacent to the developing

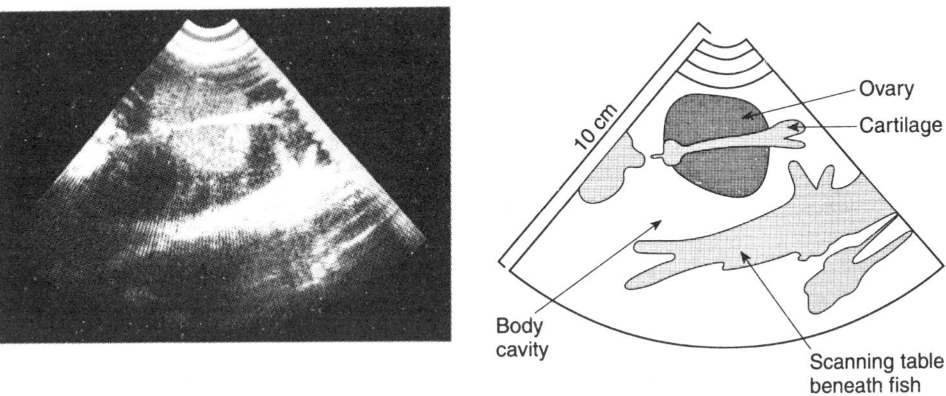

Fig. 13.3. Immature female halibut ovary viewed from behind the operculum. Transverse (lateral) view.

gonad. Experience must be developed to distinguish the gonad from the adjacent liver and kidney.

Female

The bipartite ovary is located on either side of the midline skeletal structures. Development of the two halves may not be synchronous. As maturity is approached there is a dramatic increase in size of the ovary which displaces abdominal organs and enlarges caudally. The two halves become less easily separated visually. Figure 13.2 shows the typical appearance in a mature salmon, while Fig. 13.3 shows an immature female halibut. The ovarian contents become more granular in appearance as the ova become hydrated within the ovarian lumen and surrounded by fluid, and this qualitative change can be easily discerned with experience. Indeed in the early stages of development, ultrasound penetration may be poor due to the high reflectivity of the developing ova, which are yolk-filled at this stage (Fig. 13.4a). Ultrasound penetration increases only during the final maturation when ova take in water (Fig. 13.4b). Immediately prior to release, therefore, the distinctive fluid centre of the expanded ova can be recognized when scanning at high frequency. After egg collection (stripping) the proportion of hydrated ova is reduced and this change can again be discerned. Ova of different developmental stages may be identified on the lamellar supporting tissue.

Gonad diameter is readily measured and the gonadosomatic index calculated as a measure of maturity (Mattson, 1991).

Male

The distinctive male gonad presents as a finely textured grey oval structure, generally surrounded by a fluid (black) area (Fig. 13.5). In early stages of development its centre appears darker (due to a higher water content) but approaches the density (yet more finely grained) of the ovary as the fish matures. Qualitative changes following collection of milt are less easily determined than equivalent changes in the female.

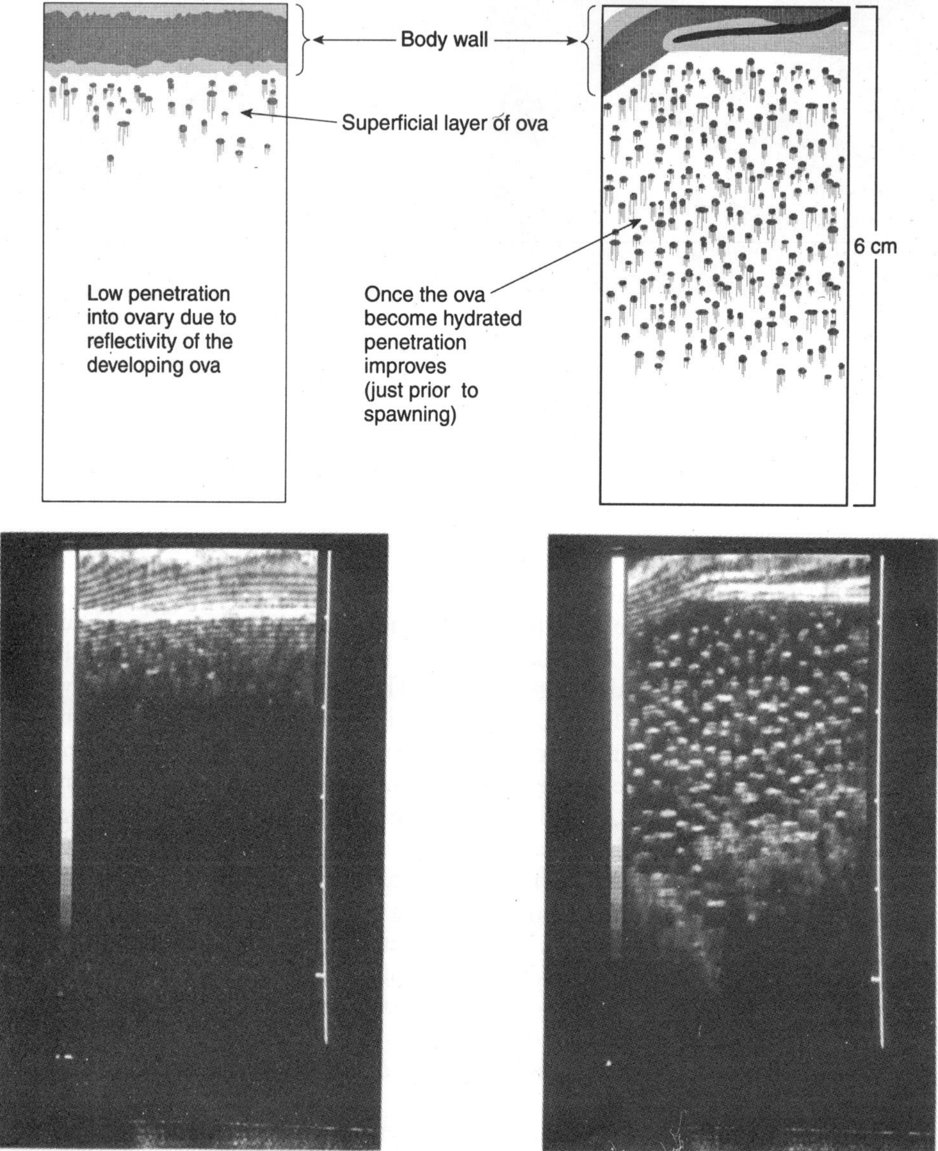

Fig. 13.4. Qualitative change in sonographic appearance of a maturing halibut ovary. Transverse (lateral) views. Sonograms courtesy of Dr R. Shields.

Bonar *et al.* (1989) found that sex determination in the Pacific herring was entirely reliable when the weight of the gonads exceeded 2.9 g, and both sexes were equally identifiable when scanning fish at 5 MHz. Other reports suggest that immature males are less easily identified than females, and may only be selected by default (i.e. not female).

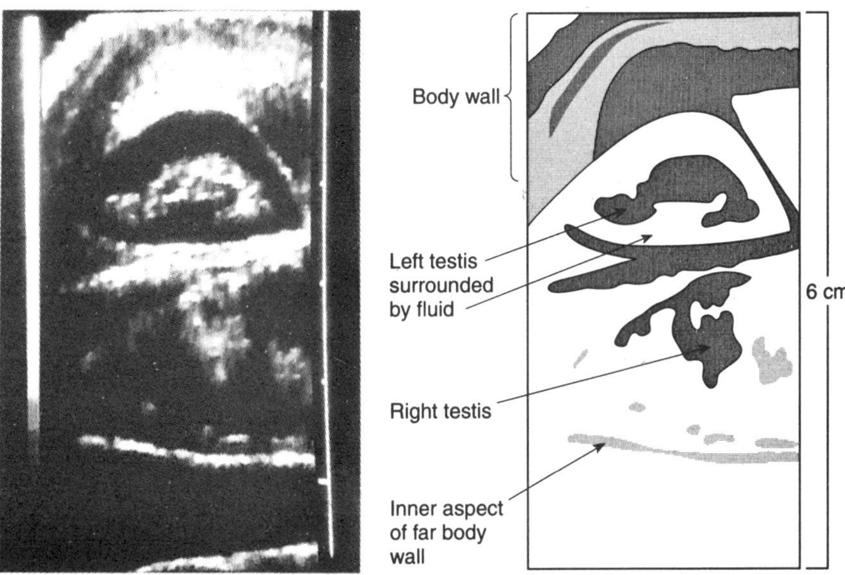

Fig. 13.5. Male gonad in a mature halibut. Transverse (lateral) view. Sonogram courtesy of Dr R. Shields.

Abdominal viscera

A number of abdominal components are readily identified and in the immature fish these occupy the majority of the body cavity, together with variable amounts of adipose tissue. Figure 13.6 presents sonograms of the liver, stomach and pyloric caecae, the latter being modifications of the mid-gut, opening into the intestine caudal to the stomach. It should be noted that the gall bladder becomes very large in non-feeding fish.

Diagnostic applications

Neoplasia

Farmed fish are harvested at a relatively young age and consequently the incidence of neoplastic conditions is low. However, hepatoma in trout caused by aflatoxicosis following feeding on mouldy feed may be seen before fish reach market weight. Rainbow trout are most sensitive and epidemics have occurred. Fish develop extremely friable livers and high mortality ensues. Enlarged livers could be seen *ante mortem* using ultrasonography.

Eyes

Ultrasonography may be valuable in the diagnosis of ophthalmic lesions in larger fish as an adjunct to conventional methods of examination, particularly when

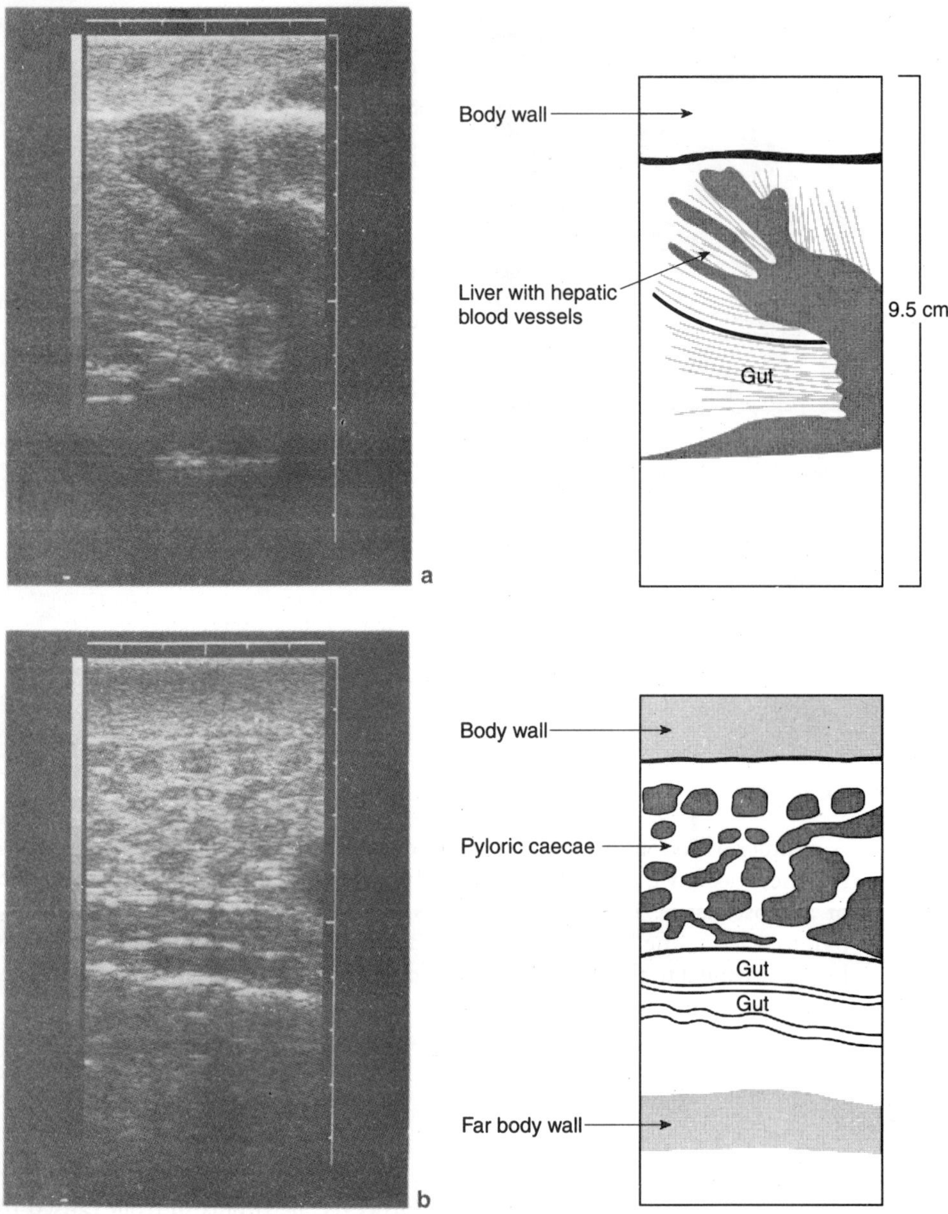

Fig. 13.6. Abdominal viscera in the salmon (**a** and **b**). The scale is the same in both scans.

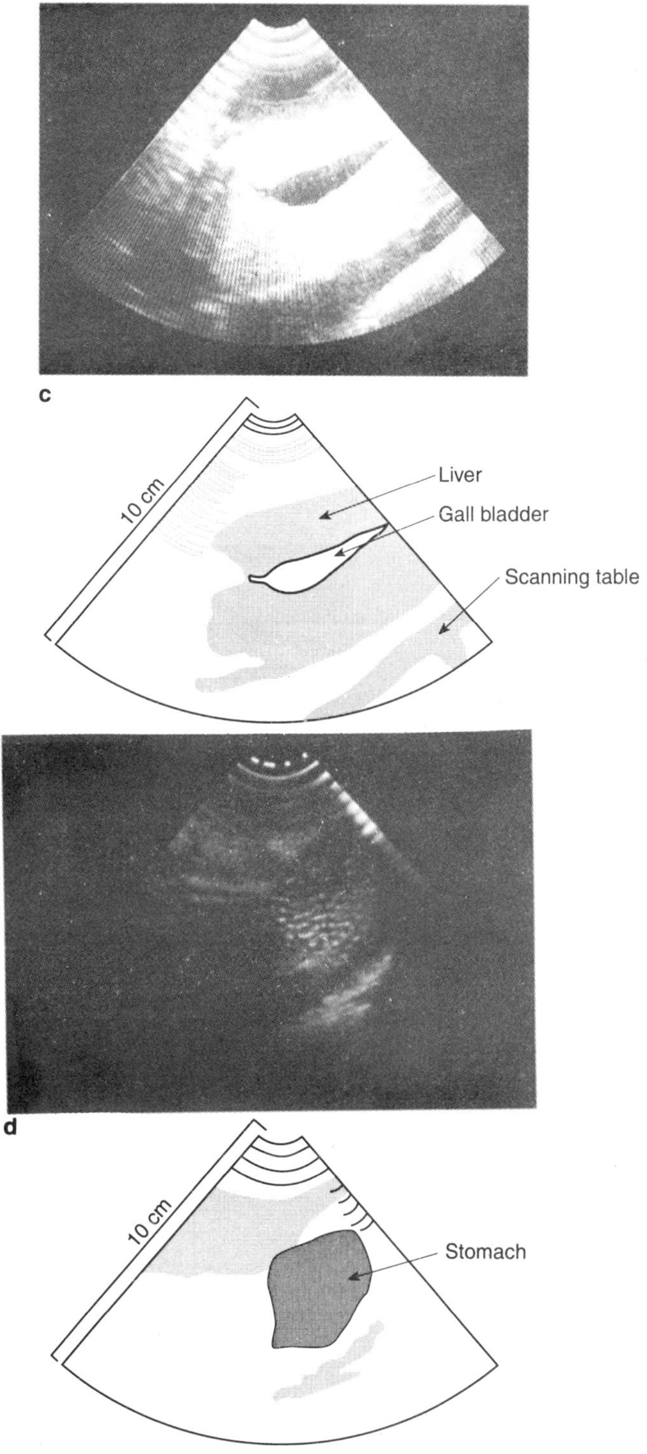

Fig. 13.6 *cont.* Abdominal viscera in the halibut (**c** and **d**).

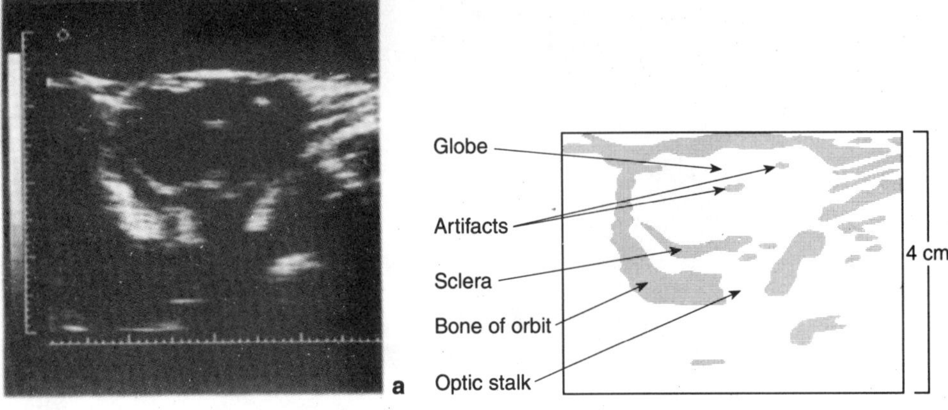

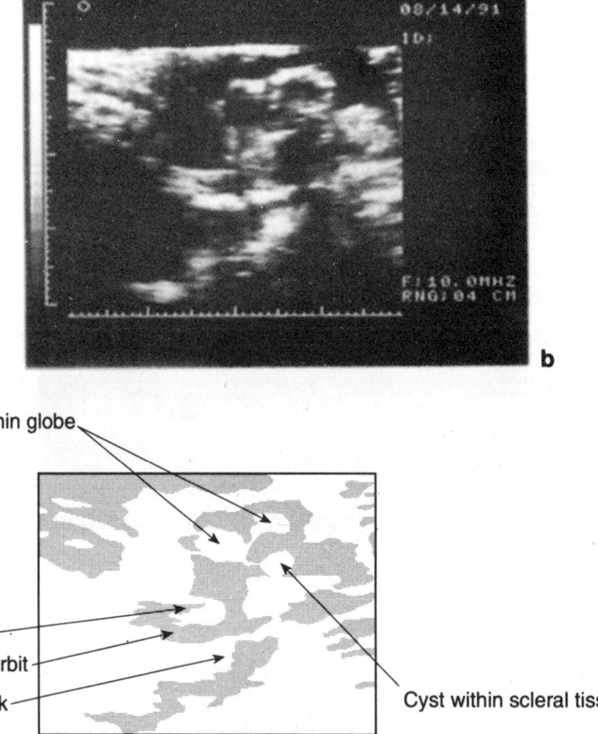

Fig. 13.7. Suspected gas bubble disease in fish eyes. **(a)** Normal eye. **(b)** Diseased eye. (Aloka ASU32WL, 10 MHz in-line oscillating sector, inbuilt stand-off.)

corneal oedema or lens defects prevent visualization of deeper structures. Eyes can be examined transcorneally or transcutaneously although the bony structures surrounding the globe may hamper sonography. As an example of this application Fig. 13.7 shows a case of suspected gas bubble disease. Corneal opacity prevented conventional ophthalmoscopy, yet *in vivo* ultrasonic examination showed cystic defects to be present behind the retina.

Swim bladder defects

The swim bladder (gas bladder) is primarily a hydrostatic organ. While it may theoretically present a problem of poor transmission of ultrasound through gases, in practice its relatively small size does not interfere with imaging. Swim bladder fibrosarcoma has been seen in cage culture of Atlantic salmon. Large neoplasms impinge on the swim bladder and cause loss of equilibrium and swimming ability. Again, diagnostic ultrasonography would aid examination of live fish. In Fig. 13.8 a sonogram from a grossly enlarged salmon with a swim bladder defect is presented. The swim bladder of salmonids is normally simple and saclike but in this case a multilocular appearance can be clearly seen.

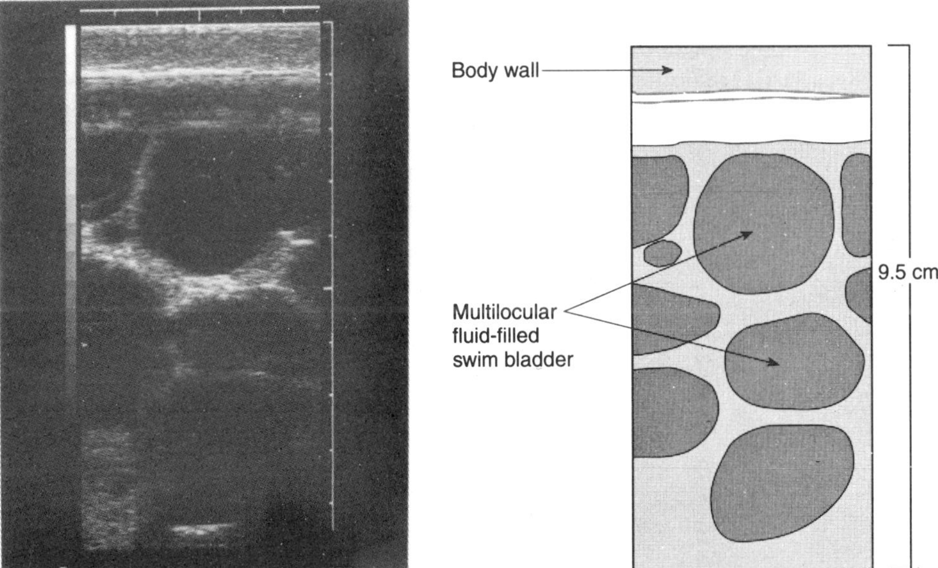

Fig. 13.8. Swim bladder in a grossly enlarged salmon.

Tissue cysts

Mention has already been made of tissue cysts. These and other economically significant lesions are potentially detectable using ultrasonography.

Acknowledgement

The advice of Peter Southgate is gratefully acknowledged.

References

Aksnes, A., Gjerde, B. and Roald, S.O. (1986) Biological, chemical and organoleptic changes during maturation of farmed atlantic salmon, *Salmo salar. Aquaculture*, 53, 7–20.

Bonar, S.A., Thomas, G.L., Pauley, G.B. and Martin, R, W. (1989) Use of ultrasonic images for nonlethal determination of sex and maturity of Pacific herring. *North American Journal of Fisheries Management*, 9, 364–366.

Boyce, N.P. (1985) Ultrasound imaging used to detect cysts of *Henneguya salminicola* (Protozoa: Myxozoa) in the flesh of whole Pacific salmon. *Canadian Journal of Aquatic Science*, 42, 1312–1314.

Harder, W. (1975) *Anatomy of Fishes.* E. Schweizerbart'sch Verlagsbuchhandlung, Stuttgart.

Lagler, K.F., Bardach, J.E., Miller, R.R. and Passino, D.R.M. (1977) *Ichthyology*, John Wiley and Sons, New York.

Mattson, N.S. (1991) A new method to determine sex and gonad size in live fishes by using ultrasonography. *Journal of Fish Biology*, 39, 673–677.

Naesje, T.F., Hansen, L.P. and Jarvi, T. (1988) Sexual dimorphism in the adipose fin of Atlantic salmon, *Salmo salar* L. *Journal of Fish Biology*, 33, 955–956.

Reimers, E., Landmark, P., Sorsdal, T., Bohmer, E. and Solum, T. (1987) Determination of salmonids' sex, maturation and size: an ultrasound and photocell approach. *Aquaculture Magazine*, November/December, 41–44.

14 Therapeutic Ultrasound

M. Porter
4350 Harrodsburg Road, Lexington, Kentucky KY 40513,
USA

Ultrasound is classified as a heating agent when used therapeutically. Therapeutic heating agents are divided into two categories: those that heat superficial tissues and those that heat deeper tissues. Those agents that produce temperature changes in the skin and subcutaneous tissue to a depth of approximately 1 cm include hot packs and warm water baths. These agents only elevate skin temperature with little change in the temperature of the underlying structures. Deep heating agents cause temperature elevations in tissues to depths of 3 cm or more, without overheating the superficial tissues. Besides ultrasound, short-wave and microwave diathermy are included in this category but of these, ultrasound is by far the most appropriately designed tool to use on a horse.

In human medicine, ultrasound is used for diagnosis (imaging of internal structures), for tissue destruction (surgery for tumour irradiation and lipostripsy), and for physical therapy (to promote deep tissue healing and restore function in joints). This chapter will discuss the therapeutic use of ultrasound. Topics will include the physics of ultrasound, the physical effects of ultrasound, the biological and therapeutic effects of ultrasound, and treatment methods, protocols, and precautions.

The Physical Principles of Therapeutic Ultrasound

In her book *Thermal Agents in Rehabilitation* (1986), Susan Michlovitz provides an eloquent description of the nature of sound. She points out that solids and liquids consist of molecules held together by elastic forces that connect each molecule to its nearest neighbour. Thus a molecule set in motion will cause its neighbour to move, and in turn *its* neighbour, until the vibration has propagated throughout the material. Propagation of this vibratory motion is the basic element of sound wave production.

The vibratory frequency of a sound wave affects its absorption into body tissues. Frequency refers to the number of vibrations a molecule in the sound wave undergoes in one second. The higher the frequency, the less the sound waves diverge. Audible sound ranges between 16 and 20,000 cycles of vibration per second. Sound waves at this frequency appear to spread out in all directions. Ultrasound waves have a frequency of greater than 20,000 cycles per second (Hz) and are well collimated. Physical therapy devices product a beam of sound at a frequency of one million cycles per second (1 MHz) that is sufficiently collimated to penetrate to selected target tissues.

As sound wave frequency increases, its absorption by the tissues increases. As absorption increases there is less sound energy available to propagate further through the tissue. Therapeutic frequencies of 1 MHz penetrate as deep as 4–6 cm into the tissues. Tissues with a high fluid content, such as blood and muscle, will absorb sound waves better than less hydrated tissues. Nerve tissue has a high coefficient of ultrasound absorption. This expands treatment possibilities to sounding nerve roots that are associated with peripheral conditions.

Heating Effects of Ultrasound

Ultrasound's primary therapeutic use is as a deep tissue heating modality. As the ultrasound wave travels through the medium, mechanical energy is converted to heat. The heat diffuses into surrounding tissues by waves reflecting off acoustic inhomogeneities such as tissue interfaces or dissolved gas bubbles.

Within the body tissues, wave reflection is greatest at interfaces of bone and soft tissue because of the great difference in their acoustical absorption. Reflected waves, called transverse or shear waves, interact with incoming longitudinal waves. Although liquids cannot sustain shear waves, solids can. Soft tissues in the body behave as liquids, and bone behaves as a solid in the way they sustain sound waves. Bone can be subjected to high ultrasound intensity as the incoming longitudinal wave is absorbed and the transverse or reflected wave is superimposed on it. Overheating of bone is thus a danger of incorrect use of ultrasound. Blood vessels and membranes in the path of the interacting waves could also suffer thermal damage. When the highly innervated periosteum is overheated, pain results. The sensation is a dull, aching pain but one which animals are not likely to react to quickly. Thermal damage could occur before overheating is appreciated by the patient or the operator. This can be avoided by using low intensities and by steadily moving the sound head over an area if bone is close to the skin surface.

Absorption of ultrasound takes place on the molecular level and protein molecules are the major absorbers (Hartley, 1991). Skin and subcutaneous fat do not absorb ultrasound well, so the skin surface may remain cool while underlying structures are heated. This unique characteristic among heating modalities makes ultrasound an ideal therapeutic tool for sports injuries. Such injuries usually occur to the nerves, ligaments, tendons, joint capsules and muscles, all tissues with a high protein component and high coefficients of ultrasound absorption.

Sound wave reflection occurs at interfaces such as nerve and nerve sheath, muscle sheath and muscle, joint capsule and joint structures, tendon and tendon sheath, and scar tissue and the tissue surrounding it. The interaction of incoming and reflected waves at these interfaces causes selective heating of **these tissues.**

Chemical Effects of Ultrasound

Ultrasound is unique among the heating modalities because of its supplementary non-thermal effects, those chemical changes that must be attributed to mechanisms other than tissue temperature increases. Ultrasound waves are made up of alternating areas of compression (areas of increased density and pressure) and rarefaction (areas of decreased density and pressure). Rarefaction causes air bubbles in the blood or tissue fluids to expand because of the decrease in pressure. During expansion gas enters the bubble. The compression phase for the wave causes the gas to flow out of the bubble. This gaseous exchange exerts mechanical stress on the surrounding cells and generates chemical activity. This phenomenon is called cavitation, a term that refers to a variety of bubble activities, ranging from stable vibration in response to the regularly repeated pressure changes induced by the sound wave, to violent implosion of the bubble under high ultrasound intensities (Dyson, 1987).

Cavitation produces some of the therapeutic benefits of ultrasound, but its precise role is still being investigated. Stable cavitation may produce an increase in protein synthesis and cell permeability. It has a sclerolytic effect, useful in the breaking up of calcified deposits and increasing the extensibility of tight capsule tissue. Cavitation can occur readily in a joint into which effusion has occurred due to the lower viscosity of the fluid.

Unstable cavitation results in the collapse of bubbles under the influence of changing pressures in an ultrasonic wave. Bubble implosion causes high temperature and pressure which can be destructive. Locally, cells are destroyed and free radicals are produced. Ultrasound administered within the therapeutic range produces stable cavitation. Higher intensities than those used therapeutically produce unstable cavitation. This should not occur if ultrasound is used properly. It also can occur if the ultrasound unit is not properly calibrated. Ultrasound machines used on the racetrack are often hand-me-down units that have known several owners. Operators should consult the manufacturer on recalibration before using such a unit.

Another non-thermal effect of ultrasound is acoustic streaming, sometimes called microstreaming. Acoustic streaming refers to liquid flow along cell membranes pushed by the pressure of the sound wave. Acoustic streaming is therapeutically valuable in facilitating diffusion of ions and metabolites across the membrane. Changes in membrane permeability to sodium ions could be involved in the altered electrical activity in nerves, resulting in pain relief. Increased membrane permeability to sodium and calcium exchange may explain the effect on contractile tissue in reduction of muscle spasm.

Therapeutic Effects of Ultrasound

The scientific literature contains many studies to support recommendations for the therapeutic use of ultrasound. Though no studies could be found using horses as subjects, the information from human studies is pertinent to ultrasound applications on horses.

Increase in joint range of motion

Periarticular connective tissue changes result from unwillingness to move the body part through its full range of motion due to pain. Stiffness and a decrease in flexibility must be addressed with stretching exercises to regain normal joint function. Stretching exercises are facilitated by the heating effects of ultrasound.

Elevating the tissue temperature before passive or active stretching will enhance the effects of the stretch. Preheating connective tissue before it is stretched produces a greater residual increase in tissue length with less potential damage (Lehmann, 1970). Heating of the deep tissues alters the elastic properties of collagen tissue and its molecular bonding. Deep tissues surrounding a joint are rich in collagen. Because ultrasound selectively heats this type of tissue, it is the ideal modality for pre-stretch heating (Fig. 14.1).

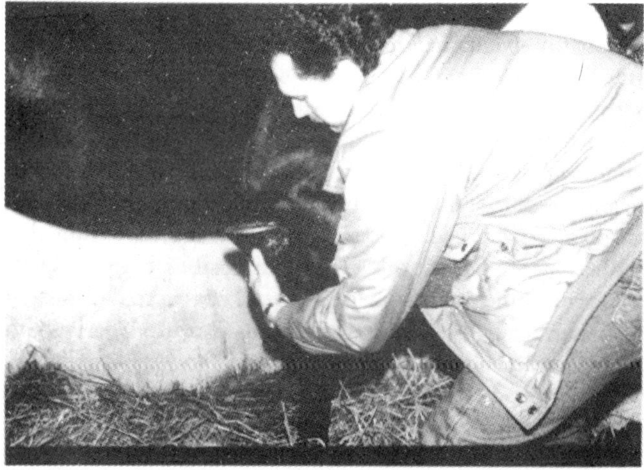

Fig. 14.1. Stretching to increase joint range of motion, following ultrasound application.

Horses respond well to sustained manual stretching in conjunction with tendon heating. When injury results in a shortened stride length or decreased joint range of motion veterinary consultation will help identify tendons that have undergone contracture. Ultrasound provides the ideal means to increase the temperature of these specific structures without overheating the skin.

Scar tissue is rich in collagen and more dense than the surrounding tissue. It can be selectively targeted by ultrasound. Scar tissue can limit movement or simply blemish the horse and reduce his sale potential. Ultrasound administered daily can reduce the size of the scar as long as the scar is under three months old. As the length of time between the injury and onset of treatment increases the results become less satisfactory.

Decrease in pain and muscle spasm

Ultrasound treatments reduce pain following injury or surgery. Researchers have sought to isolate the effects of heat on nerve fibres to determine its effects on the pain threshold of free nerve endings (Halle *et al.*, 1981). Ultrasound has an effect on nerve fibre conduction, though the physiological mechanisms responsible for this effect are not clear. It is also not entirely clear whether ultrasound increases or decreases the velocity of peripheral nerve conduction. The effect may be intensity dependent. Ultrasound administered in the middle of the therapeutic range, from 0.88 W cm^{-2} to 2.0 W cm^{-2} for five minutes decreases motor nerve conduction velocity. Increases in nerve conduction velocity occur when ultrasound is applied at intensity levels at the extremes of the therapeutic range, 0.05 W cm^{-2} and 3.0 W cm^{-2} for five minutes (Madsen and Gersten, 1961).

Other studies have looked at the effects of ultrasound on pain without raising the question of changes in nerve conduction. Bearzy (1953) reported on the administration of ultrasound at doses of 2 W cm^{-2} for five minutes to the pain site created by shoulder bursitis in 50 patients. In each instance the complaint was of pain, tenderness and limitation of motion of a duration of up to two years. On average five treatments were necessary to obtain relief of the symptoms.

Ultrasound therapy was used successfully on painful neuromas and post-operative scars (Tepperberg and Marjey, 1953). The treatment protocol used 1.5 W cm^{-2} of pulsed sound for about six minutes administered to the pain site. Though most of these patients had received other forms of therapy including nerve resections without obtaining relief, ultrasound did reduce the pain within ten treatments, or less.

Back pain is a common occurrence in humans and horses. Symptoms include localized muscle spasm, lack of mobility and discomfort. Aldes and Grabin (1958) presented a large case study of patients suffering low back pain secondary to herniated intervertebral disc syndrome. Ultrasound was successful in 86% of the cases. The treatment protocol used low intensities ranging from 0.3 to 0.8 W cm^{-2} given in 12-minute sessions over the pain site. Hot packs and massage were also used.

Calcium deposits

Exostosis of the interosseous ligament between the second and third, or third and fourth metacarpal bones responds to ultrasound treatment. Called a splint, this condition is caused by new bone formation in response to trauma from a blow or from weight bearing on imperfectly positioned bone. It is thought by some that ultrasound can be used to stimulate the resorption of calcium deposits. No controlled studies have been published to date to validate this use of ultrasound.

Reduction in splint size is probably due to a reduction in the swelling in the soft tissue and a resolution of the scar tissue around the injury. The most satisfying results would be obtained from treatment that was begun at the first sign of inflammation.

Wound healing

Wound closure is more rapid when wounds are treated with ultrasound (Dyson and Suckling, 1978). Interestingly, the skin temperature rise observed was considered to be too small for heating to be responsible for the effects. Acoustic streaming may play a part in tissue repair.

Ultrasound promotes the healing of pressure sores (Paul *et al.*, 1960). Pressure wounds that showed a reluctance to heal responded to ultrasound with an increased rate of replacement of tissue. Experimental evidence indicates that ultrasound can increase the rate of protein synthesis by fibroblasts that are responsible for the repair of injured tissue. Harvey *et al.* (1975) have shown an increase in the rate of protein synthesis by fibroblasts exposed to ultrasound. There was also evidence of increased lysosomal permeability that enhances protein synthesis.

Studies of tendon repair indicated that the stage of the healing process at which ultrasound is applied is very important (Rutherford and Harris, 1982). Ultrasound applications begun too early in the repair process could retard healing. Ultrasound applied to soft tissue within the first week of injury or surgical repair could hinder initiation of the healing process. Ultrasound applied at low intensities two weeks after the injury, when collagen formation and fibroblast infiltration has begun, will be beneficial.

Treatment Methods and Protocols

The opportunity for misuse of ultrasound will increase as the popularity of this therapeutic modality grows in the horse industry. Overdosing with ultrasound can result in deep tissue damage. Overdosing means an application schedule that is too high in intensity level or too frequent or prolonged. Beneficial results should be noted by three treatments. If there is no improvement, reassess the lesion and the dosage. Limit total treatments to twelve unless continued progress is documented.

As with any therapeutic treatment, it is important to evaluate the type and extent of the injury before any treatment is begun. The age and health status of the horse should be considered in determining dosage levels. To begin an ultrasound treatment, assemble the transmission gel, a sponge and clean water to wet the hair coat. Remove the gel and towel-dry the horse after treatment. Once the treatment has begun the therapist must keep the sound head moving slowly and steadily over the target area. Avoid holding the sound head stationary since this will produce hot spots with the potential for tissue damage. The sweep should cover about 4 cm sec^{-1}. The purpose of the motion is to distribute energy as evenly as possible throughout the tissue. The horse should be completely relaxed. Restraint such as twitching is never necessary with ultrasound. Horses apparently feel a very pleasant sensation during treatment. Although you may provide some hay to eat, a horse will usually stand quietly enjoying the ultrasound treatment. Treatment should take place in a clean, dry stall with good lighting.

Position the unit so that it is in a clean, dust-free area, with the intensity indicator easily visible and the controls easily accessible (Fig. 14.2). Have plenty of gel available for reapplication whenever needed. Fresh gel is needed when a decrease in wattage output is seen or when air bubbles become mixed into the gel. An accumulation of air bubbles in the gel or an inadequate amount of gel will result in poor transmission of sound waves into the tissue. Although air is necessary for the transfer of audible sound, it is the anathema of ultrasound transmission. Due to lack of molecular density ultrasound cannot pass through a layer of air as thin as one hundredth of a millimetre. Therefore, the sound head should never be held away or tilted away from the horse while the unit is on, since ultrasound will be reflected back into the transducer, leading to overheating and damage.

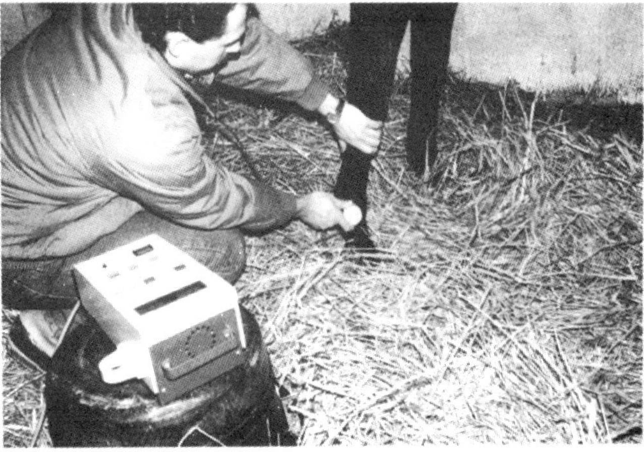

Fig. 14.2. Proper set-up for ultrasound application involves positioning the unit so controls are visible.

Use of the underwater technique, or immersion, is recommended where body curvature or bony prominences make it difficult to keep the sound head flat on the skin surface (Fig. 14.3). Ultrasound can be administered by the immersion technique when the hoof is to be treated. For the immersion technique, the sound head is held 0.5 to 3.0 cm from the surface of the area to be treated. As air bubbles accumulate on the skin surface or on the face of the sound head they must be wiped away.

Phonophoresis

Phonophoresis is a special use of ultrasound in which the sound waves aid in the transport of medications through tissue membranes. The sound wave drives whole molecules subcutaneously. Although it is a topic of scientific debate, researchers have reported penetration depths of up to 6 cm using phonophoresis.

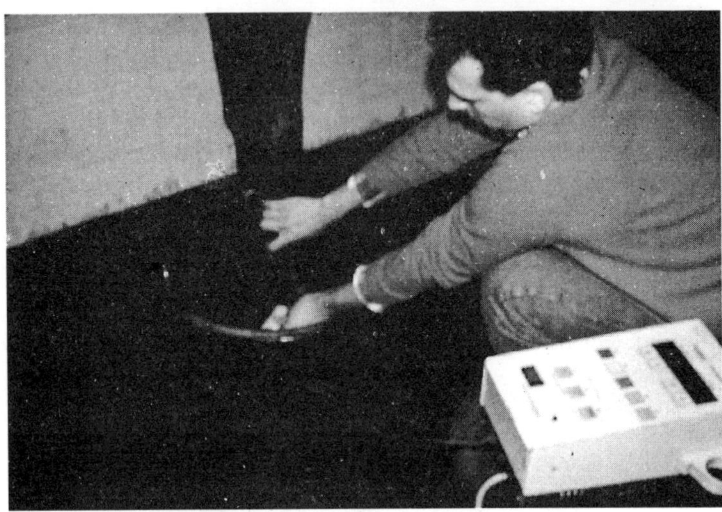

Fig. 14.3. When the sound head cannot be kept flat on the skin surface, ultrasound can be applied underwater.

The medications used in phonophoresis are anti-inflammatory agents and anaesthetics. Hydrocortisone is the drug used most often in the treatment of tendonitis, epicondylitis, bursitis and other myofacial pathologies.

The efficiency of ultrasound in driving cortisol through the skin to underlying muscle and nerve tissue was reported by Griffin and Touchstone (1963). The intensity level used in the study was 1 W cm^{-2}, somewhat higher than conservative recommendations. Cortisol levels in the muscle increased three-fold, with concentrations in the nerve increasing four-fold following the use of phonophoresis.

For this technique, mix the drug in proportions of 5% to 10% into the transmission gel. Use the continuous wave mode and an intensity range of 0.3–0.5 W cm^{-2}. The duration of application is up to ten minutes for a 5 cm^2 area.

Continuous versus Pulsed Wave

Most ultrasound units offer a choice of wave modes, the continuous wave and the pulsed wave. These mode choices allow the therapist to treat a broader range of conditions and offer the opportunity to produce a greater range of effects.

Use the continuous wave form when heating is desired. This mode delivers an uninterrupted train of sound waves and is useful for treating heavily muscled areas such as the gluteus, the back, or the shoulder muscles. Muscle blood flow provides a cooling mechanism so tissue interfaces are not overheated in such areas as long as the sound head is moved steadily.

The wave train is interrupted at specific intervals in the pulsed mode. This reduces the total number of waves produced in any second of treatment. The output may be interrupted or have an off-time of 50% or 80%. Breaks in the wave train occur so that heat can be dissipated by circulation. Use pulsed ultrasound when effects other than heat are desired. The non-thermal effects of ultrasound include acoustic streaming, which enhances the process of diffusion. In this regard, pulsed ultrasound would be effective in reducing the oedema associated with recent soft tissue injuries. Pulsed ultrasound is also useful when the area to be treated is small and there is little room for sound head movement.

Dosage

Ultrasound dosage must be sufficient to create a biological change yet not fall into the range of over exposure. To arrive at the appropriate dosage, consider the power output intensity (watts), the duration of exposure, and the size of the surface area over the structures to be treated.

The intensity dosage is determined by the amount of soft tissue in the target area. When using the continuous mode to elevate tissue temperature in an area such as the horses's hip or back, intensities as high as 1.5 to 2.0 W cm^{-2} of the sound head are used. Use lower intensities of 0.5 to 1.0 W cm^{-2} of the sound head over areas where there is less soft tissue coverage and where bone is closer to the skin surface. Higher intensities are chosen when the desired effect is tissue heating such as before stretching exercises. Use lower intensities for pain reduction, spasm relief and oedema dispersal. Lower intensities still (0.3 to 0.5 W cm^{-2} of the sound head) are most suitable for wound repair or for use on the lower leg of the horse.

Duration of treatment depends on the condition treated and the size of the treatment site. The size of the area to be treated is two to three times the size of the surface of the sound head. An area of this size should be sonated for five minutes. If treatment must extend over a larger area it should be subdivided into small treatment areas, each treated for five minutes.

Treatment Precautions

Ultrasound is not dangerous if the operator carefully follows the treatment rules and endeavours to understand the capabilities of this therapeutic modality. Contraindications for the use of ultrasound do exist. Studies have shown that ultrasound applications just above the therapeutic dosage cause a variety of pathological effects (Oakley, 1978). The occurrence of pain during treatment can be attributed to overheating of superficial compact bone. This may lead to the eventual thinning of bone. It is caused by prolonged use or use at too high an intensity.

The uterus should not be exposed to therapeutic ultrasound during pregnancy because of the possibility of cavitation in the amniotic fluid. The heart should not be directly sonated at therapeutic levels because the possibility exists that it may change action potentials and contractile properties of the myocardium. Ultrasound should not be used repeatedly over or near growth centres of bone until bone growth is essentially complete. Laboratory experiments demonstrate that a high number of exposures at therapeutic levels or a low number of exposures at high levels of intensity result in damage to the epiphyseal cartilage. Widening of the epiphyseal plate and premature closure were seen with lower doses of ultrasound while displacement of the epiphyseal plate was seen with higher doses (DeForest *et al.*, 1953). The number of treatments should be kept under ten with low intensity when administering ultrasound to the epiphyseal regions of a horse with bones still in the growth stage.

Because of its heating effects ultrasound should not be used on an injured area immediately after exercise. Irritation from the exercise would be increased by ultrasound.

Conclusion

Tissue reactions to ultrasound are due to heating and to the mechanical action the sound wave vibrations produce. Ultrasound does not appreciably heat skin but can significantly heat deeper tissues such as tendon, muscle, nerve and bone. No other modality can be substituted for ultrasound and produce the same results.

It is important to know how to apply ultrasound to cause a temperature rise in the target tissues without overheating tissue interfaces and bone. A principle that applies to ultrasound is that too small an amount of energy produces no useful reaction, too much energy destroys tissue, but the appropriate amount of energy provides the desired response.

References

Aldes, J.H. and Grabin, S. (1958) Ultrasound in the treatment of intervertebral disc syndrome. *American Journal of Physical Medicine*, 37, 199.

Bearzy, H.J. (1953) Clinical applications of ultrasonic energy in treatment of acute and chronic subacromial bursitis. *Archives of Physical Medicine and Rehabilitation*, 34, 228–231.

DeForest, R.E. Herrick, J.F., Janes, J.M., and Krusen, F.H. (1953) Effects of ultrasound on growing bone: an experimental study. *Archives of Physical Medicine and Rehabilitation*, 34, 21–31.

Dyson, M. (1987) Mechanisms involved in therapeutic ultrasound. *Physiotherapy*, 73, 116–120.

Dyson, M. and Suckling, J. (1978) Stimulation of tissue repair by ultrasound. *Physiotherapy*, 64, 105–108.

Griffin, J. and Touchstone, J. (1963) Ultrasonic movement of cortisol into a pig: I. Movement into skeletal muscle. *American Journal of Physical Medicine*, 42, 77–85.

Halle, J.S., Scoville, C.R., and Greathouse, D.G. (1981) Ultrasound's effect on the conduction latency of the superficial radial nerve in man. *Physical Therapy*, 61, 345–350.

Hartley, A. (1991) *Ultrasound*. Anne Hartley, Canada, p. 8.

Harvey, W., Dyson, M., Pond, J.B., and Grahame, R. (1975) Stimulation of protein synthesis in human fibroblasts by therapeutic ultrasound. *Rheumatology and Rehabilitation*, 14, 237.

Lehmann, J.F. (1970) Effects of therapeutic temperatures on tendon extensibility. *Archives of Physical Medicine and Rehabilitation*, 51, 481–487.

Madsen, P.W. and Gersten, J.W. (1961) Effect of ultrasound on conduction velocity of peripheral nerves. *Archives of Physical Medicine and Rehabilitation*, 42, 645–649.

Michlovitz, S.L. (1986) *Thermal Agents in Rehabilitation*, F.A. Davis Company, Philadelphia, p. 142.

Oakley, E.M. (1978) Dangers and contra-indications of therapeutic ultrasound. *Physiotherapy*, 64, 171–174.

Paul, B.J., Lafratta, C., Dawson, A.R., Baab, E. and Bullock, F. (1960) Use of ultrasound in the treatment of pressure sores in patients with spinal cord injury. *Archives of Physical Medicine and Rehabilitation*, 41, 438–440.

Rutherford, J.H., and Harris, D. (1982) The effect of ultrasound on flexor tendon repairs in the rabbit. *Hand*, 14, 17–20.

Tepperberg, I. and Marjey, E.J. (1953) Ultrasound therapy of painful post-operative neurofibromas. *American Journal of Physical Medicine*, 32, 27–30.

15 Ultrasonography and Body Composition in Sheep

A.J.F. Russel
The Macaulay Land Use Research Institute, Hartwood Research Station, Hartwood, Shotts, Lanarkshire ML7 4JY, UK

Introduction

Ultrasonography is one of a number of technologies used to predict the quantities or proportions of lean meat and fat in live sheep and in sheep carcasses. The demand for objective information on these parameters stems from the increasing preference by consumers for leaner meat on grounds of both human health considerations and taste (Woodward and Wheelock, 1990).

Ultrasound has two principal uses in the production of leaner sheepmeat. The first is as a tool in genetic improvement programmes as described, for example, by Simm (1992). In this approach ultrasound is used to identify individual animals, generally rams, which are superior in terms of having low levels of fat and high proportions of lean meat, to be parents of the next generation. The measurement of these traits in the live animal is of considerable benefit in that it avoids the time and expense of progeny testing in which a ram's genetic worth is assessed following measurement of the carcass composition of its progeny. It is probable that techniques such as X-ray tomography and nuclear magnetic resonance have the potential to provide more precise *in vivo* estimates of body composition than can be achieved using ultrasonography (Simm, 1989), but the equipment is many times more expensive than the ultrasonic instruments which are being increasingly used as tools in sheep breed improvement programmes.

The second main application of ultrasound in the production of lean sheepmeat is in the identification of lambs which have attained the optimum level of fatness for slaughter. In theory the technology used in breeding programmes could also be applied to the selection of lambs for slaughter, but in practice the rate of throughput is too low, and the cost consequently too high, for current ultrasonic equipment to be used for this purpose.

The different technological requirements of instruments for the two applications of ultrasound to the estimation of body and carcass composition are considered in more detail later in this chapter.

"

Instruments

Two different principles, both using ultrasound, have been applied to the *in vivo* measurements of body composition in sheep. These are the pulse–echo and transmission or velocity of ultrasound (VOS) techniques. The more commonly employed approach is based on pulse–echo technology using A-mode, B-mode and real-time scanning instruments (see Chapter 1) to image tissue interfaces. Simple A-mode instruments have been used very successfully for more than 30 years in the pig industry to measure subcutaneous fat depth at a single point, generally on the loin area, in the live animal (Wilson, 1992). More recently developed instruments also measure the distance to the next tissue interface to provide an estimate of eye muscle depth.

A-mode instruments have never proved as successful in use on sheep as they have with pigs. One reason which has been advanced for this failure is the greater difficulty of achieving good acoustic coupling because of the sheep's dense fleece and waxy skin surface, as opposed to the pig's sparse covering of bristles. The excellent quality images which can be obtained on sheep with B-mode instruments suggest, however, that some other factor is responsible for the lack of success with A-mode technology in sheep. It is more likely that the reason lies in the greater difficulty of measuring the generally lesser depths of subcutaneous fat in sheep.

The layering of the subcutaneous fatty tissue in sheep can also lead to problems when using A-mode instruments, in that the first returning signal may come from the boundary between two fat layers rather than from the fat–muscle interface. This difficulty is overcome with the aid of the visual image provided by real-time instruments.

Two-dimensional B-mode and real-time scanning instruments, generally with linear array probes and less commonly with sector probes, have been used successfully for *in vivo* body composition studies in sheep. Unlike the A-mode instruments used in pigs, the scanners used in studies with sheep have not been developed specifically for measurement of superficial tissues but have been designed to examine deeper tissues and for the diagnosis of pregnancy and the determination of fetal numbers. The focusing of the ultrasonic beam in these instruments is generally concentrated on the mid-field (about 30–100 mm) and thus the images of the tissues lying in roughly the first 20 mm of the field do not have the highest quality definition. This difficulty has been overcome in some instances by the use an offset or stand-off to bring the subcutaneous fat and eye muscle tissues into the range of optimum resolution. Water-filled latex bags are particularly useful in this respect as they also help to prevent distortion of the tissues by pressure applied via the probe (McEwan *et al.*, 1989).

To date, the use of ultrasonic scanners for estimating body tissue depths and areas in sheep has been confined almost exclusively to identifying superior individuals for use in breeding programmes rather than in selecting lambs for slaughter at the optimum level of fat cover. Measurements of fat and muscle depth can be made with existing instruments only on screen, using in-built cursors or callipers, or from images captured on Polaroid film or stored on videotape, and which are interpreted and measured at some later time. No instrument is currently available which satisfactorily processes the real-time image and gives the immediate display of values, linear measurements or areas which the commercial selection of finished lamb requires.

The ultrasound transmission technique (VOS) for estimating body composition operates on a different principle from the pulse–echo approach. This alternative technique is based on the fact that at normal body temperature the speed of transmission of ultrasound through muscular tissue is some 10% greater than through fat. Measurement of the speed of ultrasound through soft tissue can therefore be used to estimate the proportions of muscle and fat in that tissue. The technique has been used successfully in cattle *in vivo* (Miles *et al.*, 1983, 1984).

For some time it appeared that this technique was not suitable for sheep because the difficulty of finding suitable bone-free areas through which the velocity of ultrasound could be measured. Recently, however, Chadwick *et al.* (1993) reported that the technique could be used in the shoulder and loin areas and that it provided estimates of body composition of comparable accuracy to that obtained using real-time linear array instruments.

Measurement Sites

The two main criteria for the selection of body sites at which to make ultrasonic measurements are, firstly, that they can be readily and repeatably identified anatomically from external landmarks and, secondly, that the measurements of tissue depths and areas made at these points are themselves good indices of whole body or carcass composition.

The sites favoured by most workers using A-mode or real-time ultrasonic instruments are in the region of the 12th rib and in the lumbar area. Some workers have a preference for making measurements directly over a specific rib, frequently the 12th (e.g. Hopkins, 1990b) or lumbar vertebra, generally the third (e.g. Simm, 1992), presumably because these sites are easily and repeatably located. Others, however, prefer to make measurements between the 11th and 12th or 12th and 13th ribs (e.g. Wood and MacFie, 1980) or between the third and fourth lumbar vertebrae as these sites repeat more faithfully the locations of measurements made on the cut surfaces of carcasses which are split between, rather than through, ribs and vertebrae.

The most commonly made linear measurements are those described by Wood and MacFie (1980) and made between the last and second last rib, and by Simm (1992) at the third lumbar vertebra:

A = the maximum width of the eye muscle (*m. longissimus thoracis* in the rib region or *m. longissimus lumborum* in the loin);
B = the maximum depth of the eye muscle measured at right angles to A;
C = the depth of the layer of subcutaneous fatty tissue directly over measurement B.

Eye muscle area is frequently calculated as the product $A \times B$; alternatively the actual area may be measured on a frozen screen image or from a Polaroid photograph or videotaped image.

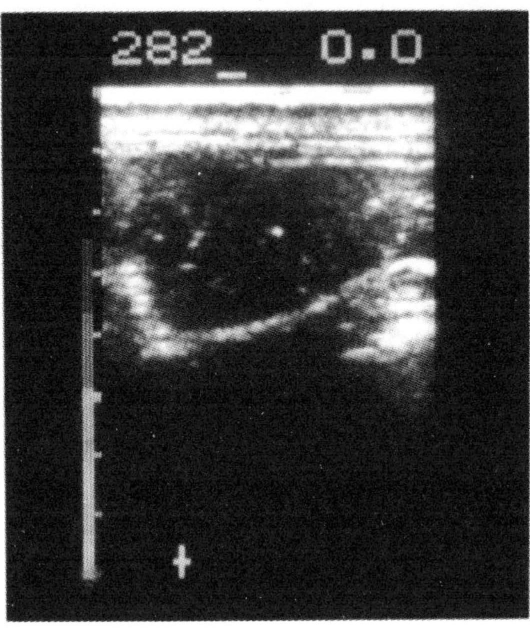

Fig. 15.1. A typical image of tissues lying above the third lumbar vertebra, from a real-time instrument with a 3.5 MHz linear array probe. (Reproduced by kind permission of Dr G. Simm.)

A typical image of subcutaneous fat and the eye muscle at the third lumbar vertebra, obtained with a real-time scanner with a linear array probe, is illustrated in Fig. 15.1.

A site that is being used increasingly, particularly by workers in Australasia (McEwan *et al.*, 1989; Hopkins, 1990a) is the GR measurement of tissue depth (i.e. skin + subcutaneous fatty tissue + muscular tissue) described by Kirton and Johnson (1979). This is a measurement made at the 12th rib (or occasionally between the 11th and 12th or 12th and 13th ribs) at a point 110 mm lateral to the midline. Although the GR measurement is of total tissue depth, and not only of fat, it is favoured by, among others, Hopkins (1990a), who showed that the distribution of C measurements tends to be highly skewed, but that near normality could be achieved by a square root transformation. Hopkins (1990a) further showed that the GR measurement was approximately $3 \times C^{0.5}$ and very highly correlated to C, but that the precise relationship between the two measurements was breed and weight dependent.

In the UK, the Meat and Livestock Commission calculate fat depth as the mean of three measurements made at C and at two points 10 and 20 mm lateral to C (M.G. Owen, 1993, personal communication). This would appear to have at least two advantages. Firstly, a mean of three measurements will give a more accurate estimate of fat depth than will a single measurement, if all are made with the same degree of precision. Secondly, because as sheep fatten the increase in fat depth is greater towards the outer margin of the eye muscle than it is nearer the midline, differences in fat depth between individuals will be more readily detected at the more lateral points. The commonly made linear measurements of fat depth and eye muscle dimensions are illustrated in Fig. 15.2.

The VOS technique estimates the proportions of fatty and muscular tissues in the areas through which ultrasound is transmitted, and cannot be used to estimate fat depths or muscle depths and areas at the sites noted above. The areas of the body on which successful measurements have been made in sheep are bone-free parts of the shoulder and the loin (Chadwick *et al.*, 1993).

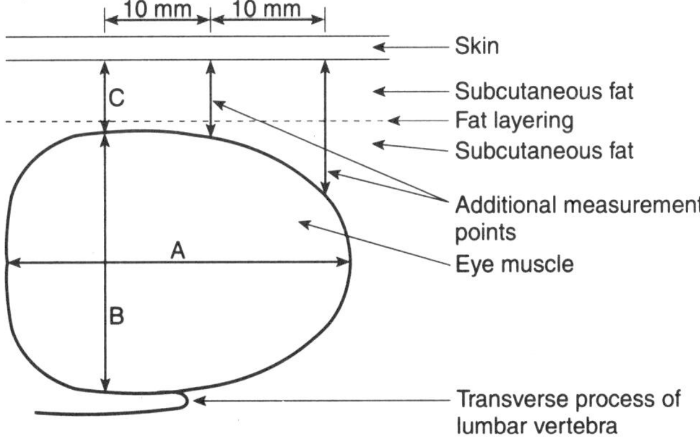

Fig. 15.2. Diagram showing linear measurements of fat depth and eye muscle characteristics made in the lumbar region.

Precision of Estimation of *In Vivo* Composition

The scientific literature contains many reports of the precision with which ultrasound can be used to predict the fat and lean contents of live adult sheep and of lamb carcasses (see reviews by Houghton and Turlington, 1992; Simm, 1992; Wilson, 1992). The results are generally reported as correlation coefficients relating the ultrasonic measurement to, and as residual standard deviations of, the predicted variate. At first sight the reported levels of prediction appear to be highly variable. Although some of this variation is undoubtedly due to differences in operator skill and to technical limitations of different instruments, the principal reasons for the apparent differences in level of prediction lie in the traits predicted and in the animal populations on which the trials were conducted.

Where the ultrasonic measurement is used to predict the same trait in the carcass the correlations are generally high (of the order of 0.8 or more) and the residual standard deviations low. Where, however, the predicted measurement is itself being used as an index of body composition the relationship between the variables will necessarily be less close. Ultrasonically measured fat depth would, for example, be expected to be closely correlated with the actual measurement made at or near the same location on the carcass but would not be as closely related to the proportions of fat in the carcass.

Similarly, correlation coefficients would be expected to vary with the degree of variation in the estimated and actual *in vivo* and carcass measurements. Where the level of fatness in a group of animals is highly variable, a closer correlation between estimated and actual measurements would be expected than in, say, a group of lambs which had been selected on the basis of subjectively assessed body conditions as being in a particular fat class or grade. Correlation coefficients are thus not an adequate criterion of the accuracy of prediction of *in vivo* body or carcass composition.

In theory, variation in the level of fatness of the group of animals on which the *in vivo* predictions of compositions are made should not affect the residual standard deviation of the predicted variate. In practice, however, it may, because the precision with which fat depth can be measured (perhaps ±1 mm) will be proportionately greater in, for example, a group of relatively lean lambs than in a group of ewes in good body condition. None the less, the residual standard deviation is likely to be less affected than the correlation coefficient by the variance of fatness in the population and is the parameter of choice in comparing results obtained in different trials.

In a group of sheep of the same breed and sex and of similar age, the heavier animals will be the fatter. If prediction equations for that breed and sex have been established, body weight alone may give an acceptable estimate of carcass fatness. The usefulness of ultrasonics in the estimation of *in vivo* composition has therefore to be assessed in terms of the additional information which is supplied over and above that provided by the more easily and less expensively obtained measurement of body weight. Most reports in the literature indicate that ultrasonic measurements, particularly of fat depth C or tissue depth GR, add significantly to the predictive information supplied by live weight. For example Simm (1987) found that the residual standard deviation of lean prediction was reduced from 2.9 to 2.4% after adding ultrasonic measurements to live weight. McEwan *et al.* (1989) also reported that ultrasonic measurements of C and GR reduced the residual standard deviation of percentage chemical fat in the carcass from the 3.04% achieved by live weight to 2.36 and 2.87% respectively, although in this study the inclusion of live weight in the prediction equations added no significant information to that obtained from either of the ultrasonic measurements on its own.

It might be thought that the best estimates of the weight or proportion of fatty tissue in the body or carcass would be provided by measurements of fat depth (e.g. measurement C) and that muscular tissue or lean would be best predicted by estimates of eye muscle dimensions (A or B or some combination of the two). In practice, however, because the proportions of fatty and muscular tissues are strongly and negatively correlated, measurements of fat depth are generally better indices of lean content than are measurements of eye muscle dimensions. Hopkins (1990b) reported that percentage lean in lamb carcasses was best estimated from a combination of live weight and measurement C (fat depth) and concluded that eye muscle area *per se* was of no value. Ward *et al.* (1992) concluded, however, that measurement *B* (eye muscle depth) and estimates of eye muscle area can provide limited but none the less useful information on lamb leg muscularity, while Waldron *et al.* (1992) calculated that measurement *A* (eye muscle width) provided the greatest economic response to selection for muscularity.

The precision of estimation of *in vivo* body composition by ultrasonography would be expected to be influenced by the skill and experience of the operator. Nicol *et al.* (1988) found, for example, that the second of two measurements of fat depth made at the same site with an A-mode instrument was more closely correlated with the corresponding carcass fat measurement and with the percentage carcass fat than was the first. They also noted that measurements made on the side of the animal opposite to the operator were more accurate than those taken on the same side. More recent work from the same centre (Young *et al.*, 1992) concluded, however, that tissue depths estimated with a real-time B-mode instrument could be assessed accurately from a single measurement; it was also found that fat depth could be estimated with equal accuracy by two operators with different levels of experience, but that muscle depth was measured with greater accuracy by the more experienced operator.

Operators experienced in body condition scoring (Russel *et al.*, 1969) can make subjective assessments of fatness which are comparable in terms of accuracy to those obtained from live weight and ultrasonic measurements (Bass *et al.*, 1982) but in practice there is likely to be considerable difficulty in achieving standardization between operators.

Future Developments

The use of ultrasonics to estimate *in vivo* body composition is still confined mainly to those engaged in research. The technique will, however, eventually find wider commercial use, and it would be helpful if, before that stage is reached, there was a greater consensus regarding the optimum site at which measurements are made. Some workers clearly prefer to make their measurements in the rib area, using either the 11th, 12th or 13th rib or the intercostal spaces between two of these rib pairs; some measure only *C*, others measure *C* plus two further fat depths lateral to *C*, and others also measure *A* and *B* on the eye muscle; some rely only on the overall GR tissue depth; some prefer to concentrate on the loin area and make measurements of *C*, *C* and *B*, or *C*, *B* and *A* directly over the third lumbar vertebra, while others favour the point between the third and fourth vertebrae. There is scope for a definitive study which would lead to standardization of measurements at a specific site.

While it is desirable that any standardized protocol gives the best prediction of *in vivo* composition, it is also important that the measurement site be easily accessible and readily and repeatably identified so that it can be used effectively and quickly in commercial practice on large numbers of animals.

Technically there is a need for an ultrasonic instrument designed specifically to make measurements of those characteristics in the live animal which are the best indices of carcass composition. The ideal attributes of such an instrument are that it is sufficiently small and lightweight to be hand-held and that it gives a readout of fat and eye muscle depths (in millimetres); it must have high resolution in the near field; and it should incorporate a screen showing a real-time display of the tissues imaged, to enable the operator to confirm that the probe is correctly located, that the contact is good and that the image to be analysed is of satisfactory quality, e.g. that the appropriate tissue interfaces are continuous and not broken. Finally, the instrument should be capable of making a number of estimates of fat depth, most probably from site C to a point some 20 mm laterally and of presenting a mean fat depth over this range.

An instrument such as that prescribed above would have immediate application in the objective selection of lambs at the optimum degree of finish for slaughter. It would be particularly useful in the recently developed and rapidly expanding method of selling lambs 'sight unseen' by 'electronic auction' in which an objective and reliable description of the animals is invaluable.

A more sophisticated model of such an instrument would find a place in the more limited market of research use. The additional facilities required for use in, e.g. breed improvement programmes, would include the ability to input the animal's identification and possibly live weight, and a memory to store data for later downloading on to disk.

It is only in comparatively recent years that ultrasonography has been widely and routinely applied to work on animals. It has, however, proved to be an invaluable technology in this area and its uptake has been rapid. It is estimated that within a decade of the first trials being carried out, some ten million ewes in the UK, about half the national flock, are routinely scanned for the diagnosis of pregnancy and the determination of fetal numbers. Given the development of the appropriate instruments, which is already technically possible, a similar degree of use in the *in vivo* estimation of body composition is not only possible, but is highly probable.

References

Bass, J.J., Woods, E.G. and Paulson, W.D. (1982) A comparison of three ultrasonic machines (Danscan, AIDD (NZ) and body composition meter) and subjective fat and conformation scores for predicting chemical composition of live sheep. *Journal of Agricultural Science*, 99, 529–532.

Chadwick, J.P., Yates, C.M. and Owen, M.G. (1993) Comparison of four ultrasonic techniques for *in vivo* estimation of sheep carcass composition. *Animal Production*, 56, 426.

Hopkins, D.L. (1990a) Determining GR from subcutaneous fat depth over the eye muscle. *Proceedings of the Australian Society of Animal Production*, 18, 492.

Hopkins, D.L. (1990b) The usefulness of eye muscle area as a predictor of lamb composition. *Proceedings of the Australian Society of Animal Production*, 18, 493.

Houghton, P.L. and Turlington, L.M. (1992) Application of ultrasound for feeding and finishing animals: a review. *Journal of Animal Science*, 70, 930–941.

Kirton, A.H. and Johnson, D.L. (1979) Interrelationships between GR and other lambs carcass fatness measurements. *Proceedings of the New Zealand Society of Animal Production*, 39, 194–201.

McEwan, J.C., Clarke, J.N., Knowler, M.A. and Wheeler, M. (1989) Ultrasonic fat depths in Romney lambs and hoggets from lines selected for different production traits. *Proceedings of the New Zealand Society of Animal Production*, 49, 113–119.

Miles, C.A., Fursey, G.A.J. and Pomeroy, R.W. (1983) Ultrasonic evaluation of cattle. *Animal Production*, 36, 363–370.

Miles, C.A., Fursey, G.A.J. and York, R.W.R. (1984) New equipment for measuring the speed of ultrasound and its application in the estimation of body composition of farm livestock. In: Lister, D. (ed.) In Vivo *Measurement of Body Composition in Meat Animals*. Elsevier, London, pp. 93–105.

Nicol, A.M., Jay, N.P. and Beatson, P.R. (1988) A comparison of ultrasound backfat measurements on sheep. *Proceedings of the New Zealand Society of Animal Production*, 48, 33–36.

Russel, A.J.F., Doney, J.M. and Gunn, R.G. (1969) Subjective assessment of body fat in live sheep. *Journal of Agricultural Science*, 72, 451–454.

Simm, G. (1987) Carcass evaluation in sheep breeding programmes. In: Maral, I.F.M. and Owen, J.F. (eds) *New Techniques in Sheep Production*. Butterworths, London, pp. 125–144.

Simm, G. (1989) Current and possible future applications of *in vivo* assessment in sheep breeding programmes. In: Kalliweit E., Henning, M. and Groenevald E., (eds) *Application of NMR Techniques on the Body Composition of Live Animals*. Elsevier, London, pp. 149–159.

Simm, G. (1992) Selection for lean meat production in sheep. In: Speedy, A.W. (ed.) *Progress in Sheep and Goat Research*. CAB International, Wallingford, UK, pp. 193–215.

Waldron, D.F., Clarke, J.N., Rae, A.L. and Woods, E.G. (1992) Expected responses in carcass composition to selection for muscularity in sheep. *Proceedings of the New Zealand Society of Animal Production*, 52, 29–31.

Ward, B.G., Purchas, R.W. and Abdullah, A.Y. (1992) The value of ultrasound in assessing leg muscling of lambs. *Proceedings of the New Zealand Society of Animal Production*, 52, 33–36.

Wilson, D.E. (1992) Application of ultrasound for genetic improvement. *Journal of Animal Science*, 70, 973–983.

Wood, J.D. and MacFie, H.J.H. (1980) The significance of breed in the prediction of lamb carcass composition from fat thickness measurements. *Animal Production*, 31, 315–319.

Woodward, J. and Wheelock, V. (1990) Consumer attitudes to fat in meat. In: Wood, J.D. and Fisher, A.V. (eds) *Reducing Fat in Meat Animals*. Elsevier, London, pp. 66–100.

Young, M.J., Deaker, J.M. and Logal, C.M. (1992) Factors affecting repeatability of tissue depth determination by real-time ultrasound in sheep. *Proceedings of the New Zealand Society of Animal Production*, 52, 37–39.

Index

M-mode ultrasound 8, 88, 105–106, 108,
        111, 113–115, 126, 127, 131–132,
        142–149, 158, 159, 203

neoplasia
        abdominal 47, 201–203
        adrenal 25, 45–46
        bladder 47
        gastric 46, 194, 203
        hepatic 35–39, 188, 297
        in fish 291, 297
        intestinal 47
        mesenteric 47
        neuroma 307
        ocular 92, 98, 100
        ovarian 70–71, 202–203
        pancreatic 46
        prostatic 79
        renal 43, 194
        splenic 41, 42, 190–191
        testicular 73–75
        uterine 59
Nyquist limit 107

ocular ultrasonography 87–104, 297–301
        abnormalities
            anterior chamber 91–93
            posterior segment 93–98
        indications for use 89–90
        measurement (biometry) 87, 89, 90
        normal structures 90–91
optic nerve 91, 101
orbit 98–100
ovary
        abnormal 70–71, 249–250, 285
        absence of, confirmation 71
        cyclic events 67–70, 167–170,
            237–241, 249, 269–270
        follicular aspiration 252–255
        normal 67–71, 235, 237–241,
            269–270, 281
        in pregnancy 244

pancreas
        abnormal 41, 46
        normal 31–33
pastern, normal 214–217
peritoneal fluid 23, 27, 35, 46, 47, 194,
        196
peritoneum
        abnormal 47, 194, 196, 199

normal 33
peroneus tertius, normal 220
phonophoresis 309–310
piezoelectric effect 2, 9, 11
placenta
        abnormal 182, 203
        normal 62, 283
        retention 67
placentomes 244, 261, 265–266, 268
portal vein 27
pregnancy
        accuracy of diagnosis 64, 273,
            278–279, 280, 283–284
        bovine 244–248
        camelid 262, 264, 266, 270
        canine 59–63
            abnormalities of 64–67
        caprine 264, 265–268
        cervine 261–262, 264
        equine 172, 176–177
            embryonic/fetal loss 176, 181–182
            twinning 177–180, 203
        feline 63
        ovine 257–259, 261–269
        porcine 275–284
            embryonic loss 276
probe *see* transducer
prostate gland
        abnormal 78–80
        normal 77–78
        paraprostatic cyst 47, 80

radiography 21, 22, 23, 42, 43, 194, 207,
        258
resolution 12, 260
        axial 2, 4, 9
        lateral 4, 6
        power of 15

safety 11–14, 281, 291, 305, 311–312
scatter 5–6, 24, 236, 243
scrotum 76
sector scanner 3, 10–11, 105, 131,
        185–186, 194, 208, 234, 259, 260,
        261, 281, 291
sex determination
        fetus 181, 251–252
        fish 289–290, 294
specular reflectors 5, 23, 60, 176; 236, 244,
        292